Movement disorders in children:
a clinical update with video recordings

Fondazione Pierfranco e Luisa Mariani ONLUS
viale Bianca Maria 28
20129 Milan, Italy

Telephone: +39 02 795458
Fax: +39 02 76009582
Publications coordinator: Valeria Basilico
e-mail: publications@fondazione-mariani.org
www.fondazione-mariani.org

Movement disorders in children: a clinical update with video recordings

Edited by

N. Nardocci and E. Fernandez-Alvarez

Mariani Foundation Paediatric Neurology Series: 17
Series Editor: Maria Majno

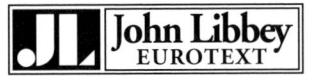

ISSN: 0969-0301
ISBN: 978-2-74-200657-1

Cover illustration: 'Sections of my destiny' by Marlene Healey. The kind permission of the Artist is gratefully acknowledged.
www.healeyartgroup.com
Design elaboration by Costanza Magnocavallo.
Technical and language editor: Oliver Brooke.

Published by

Éditions John Libbey Eurotext
127, avenue de la République, 92120 Montrouge, France.
Tél.: 33 (0)1 46 73 06 60; Fax: 33 (0)1 40 84 09 99
e-mail: contact@jle.com
http//www.jle.com

© 2007 John Libbey Eurotext. All rights reserved.

Unauthorized duplication contravenes applicable laws.

Il est interdit de reproduire intégralement ou partiellement le présent ouvrage sans autorisation de l'éditeur ou du Centre Français d'Exploitation du Droit de Copie, 20, rue des Grands-Augustins, 75006 Paris.

Contents

Chapter 1	Nosography and semiology of movement disorders in childhood *Lucia Angelini, Giovanna Zorzi and Nardo Nardocci*	1
Chapter 2	The genetics of dystonia *Barbara Garavaglia and Chiara Barzaghi*	7
Chapter 3	Neuroradiological findings in paediatric movement disorders *Luisa Chiapparini, Marina Grisoli and Mario Savoiardo*	19
Chapter 4	Neurophysiological investigations in movement disorders *Silvana Franceschetti, Laura Canafoglia, Flavia Tripaldi, Claudia Ciano and Ferruccio Panzica*	35
Chapter 5	Quantitative assessment of paediatric movement disorders *Renata Bono, Emanuela Pagliano, Elena Andreucci, Simona Malinverni and Alice Corlatti* video 1	49
Chapter 6	Primary dystonia *Nardo Nardocci, Federica Zibordi, Caterina Costa and Giovanna Zorzi* video 2	59
Chapter 7	Update on myoclonus-dystonia *Enza Maria Valente and Bruno Dallapiccola*	67
Chapter 8	Pharmacological treatment of childhood dystonia *Agathe Roubertie, Julie Leydet, Nathalie Demonceau and Bernard Echenne*	77

Chapter 9	Deep brain stimulation of the globus pallidus internus for the treatment of childhood-onset dystonia *Giovanni Broggi, Carlo Marras, Angelo Franzini, Giovanna Zorzi, Luigi Romito, Dario Caldiroli, Luisa Chiapparini and Nardo Nardocci* video 3	83
Chapter 10	Dopa-responsive dystonias/dyskinesias (DRDs): diagnosis and monitoring of the treatment *Vincenzo Leuzzi, Teresa Giovanniello, Carla Carducci, Claudia Carducci and Italo Antonozzi*	91
Chapter 11	Clinical and aetiological spectrum of dopa-responsive syndromes *Giovanna Zorzi, Federica Zibordi, Daniele Ghezzi, Chiara Barzaghi, Barbara Garavaglia and Nardo Nardocci* video 4	105
Chapter 12	Sydenham's chorea *Francisco Cardoso* video 5	113
Chapter 13	Opsoclonus-myoclonus syndrome *Michael R. Pranzatelli*	125
Chapter 14	Pantothenate kinase-associated neurodegeneration *Susan J. Hayflick* video 6	139
Chapter 15	Functional (psychogenic) movement disorders in childhood *Robert Surtees*	145
Chapter 16	Movement disorders in Rett syndrome *Teresa Temudo* video 7	153
Chapter 17	Rapid-onset dystonia-parkinsonism *Andrew McKeon and Mary D. King*	167
Chapter 18	Alternating hemiplegia of childhood (AHC) *Giuseppe Gobbi, Melania Giannotta, Tiziana Granata, Fiorella Gurrieri, Edvige Veneselli, Federico Vigevano, Claudio Zucca, Nardo Nardocci and Emilio Fernandez-Alvarez* video 8	173

Chapter 1

Nosography and semiology of movement disorders in childhood

Lucia Angelini, Giovanna Zorzi and Nardo Nardocci

*Unit of Child Neuropsichiatry, Fondazione IRCCS Istituto Neurologico 'C. Besta',
via Celoria 11, 20133 Milan, Italy*
langelini@istituto-besta.it

Summary

Movement disorders can be defined as neurological syndromes characterized by excess of movement or slowness or poverty of movement unrelated to weakness or spasticity. Classification is primarily based on the clinical description of the phenomenology observed. Movement disorders can be divided into two main groups: *hyperkinesias* and *hypokinesias*. The most important hyperkinesias are represented by chorea, dystonia, tremor, myoclonus, and tics; hypokinesias are mainly represented by parkinsonism (hypokinetic-rigid syndrome). The diagnostic approach to movement disorders is a multistep process: (1) identify the most pertinent category in which the observed phenomena can be included; (2) distinguish between primary (without recognizable cause) and secondary (caused by an established disease) – this distinction is supported by an accurate investigation into family and personal history and by general and neurological evaluation of the patient; (3) plan the diagnostic investigations depending on information derived from the above steps.

Definition and classification of movement disorders

Movement disorders can be defined as neurological syndromes characterized by excess of movement or slowness or poverty of movement unrelated to weakness or spasticity. The term 'movement disorder' has replaced the previous terms 'basal ganglia disorder' and 'extrapyramidal disorder', but unfortunately the latter are still used synonymously, notwithstanding their inability to include all the syndromes considered under the spectrum of movement disorders (Jancovic & Lang, 2004).

Movement disorders can be divided into two main groups: *hyperkinesias* and *hypokinesias*. A comprehensive list of movement disorders in alphabetical order is given in Table 1. Hyperkinesias (also referred to as dyskinesias or abnormal involuntary movements) are mainly represented by chorea, dystonia, myoclonus, tics, and tremor; parkinsonism is the most common cause of hypokinesia.

Table 1. List of movement disorders

HYPOKINESIAS
Akinesia/bradykinesia (parkinsonism)
Apraxia
Blocking tics
Catatonia, psychomotor depression, obsessional slowness
Freezing phenomenon
Hesitant gaits
Hypothyroid slowness
Rigidity
Stiff muscles
HYPERKINESIAS
Abdominal dyskinesias
Akathisic movements
Asynergia/ataxia
Athetosis
Ballismus
Chorea
Dysmetria
Dystonia
Hemifacial spasm
Hyperplexia
Jumpy stumps
Moving toes/fingers
Myoclonus
Myokimia
Myorhythmia
Paroxysmal dyskinesias
Restless legs
Stereotypy
Tics
Tremor

From: Fahn, 1999

Clinical approach

The clinical approach to movement disorders differs from the traditional approach used in other neurological fields, which is focused on the topography and underlying aetiology of the symptoms. The approach to movement disorders involves three diagnostic steps.

The first step is to identify the most pertinent category in which the phenomenology observed can be included, based on knowledge and specific experience. Movement disorders may be unusual or bizarre and therefore difficult to categorize. Mistakes of definition are still frequent despite a greater consensus obtained in this field. The consequence of an inappropriate categorization is not only a misinterpretation of the clinical, genetic, and epidemiological data, but also a distortion of the diagnostic work-up. Video recording has become a working tool for comparing opinions and discussing the appropriate classification of movement disorders.

The second step is to distinguish between primary disorders (without recognizable cause) and secondary disorders (caused by an established disease). This distinction is supported by an accurate investigation of both family and personal history. Ethnic origin and parental consanguinity must be considered. It is very important to take into account that movement disorders other than those observed in the patient may be present in other family members. A history of birth problems, particularly anoxia and kernicterus, must be sought. Previous encephalitis, recreational drug use, or exposure to toxins (especially those relevant to the aetiology of movement disorders) must be ruled out. An accurate general and neurological evaluation will identify other possibly relevant neurological or physical signs and symptoms.

The third step is to plan the diagnostic investigations, depending on the information derived from the first two steps (Jancovic & Lang, 2004).

The clinical features of, and the diagnostic approach to, parkinsonism and dystonia – as examples of hypokinesias and hyperkinesias, respectively – will be described in detail; the other movement disorders will be outlined elsewhere in this volume.

Parkinsonism

Parkinsonism is a syndrome characterized by any association of the following six cardinal features: bradykinesia, rigidity, tremor at rest, loss of postural reflexes, flexed posture, and motor block (freezing) (Jancovic, 2003). Combinations of these signs enable the diagnosis of clinically definite, probable, and possible parkinsonism to be made (Table 2).

Table 2. Diagnostic criteria of parkinsonism

Cardinal features
1. Tremor at rest
2. Akinesia/bradykinesia
3. Rigidity
4. Loss of postural reflexes
5. Flexed posture
6. Freezing (motor blocks)

Definite parkinsonism: two of the above features must be present, with one of them being 1 or 2
Probable parkinsonism: features 1 or 2 alone are present
Possible parkinsonism: at least two of features 3–6 must be present

From: Fahn, 1999

Classification

Parkinsonism can be subdivided into four main categories: *primary, parkinsonism-plus syndromes, heredo-degenerative and secondary* (Table 3).

Table 3. Classification of parkinsonism

I. Primary parkinsonism
- Parkinson's disease
- Genetic parkinsonism

II. Multisystem degenerations ('parkinsonism-plus')
- Progressive supranuclear palsy
- Multiple system atrophy
- Corticobasal degeneration
- Progressive pallidal atrophy
- Parkinsonism-dementia complex
- Pallidopyramidal disease

III. Heredo-degenerative parkinsonism
- Hereditary juvenile-dystonia-parkinsonism
- Autosomal dominant Lewy body disease
- Huntington's disease
- Pantothenate kinase associated neurodegeneration
- Olivopontocerebellar and spinocerebellar atrophies and Machado-Joseph
- Ceroidolipofuscinosis, neuroacanthocytosis, gangliosidosis

IV. Secondary (acquired or symptomatic)
- Post-infectious
- Drugs (D2-receptor blocking agents) and toxins
- Vascular, traumatic, others.

Modified from Jancovic & Lang, 2004

The most frequent akinetic-rigid syndrome is Parkinson's disease, or primary idiopathic parkinsonism. Advances in genetics have drawn attention to different genetic causes of primary parkinsonism, such as mutations in the genes coding for α-synuclein (a rare cause of parkinsonism) or Parkin protein (responsible of up to 50 per cent of cases of early-onset parkinsonism). Other causes of parkinsonism are multiple system degeneration (also called parkinsonism-plus syndromes), secondary parkinsonism, and heredo-degenerative parkinsonism. Several clinical features may be useful in differentiating primary parkinsonism from secondary and heredo-degenerative conditions: absence or paucity of tremor, postural instability, pyramidal tract signs, and a poor response to L-dopa treatment (Jancovic, 2003).

Phenomenology of parkinsonism

The clinical features of parkinsonism, as exemplified by Parkinson disease, include motor, behavioural, and autonomic disturbances and are described in table 4.

Table 4. Clinical features of parkinsonism

Motor disturbances
1. Akinesia: absence or paucity of movement
Cranial: Reduction of facial expression, decreased frequency of blinking, drooling of saliva, diplopia
Arms: Reduction in arm swing while walking, micrographia
Legs: short stepped, shuffling gait
Trunk: difficulty in rising from a chair or turning in bed
2. Bradykinesia: slowness of voluntary movement
Loss of automatic movements, slowness in initiating movement, etc.
3. Speech disturbances → hypophonia, aprosody, stuttering, palilalia, ecolalia
4. Rigidity: increased resistance throughout the range of movement by passive flexing. In advanced stages, flexed postures appear, particularly of the neck, thorax, elbows, hips, and knees; 'striatal hand'
5. Loss of postural reflexes
6. Tremor: rest tremor in distal parts of extremities ('pill-rolling'), lips, tongue, chin, head
7. Freezing: start-hesitation of gait, stopping before reaching the final destination
Behavioural disturbances
1. Bradyphrenia: slowness of thought, inattentiveness, slowness in responding to questions
2. Mood disorders: depression, anxiety
3. Fatigue, apathy, abulia
Autonomic and sensory disturbances
Constipation, impaired olfactory function, orthostatic hypotension, sphincter dysfunction, seborrhoea

Modified from Jancovic & Lang, 2004

Dystonia

Dystonia is a clinical syndrome characterized by sustained muscle contractions, often causing twisting and repetitive movements or abnormal postures. The term dystonia has been used to describe both the specific motor phenomena and a specific disease entity, today known as primary dystonia. To clarify the term, the definition of dystonia given above was proposed in 1976 by an ad hoc committee and is now universally accepted (Fahn *et al.*, 1987).

Phenomenology of dystonia

The main characteristic of dystonic movements is their relatively long duration, resulting in twisting of the affected body part and the continual involvement of the same muscle groups.

The duration of dystonic movements can be very variable, from very short contractions to prolonged spasms.

Dystonic movements are often aggravated by voluntary actions. When dystonia appears in association with specific voluntary actions (task-specific), it is termed 'action dystonia' – for example, hand dystonia occurring only while writing or playing an instrument; leg dystonia occurring only when walking forward and not when walking backwards. Action dystonia is a typical feature of primary dystonia. With the progression of dystonia, the dystonic movements may be elicited by less specific voluntary actions or by voluntary actions of other body parts ('overflow' – for example, the appearance of a dystonic movement of the leg or arm while talking). Occasionally, dystonic postures may appear at rest; these can involve any body part: arm (hyperpronation of wrists, hyperextension of fingers), neck (retrocollis, torticollis, opisthotonus), pelvis (tortipelvis), cranial muscles (dysphonia, oromandibular dystonia, blepharospasm), or leg (intrarotation or hyperextension of the feet).

Dystonia is worsened by stress, fatigue, and fever, tends to be relieved by relaxation, and disappears during deep sleep. A unique characteristic of dystonia is the possibility that it may be reduced by a *'sensory trick'* – that is, a proprioceptive or tactile stimulus. For example, a patient can reduce oromandibular dystonia by touching the lips or the chin. Some patients are able to reduce dystonia simply by thinking about a sensory trick. Another way of relieving dystonia is represented by the phenomenon of *paradoxical dystonia*, where a voluntary movement can reduce dystonia (for example, blepharospasm may be reduced by talking).

Classification of dystonia and the clinical approach

The classification of dystonia takes account of the age at onset, distribution, course, and aetiology (Table 5).

Table 5. Classification of dystonia

Age at onset	Distribution	Time course	Aetiology
Early-onset (0–12 y)	Focal	Static	Primary
Adolescent onset (13–20 y)	Segmental	Progressive	Dystonia plus
Adult onset (> 1 y)	Multifocal Generalized	Paroxysmal Fluctuating	Secondary Heredo-degenerative

Age at onset is the best prognostic factor in primary dystonia – the earlier the onset, the greater the possibility that the dystonia will become generalised. Primary adolescent or adult-onset dystonias tend to remain focal or segmental. The distribution of dystonia is useful as an indicator of its severity, and for therapeutic decision-making. A unilateral distribution in usually associated with acquired lesions of the contralateral basal ganglia.

The course of dystonia needs to be taken into account as well. Paroxysmal and fluctuating dystonias are highly suggestive of specific clinical entities, such as paroxysmal dyskinesia and dopa-responsive dystonia; a progressive course is usually seen in early-onset primary dystonia or in heredo-degenerative disorders.

An aetiological classification is the ultimate aim of the clinical evaluation of patients with dystonia. The current classification distinguishes between *primary, dystonia-plus, secondary*, and *heredo-degenerative* dystonia. Primary dystonia is characterized by dystonia as the only neurological abnormality with the exception of tremor. Dystonia-plus is defined as the association of dystonia with parkinsonism or myoclonus. Secondary dystonia is caused by acquired brain lesions, mainly involving the basal ganglia. Heredo-degenerative dystonias are associated with many progressive neurological conditions caused by metabolic or degenerative CNS processes (Fahn et al., 1987; Fahn et al., 1998).

In clinical practice, the approach to dystonic patients requires as a first step the distinction between primary and secondary dystonia. This distinction is essential for planning any subsequent diagnostic investigations, for genetic counselling, for giving a prognosis, and for therapeutic decisions.

In secondary and heredo-degenerative dystonias, other signs and symptoms (pyramidal tract signs, dementia, epilepsy) are generally found in association with the abnormal movements. The phenomenology and the type of dystonia may also be extremely useful in distinguishing between a primary and a secondary condition, as illustrated in Table 6.

Table 6. Clinical features of primary *versus* secondary dystonia

	Primary dystonia	**Symptomatic dystonia**
Action dystonia	+	–
Dystonic spasms	+	+++
Speech disturbances	± (dysphonia)	++ (aphonia)
Swallowing disturbances	–	+
Oromandibular dystonia	+	++
Inappropriate facial expression	–	++
Loss of postural reflexes	–	++
Paradoxical dystonia	+	–
Sensory tricks	+	–
Early appearance of dystonic postures at rest, and fixed dystonia	–	+

References

Fahn, S. (1999): A comprehensive review of movement disorders for the clinical practitioner. 9th Annual Course, July 30-August 2, 1999, Aspen, Colorado.

Fahn, S., Bressman, S. & Marsden, C.D. (1998): Classification of dystonia. *Adv. Neurol.* **78**, 1–10.

Fahn, S., Marsden, C.D. & Calne, D.B. (1987): Classification and investigation of dystonia. In: *Movement disorders 2*, eds. C.D. Marsden & S. Fahn, pp. 332–358. London: Butterworth.

Jancovic, J. & Lang, A.E. (2004): Movement disorders: diagnosis and assessment. In: *Neurology in clinical practise*, 4th ed., eds. W.G. Bradley, R.B. Daroff, G.M. Fenichel & J. Jankovic, pp. 293–322. Philadelphia: Butterworth Heinemann.

Jancovic, J. (2003): Pathophysiology and assessment of Parkinsonian signs and symptoms. In: *Handbook of Parkinson's disease*, eds. R. Pahawa, K. Lyons & W.C. Koller. New York: Marcel Dekker.

Chapter 2

The genetics of dystonia

Barbara Garavaglia and Chiara Barzaghi

Molecular Neurogenetics Unit, Department of Experimental Research and Diagnostic, Fondazione IRCCS Istituto Neurologico 'C. Besta', via Temolo 4, 20126 Milan, Italy
garavaglia@istituto-besta.it

Summary

Dystonia is a movement disorder characterized by sustained muscle contractions affecting one or more sites of the body, frequently causing twisting and repetitive movements, or abnormal postures. Primary forms of dystonia can be distinguished from secondary forms. Primary dystonia occurs either in a familial or a sporadic pattern, with dystonia as the unique or major symptom. In contrast, secondary dystonia refers to dystonia in the context of a neurological disease in which dystonia is usually one of several symptoms (heredodegenerative diseases), or in which dystonia is the result of an environmental insult. Both primary dystonias and heredodegenerative diseases have a strong inherited basis. In this chapter we describe recent advances in the genetics and molecular mechanisms of dystonic syndromes. Conditions discussed in detail include idiopathic torsion dystonia *(DYT1)*, dopa-responsive dystonia *(DYT5)*, myoclonus-dystonia *(DYT11)*, autosomal recessive parkinsonism (Parkin disease), and pantothenate-kinase-associated neurodegeneration *(PKAN)*.

Introduction

Dystonia is a movement disorder characterized by 'involuntary, sustained muscle contractions affecting one or more sites of the body, frequently causing twisting and repetitive movements, or abnormal postures' (Fahn *et al.*, 1987). Primary forms of dystonia can be distinguished from secondary forms. Primary dystonia occurs either in a familial or a sporadic pattern, with dystonia as the unique or major symptom. By contrast, secondary dystonia refers to dystonia in the context of a neurological disease in which this symptom is usually one of several (heredodegenerative diseases), or in which dystonia is the result of an environmental insult (for example, peripheral and central trauma or cerebrovascular, infectious, demyelinating, or neoplastic disease).

Primary dystonias

The prevalence estimates for primary dystonia range from 2 to 50 cases per million for childhood dystonia and from 30 to 7,320 cases per million for adult-onset dystonia (Defazio *et al.*, 2004).

Until recently, primary dystonias were classified on the basis of clinical criteria, such as the age of onset or the distribution of the body parts affected by dystonia. In many cases conclusive assignment of a given phenotype has not been possible owing to the phenotypic variability in dystonia. Advances in molecular genetics have enabled the definitive distinction of many forms based on genetic criteria. At present, 15 different forms of dystonia are known to have a genetic origin (Table 1). In several cases, the underlying gene defect has been identified. In most of the other forms, the gene has been mapped to a particular chromosomal location, although the gene itself remains unknown. Three of the more common forms of genetic primary dystonia are described below.

Dystonia 1

Dystonia 1 or idiopathic torsion dystonia (ITD) is an autosomal dominant disease with reduced penetrance (30 per cent). Currently, the only identified ITD gene is the *DYT1* gene on chromosome 9q32-34 which encodes the TorsinA protein (Ozelius et al., 1997). Onset is usually in childhood, but it has been described in middle life (Bressman et al., 2000). The most common presentation of ITD is early limb-onset generalized dystonia, sparing the cranial muscles; however, different phenotypes have been reported, albeit less frequently (Kabakci et al., 2004). Phenotypic variability can be present even in the same family (Opal et al., 2002). A unique 3 bp (GAG) deletion in the *DYT1* gene – resulting in the loss of a glutamic acid residue in a conserved region of the protein (Ozelius et al., 1997) – was found to be the causative mutation for ITD. An additional mutation in the *DYT1* gene, a 18 bp deletion (966–983del) in exon 5, was identified in a patient with early-onset dystonia and myoclonic features (Leung et al., 2001). This patient was later found to have a mutation in the *SGCE* gene, associated with myoclonus dystonia or dystonia 11 (Klein et al., 2002).

The frequency of GAG deletion in patients with early-onset limb dystonia is 90 per cent in Jewish population, owing to a founder effect (Risch et al., 1995). Phenotypic spectra characterized by a wide variability and frequency of GAG deletions have been described in North American (Ozelius et al., 1997), British (Valente et al., 1998), French (Lebre et al., 1999), German (Leube et al., 1999), Russian (Slominsky et al., 1999), and Italian populations (Zorzi et al., 2002).

The protein TorsinA is 332 amino-acids long, with potential sites of glycosylation and phosphorylation, as well as a signal sequence and membrane spanning region at the amino-terminus consistent with membrane translocation and targeting. Analysis of the primary amino-acid sequence of the Torsin proteins revealed similarity to the AAA superfamily of ATPases (Ozelius et al., 1997). The function of TorsinA remains unknown. Based on its homology to known proteins, it has been suggested that it might function as a molecular chaperone in cells (Ozelius et al., 1997; Breakefield et al., 2001). Both TorsinA and its mRNA are widely distributed throughout the neurons and neural processes of the human brain. The most intense expression is localized in dopaminergic neurons of the substantia nigra *pars compacta* (Augood et al., 1998, Konakova et al., 2001) suggesting a role in dopamine transmission. Torres and collaborators showed that TorsinA can regulate the cellular trafficking of the dopamine transporter, as well as other polytopic membrane-bound proteins and ion channels; this effect was prevented by mutating the ATP binding site of TorsinA (Torres et al., 2004).

Table 1. Genetic classification of primary dystonias

Designation	OMIM Ref. No.	Age of onset	Inheritance pattern	Chromosome location	Gene	Protein	Gene test available
Dystonia 1 AD early-onset dystonia; IDT; Oppenheim's dystonia	128100	Usually childhood, may be later (< 26 years in most cases)	AD, incomplete penetrance	9q34	DYT1	TorsinA	Yes
Dystonia 2 AR dystonia (unconfirmed)	224500	/	AR	/	/	/	No
Dystonia 3 X-linked dystonia, parkinsonism (XP); also known as Lubag Disease	314250	Adults (average 35 years)	XR	Xq13.1	/	/	Yes
Dystonia 4 Torsion dystonia 4	128101	13–37 years	AD	/	/	/	No
Dystonia 5 Hereditary progressive dystonia with marked diurnal fluctuation (HPD); Segawa syndrome; dopa-responsive dystonia (DRD)	128230	Variable, often childhood	AD, incomplete penetrance	14q22.1-q22.2	GCH1	GTP-cyclo-hydrolase1	Yes
Dystonia 6 Adult onset ITD of mixed type	602629	Average 19 years	AD	8p21-p22	/	/	No
Dystonia 7 Adult onset ITD; idiopathic focal dystonia (IFD); AD late-onset dystonia	602124	28–70 years	AD, incomplete penetrance	18p	/	/	No
Dystonia 8 Paroxysmal non-kinesigenic dyskinesia (PNKD); paroxysmal dystonic choreoathetosis (PDC); familial paroxysmal dyskinesia; Mount-Reback syndrome	118800	Variable: early childhood, adolescence or early adulthood	AD, incomplete penetrance	2q33-q35	MR-1	Myofibrillogenesis regulator 1	Yes
Dystonia 9 Choreoathetosis, spasticity and episodic ataxia	601042	2–15 years	AD	1p	/	/	No
Dystonia 10 Paroxysmal kinesigenic choreoathetosis	128200	6–16 years	AD, incomplete penetrance	16p11.2-q12.1	/	/	No
Dystonia 11 Myoclonic dystonia; alcohol-responsive dystonia	159900	Variable but may be in early childhood	AD, incomplete penetrance	7q21	SGCE	Epsilon-sarcoglycan	Yes
Dystonia 12 Rapid-onset dystonia with parkinsonism (RDP)	128235	Childhood, adolescence or adulthood	AD, incomplete penetrance	19q12-q13.2	ATP1A3	ATPase (alpha3)	Yes
Dystonia 13 Focal dystonia with cranio-cervical features	607671	5 years to adult	AD, incomplete penetrance	1p36.13-36.32	/	/	No
Dystonia 14	607195	Childhood	AD	14q13	/	/	No
Dystonia 15 Inherited myoclonus-dystonia	607488	6 years	AD	18p11	/	/	No

AD, autosomal dominant; AR, autosomal recessive; XR, X-linked recessive; OMIM, Online Mendelian Inheritance in Man (http://www.ncbi.nlm.nih.gov:80/entrez/query.fcgi?db=OMIM).

Dystonia 5

Dystonia 5 is caused by mutations in the *GCH1* gene located on 14q22-q22.2. Patients heterozygous for *GCH1* mutations develop dopa-responsive dystonia, also called dominantly inherited GTP cyclohydrolase I (GTPCH1) deficiency, whereas patients who are homozygous or compound heterozygous for *GCH1* mutations develop the recessive form (Blau *et al.*, 2001).

Dopa-responsive dystonia (DRD) is characterized by dystonia, concurrent or subsequent parkinsonism, a dramatic therapeutic response to L-dopa in most patients, and diurnal worsening of symptoms in about 75 per cent of index cases (Nygaard *et al.*, 1991). Symptoms and age of onset vary considerably between patients even within the same family. Although the onset is usually during childhood or adolescence, adult onset does occur (Blau *et al.*, 2001). There is incomplete penetrance (~ 30 per cent) (Nygaard *et al.*, 1990), but if subtle signs and typical symptoms are taken into account the penetrance can range from 40 to 100 per cent (Steinberger *et al.*, 1998). Females are affected two to four times more often than males (Blau *et al.*, 2001).

The recessive GTPCH1 form is a rare disease with fewer than 20 patients listed in the international database of BH4 deficiency (http://www.bh4.org). The clinical picture is characterized by neonatal onset with poor sucking and swallowing difficulties, severe hypotonia, seizures, and psychomotor retardation. In the course of the disease, recurrent hyperthermia and abnormal ocular movements have been observed. Plasma hyperphenylalaninaemia is usually detected on neonatal screening. Treatment with L-dopa/carbidopa, BH4, and 5-hydroxytryptophan can improve the neurological symptoms but does not prevent development of severe encephalopathy (Blau *et al.*, 2001). Three additional patients with recessive GTPCH1 deficiency were reported with an isolated extrapyramidal syndrome with no hyperphenylalaninaemia and complete responsiveness to L-dopa treatment (Hwu *et al.*, 1999; Nardocci *et al.*, 2003).

GCH1 codes for GTP cyclohydrolase I enzyme (GTPCH1) (EC 3.5.4.16), which is the rate-limiting enzyme in the biosynthesis of tetrahydrobiopterin (BH4), an essential cofactor for aromatic amino-acid mono-oxygenases (Thöny *et al.*, 2000). *GCH1* is composed of six exons. More than 90 independent mutations, located throughout the exons and at intronic splice sites, have been identified so far (Blau *et al.*, 2001). The activity of GTPCH1, a homodecamer, was shown to be reduced by more than 50 per cent in lymphocytes and fibroblasts of several affected heterozygous mutation carriers, suggesting a dominant negative effect of the mutant polypeptide with the wild-type subunits, or a dominant negative effect at the transcriptional level (Hirano *et al.*, 1998; Hwu *et al.*, 2000; Bonafé *et al.*, 2001, Müller *et al.*, 2002a). Depending on the biochemical defect, affected mutation carriers' cerebrospinal fluid contains low concentrations of homovanillic acid (HVA), 5-hydroxyindoleacetic acid (HIAA) (metabolites of dopamine and serotonin, respectively), neopterin, and biopterin (Williams *et al.*, 1979; Fink *et al.*, 1988; Nygaard *et al.*, 1991; Blau *et al.*, 2001).

A simple and reliable assay for the detection and functional analysis of mutations in *GCH1* gene was devised by Mancini *et al.* in 1999, using the knock-out mutant *(fol2Δ)* of the budding yeast *Saccharomyces cerevisiae*. The human GTPCH1 has an identity of 49.6 per cent with the yeast protein. In yeast the enzyme mediates the first and committing step of the folate synthesis pathway, and the *fol2Δ* allele causes auxotrophy for folinic acid. These investigators showed that the GTPCH1, encoded by the human c-DNA, complements the yeast *fol2Δ* mutation by restoring folate prototrophy (Mancini *et al.*, 1999). Using this assay, in our laboratory we studied the mutations found in eight Italian patients affected by dominant and recessive GTPCH1 deficiency (Fig. 1) (Garavaglia *et al.*, 2004).

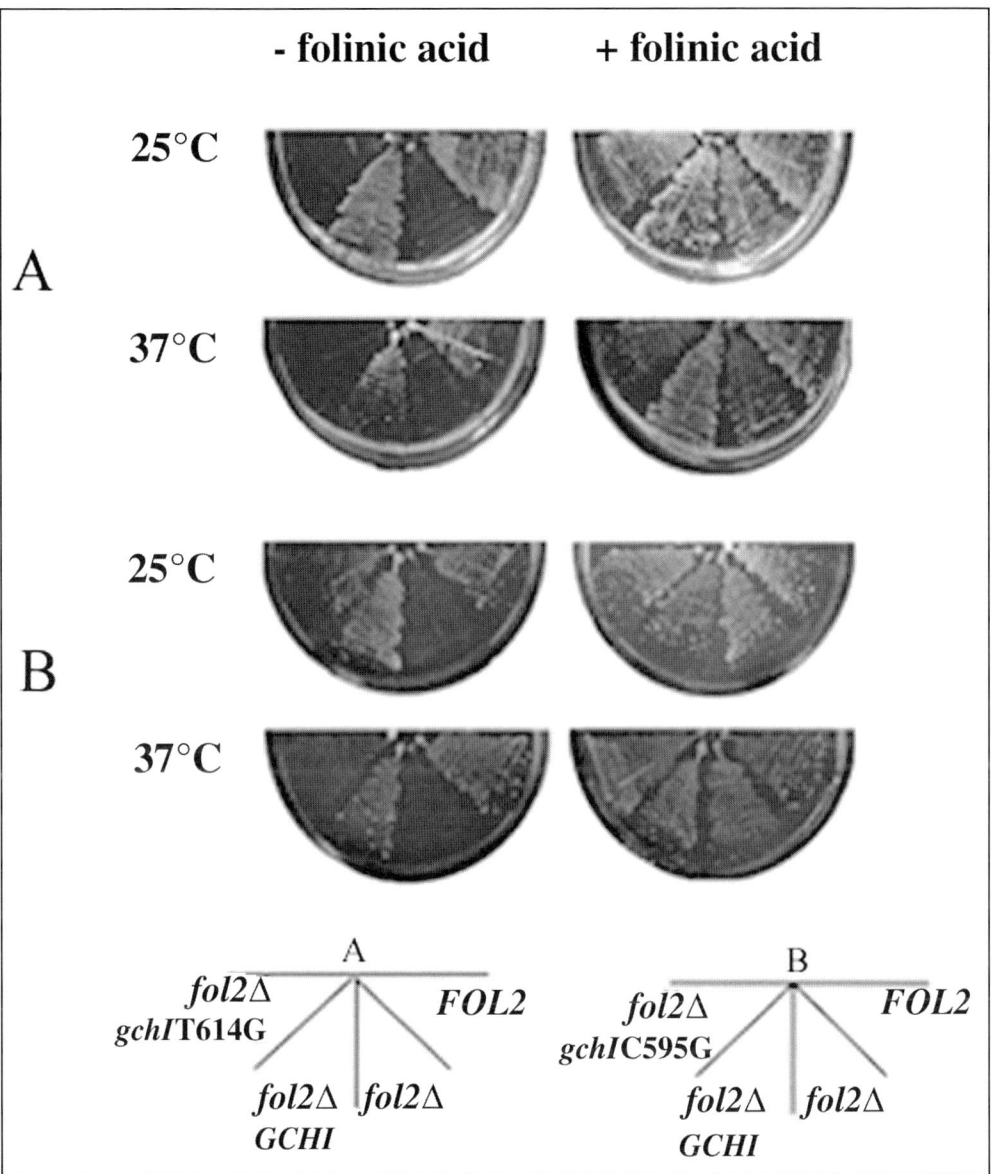

Fig. 1. Functional testing of GCH1 mutations. In panel A, the T614G mutation abolishes the enzyme function, as fol2Δ cells carrying the corresponding GCH1 allele were able to grow only on medium supplemented with folinic acid. In panel B, the C595G mutation, responsible for the recessive form, causes a conditional defect, as only a high temperature (37° C) strongly affected the capacity of the mutant GCH1 allele to complement the fol2Δ defect.

Dystonia 11

Inherited myoclonus-dystonia (MD; DYT11) is an autosomal dominant disorder characterized by bilateral, alcohol-responsive myoclonic jerks involving mainly the arms and axial muscles (Gasser, 1998). Dystonia – usually torticollis or writer's cramp, or both – occurs in most but not all affected individuals and may occasionally be the only symptom of the disease (Quinn *et al.*, 1988). In addition to these involuntary movements, psychiatric problems (for example, alcohol abuse, obsessive-compulsive disorder, and panic attacks) have often been noted in MD patients (Quinn *et al.*, 1988; Zimprich *et al.*, 2001; Saunders-Pullman *et al.*, 2002). The onset of the disorder is usually in childhood or the teenage years. In most MD families, the disease is linked to a locus on chromosome 7q21 (Nygaard *et al.*, 1999; Asmus *et al.*, 2001) and mutations in the epsilon-sarcoglycan gene *(SGCE)* are found. Epsilon-sarcoglycan protein is part of the dystrophin-glycoprotein complex that links the cytoskeleton to the extracellular matrix (Hack *et al.*, 2000). It is ubiquitously expressed, especially in the central nervous system (Nishiyama *et al.*, 2004). The human *SGCE* gene is maternally imprinted, resulting in reduced penetrance when the mutation is inherited from the mother owing to methylation of the maternal allele (Müller *et al.*, 2002b). Up to now, 72 patients with *SGCE* mutations have been described (Zimprich *et al.*, 2001; Asmus *et al.*, 2002; Doheny *et al.*, 2002a; Doheny *et al.*, 2002b; Foncke *et al.*, 2003; Han *et al.*, 2003; Hjermind *et al.*, 2003; Marechal *et al.*, 2003; Valente *et al.*, 2003). Although the *SGCE* gene seems to be the major gene responsible for autosomal dominant myoclonus-dystonia, no mutations have been found in many sporadic cases (Valente *et al.*, 2003). These data, together with the discovery of another locus for MD on chromosome 18p11 (Grimes *et al.*, 2002), are further support for the evidence for genetic heterogeneity in this clinical form.

Heredodegenerative dystonias

The heredodegenerative dystonias are the most heterogeneous group of dystonias and include autosomal dominant, autosomal recessive, and X-linked disorders (Table 2). Patients typically present with dystonia-plus syndrome and often have other neurological features such as ataxia, dysarthria, parkinsonism, choreoathetosis, and dementia. Some other diseases such as lysosomal storage disorders, amino acidurias, organic acidurias, and mitochondrial disorders can present with dystonia as a prominent feature (Fahn *et al.*, 1987). In the following section, we discuss two heredodegenerative disorders in which particular progress in molecular characterization has been made over the past few years.

Autosomal recessive, juvenile onset Parkinson's disease (AR-JP)

Autosomal recessive, juvenile onset parkinsonism (AR-JP) is a clinically and genetically distinct entity. Typical features of AR-JP include early-onset of disease (< 40 years), sustained response to levodopa, and early occurrence of levodopa-induced dyskinesias. To date, three different genes have been associated with AR-JP: the *Park2* gene (Kitada *et al.*, 1998) mapped to 6q25.2-27; the *DJ1* gene (Bonifati *et al.*, 2003); and the *Pink1* gene (Valente *et al.*, 2004) – the latter two both localized to 1p36 chromosome. While the frequency of *Park2* mutations in AR-JP patients has been estimated at 10–25 per cent (Lucking *et al.*, 2000), the *DJ1* and *Pink1* mutations seem to be rarer (Hedrich *et al.*, 2004, Valente *et al.*, 2004).

Parkin-associated AR-JP

Park2 gene encodes the Parkin protein, an E3 ubiquitin-protein ligase that targets specific substrates for degradation through the ubiquitin-proteasome pathway (Shimura *et al.*, 2000). Most *Park2* mutations are thought to be loss of function mutations, and failure of Parkin to ubiquitinate and remove substrates may lead to its accumulation and subsequent toxicity (Cookson, 2003). Exonic rearrangements as well as point mutations in the *Park2* gene have

Table 2. Genetic classification of heredodegenerative dystonias

Designation	OMIM Ref. No.	Age of onset	Inheritance pattern	Chromosome location	Gene	Protein	Gene test available
Fahr disease Idiopathic basal ganglia calcification; BGC1; IBGC; bilateral striopallidodentate calcinosis	213600	30–60 years	AD	14q	/	/	No
Aicardi-Goutière's syndrome Familial early-onset encephalopathy with calcifications of basal ganglia and chronic cerebrospinal fluid lymphocytosis	225750	Usually diagnosed shortly after birth or during early childhood	AR	3p21.3-p21.2	*TREX1*	TREX1	Yes
Pantothenate kinase-associated neurodegeneration (PKAN) Neurodegeneration with brain iron accumulation 1 NBIA1; Hallervorden-Spatz syndrome	234200	Usually 1st or 2nd decade, death by 30 years	AR	20p12.3-13	*PANK2*	Pantothenate kinase	Yes
Autosomal recessive juvenile-onset Parkinson's disease with dystonia (AR-JP; PJD)	602544	Usually < 40 years	AR	6q25.2-q27	*PARK2*	Parkin	Yes
McLeod syndrome Kell blood group precursor	314850	4th decade	XR	Xp21.2-p21.1	*XK*	Kell blood group precursor	Yes
Chorea-acanthocytosis (CHAC) Levine-Critchley syndrome; amyotrophic chorea with acanthocytosis	200150	3rd and 4th decade	AR	9q21	*VPS13A*	Chorein	Yes
X-linked deafness-dystonia-optic atrophy (Mohr-Tranebjaerg syndrome)	304700	Childhood	XR	Xq22	*TIMM8A*	Translocase of inner mitochondrial membrane 8 homolog A	Yes

AD, autosomal dominant; AR, autosomal recessive; XR, X-linked recessive; OMIM, Online Mendelian Inheritance in Man (http://www.ncbi.nlm.nih.gov:80/entrez/query.fcgi?db=OMIM).

been found in all 12 exons of the gene (Abbas et al., 1999; Lucking et al., 2000; Hedrich et al., 2001). From a clinical perspective, factors associated with mutation frequencies appear to be highly correlated with lower age of onset and a positive family history (Lucking et al., 2000). The ethnic background of the patients also affects the mutation rate, with frequencies of *Park2* mutations ranging from 66 per cent in Japanese patients (Hattori et al., 1998) to less than 4 per cent in US or Serbian populations (Chen et al., 2003; Djarmati et al., 2004). In our laboratory, we screened 320 Italian patients for *Park2* mutations – 23 with a clear autosomal recessive inheritance and 297 sporadic cases. The frequency of mutations was 39.1 per cent in familial cases and 13.8 per cent in sporadic cases. However, in sporadic cases the frequency of mutations rose with decreasing age of onset: 29.5 per cent in patients with onset < 30 years and 7.9 per cent in those with onset > 41 years (Fig. 2). The clinical Park2 phenotype is highly variable (Healy et al., 2004), but dystonia with an excellent response to levodopa can be the major clinical sign, especially in patients with a juvenile onset and can be confused with the DRD phenotype (Tassin et al., 2000).

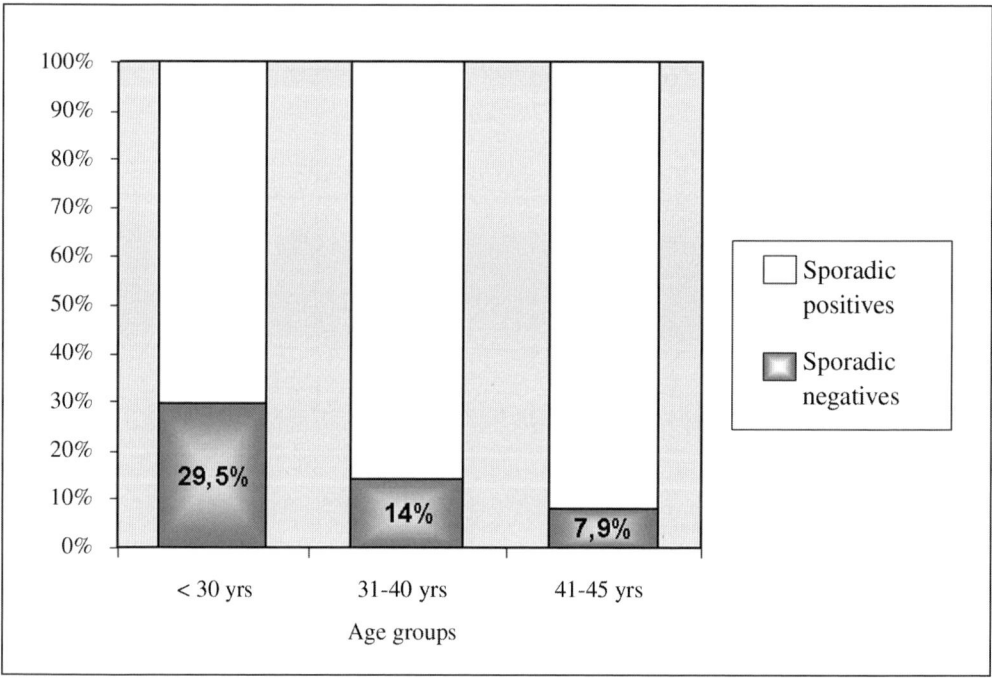

Fig. 2. *Age at onset distribution of positive and negative sporadic patients for Park2 mutations. The frequency of positives decreases progressively with increasing age of onset.*

Pantothenate kinase-associated neurodegeneration (Hallervorden-Spatz syndrome)

Pantothenate kinase-associated neurodegeneration (PKAN) is an autosomal recessive disorder associated with progressive impairment of movement, vision, and cognition (Gordon, 2002). Classic PKAN manifests in the first decade with severe extrapyramidal signs, and progresses rapidly with loss of ambulation within 15 years from onset. In atypical PKAN, the onset is in the second to third decade with less severe extrapyramidal signs, slower progression, and maintenance of independent ambulation until 15 years or more after disease onset (Hayflick et al., 2003). Linkage mapping to chromosome 20p12.3 and subsequent mutation screening in candidate genes has led to the identification of mutations in the *PANK2* gene coding for the enzyme of the initial and rate limiting step in CoA biosynthesis, the phosphorylation of pantothenate (Zhou *et al.*, 2001). *PANK2* codes for a kinase with a mitochondrial targeting sequence which directs its transport into the organelle (Hortnagel *et al.*, 2003). Altered mitochondrial CoA synthesis owing to loss of the function of the enzyme is predicted to cause mitochondrial dysfunction with subsequent degeneration of susceptible neuronal tissues, mainly the basal ganglia, the optic nerve, and the retina. The neurodegeneration is accompanied by iron accumulation, which can be demonstrated radiologically by the eye-of-the-tiger sign on magnetic resonance imaging (Angelini *et al.*, 1992). Mutations in the *PANK2* gene have been found in the entire coding region except in the part which codes for the mitochondrial target sequence, and in the 'intermediate' domains which are cleaved during maturation of the protein (Pellecchia *et al.*, 2005; Hartig *et al.*, 2006).

References

Abbas, N., Lucking, C.B., Ricard, S., Durr, A., Bonifati, V., De Michele, G., Bouley, S., Vaughan, J.R., Gasser, T., Marconi, R., Broussolle, E., Brefel-Courbon, C., Harhangi, B.S., Oostra, B.A., Fabrizio, E., Bohme, G.A., Pradier, L., Wood, N.W., Filla, A., Meco, G., Denefle, P., Agid, Y. & Brice, A. (1999): A wide variety of mutations in the Parkin gene are responsible for autosomal recessive parkinsonism in Europe. *Hum. Mol. Genet.* **8**, 567–574.

Angelini, L., Nardocci, N., Rumi, V., Zorzi, C., Strada, L. & Savoiardo, M. (1992): Hallervorden-Spatz disease: clinical and MRI study of 11 cases diagnosed in life. *J. Neurol.* **239**, 417–425.

Asmus, F., Zimprich, A., Naumann, M., Berg, D., Bertram, M., Ceballos-Baumann, A., Pruszak-Seel, R., Kabus, C., Dichgans, M., Fuchs, S., Muller-Myhsok, B. & Gasser, T. (2001): Inherited myoclonus-dystonia syndrome: narrowing the 7q21-q31 locus in German families. *Ann. Neurol.* **49**, 121–124.

Asmus, F., Zimprich, A., Tezenas Du Montcel, S., Kabus, C., Deuschl, G., Kupsch, A., Ziemann, U., Castro, M., Kuhn, A.A., Strom, T.M., Vidailhet, M., Bhatia, K.P., Durr, A., Wood, N.W., Brice, A. & Gasser, T. (2002): Myoclonus-dystonia syndrome: epsilon-sarcoglycan mutations and phenotype. *Ann. Neurol.* **52**, 489–492.

Augood, S.J., Penney, J.B., Friberg, I.K., Breakefield, X.O., Young, A.B., Ozelius, L.J. & Standaert, D.G. (1998): Expression of the early-onset torsion dystonia gene (DYT1) in human brain. *Ann. Neurol.* **43**, 669–673.

Blau, N., Thöny, B., Cotton, R.G.H. & Hyland, K. (2001): Disorders of tetrahydrobiopterin and related biogenic amines. In: *The metabolic and molecular bases of inherited disease*, 8th ed., eds. C.R. Scriver, A.L. Beaudet, W.S. Sly, D. Valle, B. Childs & B. Vogelstein, pp. 1725–1776. New York: McGraw-Hill.

Bonafé, L., Thony, B., Leimbacher, W., Kierat, L. & Blau, N. (2001): Diagnosis of Dopa-responsive dystonia and other tetrahydrobiopterin disorders by the study of biopterin metabolism in fibroblasts. *Clin. Chem.* **47**, 477–485.

Bonifati, V., Rizzu, P., van Baren, M.J., Schaap, O., Breedveld, G.J., Krieger, E., Dekker, M.C., Squitieri, F., Ibanez, P., Joosse, M., van Dongen, J.W., Vanacore, N., van Swieten, J.C., Brice, A., Meco, G., van Duijn, C.M., Oostra, B.A. & Heutink, P. (2003): Mutations in the DJ-1 gene associated with autosomal recessive early-onset parkinsonism. *Science* **299**, 256–259.

Breakefield, X.O., Kamm, C. & Hanson, P.I. (2001): TorsinA: movement at many levels. *Neuron* **31**, 9–12.

Bressman, S.B., Sabatti, C., Raymond, D., de Leon, D., Klein, C., Kramer, P.L., Brin, M.F., Fahn, S., Breakefield, X., Ozelius, L.J. & Risch, N.J. (2000): The DYT1 phenotype and guidelines for diagnostic testing. *Neurology* **54**, 1746–1752.

Chen, R., Gosavi, N.S., Langston, J.W. & Chan, P. (2003): Parkin mutations are rare in patients with young-onset parkinsonism in a US population. *Parkinsonism Relat. Disord.* **9**, 309–312.

Cookson, M.R. (2003): Parkin's substrates and the pathways leading to neuronal damage. *Neuromol. Med.* **3**, 1–13.

Defazio, G., Abbruzzese, G., Livrea, P. & Berardelli, A. (2004): Epidemiology of primary dystonia. *Lancet Neurol.* **3**, 673–678.

Djarmati, A., Hedrich, K., Svetel, M., Schafer, N., Juric, V., Vukosavic, S., Hering, R., Riess, O., Romac, S., Klein, C. & Kostic, V. (2004): Detection of Parkin (PARK2) and DJ1 (PARK7) mutations in early-onset Parkinson disease: Parkin mutation frequency depends on ethnic origin of patients. *Hum. Mutat.* **23**, 525.

Doheny, D.O., Brin, M.F., Morrison, C.E., Smith, C.J., Walker, R.H., Abbasi, S., Muller, B., Garrels, J., Liu, L., De Carvalho Aguiar, P., Schilling, K., Kramer, P., De Leon, D., Raymond, D., Saunders-Pullman, R., Klein, C., Bressman, S.B., Schmand, B., Tijssen, M.A., Ozelius, L.J. & Silverman, J.M. (2002a): Phenotypic features of myoclonus-dystonia in three kindreds. *Neurology* **59**, 1187–1196.

Doheny, D., Danisi, F., Smith, C., Morrison, C., Velickovic, M., De Leon, D., Bressman, S.B., Leung, J., Ozelius, L., Klein, C., Breakefield, X.O., Brin, M.F. & Silverman, J.M. (2002b): Clinical findings of a myoclonus-dystonia family with two distinct mutations. *Neurology* **59**, 1244–1246.

Fahn, S., Marsden, C.D. & Calne, D.B. (1987): Classification and investigation of dystonia. In: *Movement disorders 2*, eds. C.D. Marsden & S. Fahn, pp. 332–358. London: Butterworth.

Fink, J.K., Barton, N., Cohen, W., Lovenberg, W., Burns, R.S. & Hallett, M. (1988): Dystonia with marked diurnal variation associated with biopterin deficiency. *Neurology* **38**, 707–711.

Foncke, E.M., Klein, C., Koelman, J.H., Kramer, P.L., Schilling, K., Muller, B., Garrels, J., de Carvalho Aguiar, P., Liu, L., de Froe, A., Speelman, J.D., Ozelius, L.J. & Tijssen, M.A. (2003): Hereditary myoclonus-dystonia associated with epilepsy. *Neurology* **60**, 1988–1990.

Garavaglia, B., Invernizzi, F., Carbone, M.L., Viscardi, V., Saracino, F., Ghezzi, D., Zeviani, M., Zorzi, G. & Nardocci, N. (2004): GTP-cyclohydrolase I gene mutations in patients with autosomal dominant and recessive GTP-CH1 deficiency: identification and functional characterization of four novel mutations. *J. Inherit. Metab. Dis.* **27**, 455–463.

Gasser, T. (1998): Inherited myoclonus-dystonia syndrome. *Adv. Neurol.* **78**, 325–334.

Gordon, N. (2002): Pantothenate kinase-associated neurodegeneration (Hallervorden-Spatz syndrome). *Eur. J. Paediatr. Neurol.* **6**, 243–247.

Grimes, D.A., Han, F., Lang, A.E., St. George-Hyssop, P., Racacho, L. & Bulman, D.E. (2002): A novel locus for inherited myoclonus-dystonia on 18p11. *Neurology* **59**, 1183–1186.

Hack, A.A., Groh, M.E. & McNally, E.M. (2000): Sarcoglycans in muscular dystrophy. *Microsc. Res. Tech.* **48**, 167–180.

Han, F., Lang, A.E., Racacho, L., Bulman, D.E. & Grimes, D.A. (2003): Mutations in the epsilon-sarcoglycan gene found to be uncommon in seven myoclonus-dystonia families. *Neurology* **61**, 244–246.

Hartig, M.B., Hörtnagel, K., Garavaglia, B., Zorzi, G., Kmiec, T., Klopstock, T., Rostasy, K., Svetel, M., Kostic, V.S., Schuelke, M., Botz, E., Weindl, A., Novakovic, I., Nardocci, N., Prokisch, H. & Meitinger, T. (2006): Genotypic and phenotypic spectrum of PANK2 mutations in patients with brain iron accumulation. *Ann. Neurol* **59**, 248–256.

Hattori, N., Kitada, T., Matsumine, H., Asakawa, S., Yamamura, Y., Yoshino, H., Kobayashi, T., Yokochi, M., Wang, M., Yoritaka, A., Kondo, T., Kuzuhara, S., Nakamura, S., Shimizu, N. & Mizuno, Y. (1998): Molecular genetic analysis of a novel Parkin gene in Japanese families with autosomal recessive juvenile parkinsonism: evidence for variable homozygous deletions in the Parkin gene in affected individuals. *Ann. Neurol.* **44**, 935–941.

Hayflick, S.J., Westaway, S.K., Levinson, B., Zhou, B., Johnson, M.A., Ching, K.H. & Gitschier, J. (2003): Genetic, clinical, and radiographic delineation of Hallervorden-Spatz syndrome. *N. Engl. J. Med.* **348**, 33–40.

Healy, D.G., Abou-Sleiman, P.M. & Wood, N.W. (2004): PINK, PANK, or PARK? A clinicians'guide to familial parkinsonism. *Lancet Neurol.* **3**, 652–662.

Hedrich, K., Kann, M., Lanthaler, A.J., Dalski, A., Eskelson, C., Landt, O., Schwinger, E., Vieregge, P., Lang, A.E., Breakefield, X.O., Ozelius, L.J., Pramstaller, P.P. & Klein, C. (2001): The importance of gene dosage studies: mutational analysis of the Parkin gene in early-onset parkinsonism. *Hum. Mol. Genet.* **10**, 1649–1656.

Hedrich, K., Djarmati, A., Schafer, N., Hering, R., Wellenbrock, C., Weiss, P.H., Hilker, R., Vieregge, P., Ozelius, L.J., Heutink, P., Bonifati, V., Schwinger, E., Lang, A.E., Noth, J., Bressman, S.B., Pramstaller, P.P., Riess, O. & Klein, C. (2004): DJ-1 (PARK7) mutations are less frequent than Parkin (PARK2) mutations in early-onset Parkinson disease. *Neurology* **62**, 389–394.

Hirano, M., Yanagihara, T. & Ueno, S. (1998): Dominant negative effect of GTP cyclohydrolase I mutations in Dopa-responsive hereditary progressive dystonia. *Ann. Neurol.* **44**, 365–371.

Hjermind, L.E., Werdelin, L.M., Eiberg, H., Krag-Olsen, B., Dupont, E. & Sorensen, S.A. (2003): A novel mutation in the epsilon-sarcoglycan gene causing myoclonus-dystonia syndrome. *Neurology* **60**, 1536–1539.

Hortnagel, K., Prokisch, H. & Meitinger, T. (2003): An isoform of hPANK2, deficient in pantothenate kinase-associated neurodegeneration, localizes to mitochondria. *Hum. Mol. Genet.* **12**, 321–327.

Hwu, W.L., Wang, P.J., Hsiao, K.J., Wang, T.R., Chiou, Y.W. & Lee, Y.M. (1999): Dopa responsive dystonia induced by recessive GTP cyclohydrolase I mutation. *Hum. Genet.* **105**, 226–230.

Hwu, W.L., Chiou, Y.W., Lai, S.Y. & Lee, Y.M. (2000): Dopa responsive dystonia is induced by a dominant negative mechanism. *Ann. Neurol.* **48**, 609–613.

Kabakci, K., Hedrich, K., Leung, J.C., Mitterer, M., Vieregge, P., Lencer, R., Hagenah, J., Garrels, J., Witt, K., Klostermann, F., Svetel, M., Friedman, J., Kostic, V., Bressman, S.B., Breakefield, X.O., Ozelius, L.J., Pramstaller, P.P. & Klein C. (2004): Mutations in DYT1: extension of the phenotypic and mutational spectrum. *Neurology* **10**, 395–400.

Kitada, T., Asakawa, S., Hattori, N., Matsumine, H., Yamamura, Y., Minoshima, S., Yokochi, M., Mizuno, Y. & Shimizu, N. (1998): Mutations in the Parkin gene cause autosomal recessive juvenile parkinsonism. *Nature* **392**, 605–608.

Klein, C., Liu, L., Doheny, D., Kock, N., Muller, B., de Carvalho Aguiar, P., Leung, J., de Leon, D., Bressman, S.B., Silverman, J., Smith, C., Danisi, F., Morrison, C., Walker, R.H., Velickovic, M., Schwinger, E., Kramer, P.L., Breakefield, X.O., Brin, M.F. & Ozelius, L.J. (2002): Epsilon-sarcoglycan mutations found in combination with other dystonia gene mutations. *Ann. Neurol.* **52**, 675–679.

Konakova, M., Huynh, D.P., Yong, W. & Pulst, S.M. (2001): Cellular distribution of torsinA and torsinB in normal human brain. *Arch. Neurol.* **58**, 921–927.

Lebre, A.S., Durr, A., Jedynak, P., Ponsot, G., Vidailhet, M., Agid, Y. & Brice, A. (1999): DYT1 mutation in French families with idiopathic torsion dystonia. *Brain* **122**, 41–45.

Leube, B., Kessler, K.R., Ferbert, A., Ebke, M., Schwendemann, G., Erbguth, F., Benecke, R. & Auburger, G. (1999): Phenotypic variability of the DYT1 mutation in German dystonia patients. *Acta Neurol. Scand.* **99**, 248–251.

Leung, J.C., Klein, C., Friedman, J., Vieregge, P., Jacobs, H., Doheny, D., Kamm, C., DeLeon, D., Pramstaller, P.P., Penney, J.B., Eisengart, M., Jankovic, J., Gasser, T., Bressman, S.B., Corey, D.P., Kramer, P., Brin, M.F., Ozelius, L.J. & Breakefield, X.O. (2001): Novel mutation in the TOR1A (DYT1) gene in atypical, early-onset dystonia and polymorphisms in dystonia and early-onset parkinsonism. *Neurogenetics* **3**, 133–143.

Lucking, C.B., Durr, A., Bonifati, V., Vaughan, J., De Michele, G., Gasser, T., Harhangi, B.S., Meco, G., Denefle, P., Wood, N.W., Agid, Y. & Brice, A. (2000): Association between early-onset Parkinson's disease and mutations in the Parkin gene. *N. Engl. J. Med.* **342**, 1560–1567.

Mancini, R., Saracino, F., Buscemi, G., Fischer, M., Schramek, N., Bracher, A., Bacher, A., Gutlich, M. & Carbone, M.L. (1999): Complementation of the fol2 deletion in Saccharomyces cerevisiae by human and Escherichia coli genes encoding GTP cyclohydrolase I. *Biochem. Biophys. Res. Commun.* **255**, 521–527.

Marechal, L., Raux, G., Dumanchin, C., Lefebvre, G., Deslandre, E., Girard, C., Campion, D., Parain, D., Frebourg, T. & Hannequin, D. (2003): Severe myoclonus-dystonia syndrome associated with a novel epsilon-sarcoglycan gene truncating mutation. *Am. J. Med. Genet. B Neuropsychiatr. Genet.* **119**, 114–117.

Müller, U., Steinberg, D. & Topka, H. (2002a): Mutations of *GCH1* in dopa-responsive dystonia. *J. Neural Transm.* **109**, 321–328.

Müller, B., Hedrich, K., Kock, N., Dragasevic, N., Svetel, M., Garrels, J., Landt, O., Nitschke, M., Pramstaller, P.P., Reik, W., Schwinger, E., Sperner, J., Ozelius, L., Kostic, V. & Klein, C. (2002b): Evidence that paternal expression of the epsilon-sarcoglycan gene accounts for reduced penetrance in myoclonus-dystonia. *Am. J. Hum. Genet.* **71**, 1303–1311.

Nardocci, N., Zorzi, G., Blau, N., Fernandez Alvarez, E., Sesta, M., Angelini, L., Pannacci, M., Invernizzi, F. & Garavaglia, B. (2003): Neonatal dopa-responsive extrapyramidal syndrome in twins with recessive GTPCH deficiency. *Neurology* **60**, 335–337.

Nishiyama, A., Endo, T., Takeda, S. & Imamura, M. (2004): Identification and characterization of epsilon-sarcoglycans in the central nervous system. *Brain Res. Mol. Brain Res.* **125**, 1–12.

Nygaard, T.G., Trugman, J.M., de Yebenes, J.G. & Fahn, S. (1990): Dopa-responsive dystonia: the spectrum of clinical manifestations in a large North American family. *Neurology* **40**, 66–69.

Nygaard, T.G., Marsden, D. & Fahn, S. (1991): Dopa-responsive dystonia: long-term treatment response and prognosis. *Neurology* **41**, 174–181.

Nygaard, T.G., Raymond, D., Chen, C., Nishino, I., Greene, P.E., Jennings, D., Heiman, G.A., Klein, C., Saunders-Pullman, R.J., Kramer, P., Ozelius, L.J. & Bressman, S.B. (1999): Localization of a gene for myoclonus-dystonia to chromosome 7q21-q31. *Ann. Neurol.* **46**, 794–798.

Opal, P., Tintner, R., Jankovic, J., Leung, J., Breakefield, X.O., Friedman, J. & Ozelius, L. (2002): Intrafamilial phenotypic variability of the DYT1 dystonia: from asymptomatic TOR1A gene carrier status to dystonic storm. *Mov. Disord.* **17**, 339–345.

Ozelius, L.J., Hewett, J.W., Page, C.E., Bressman, S.B., Kramer, P.L., Shalish, C., de Leon, D., Brin, M.F., Raymond, D., Corey, D.P., Fahn, S., Risch, N.J., Buckler, A.J., Gusella, J.F. & Breakefield, X.O. (1997): The early-onset torsion dystonia gene (DYT1) encodes an ATP-binding protein. *Nat. Genet.* **17**, 40–48.

Pellecchia, M.T., Valente, E.M., Cif, L., Salvi, S., Albanese, A., Scarano, V., Bonuccelli, U., Bentivoglio, A.R., D'Amico, A., Marelli, C., Di Giorgio, A., Coubes, P., Barone, P. & Dallapiccola, B. (2005): The diverse phenotype and genotype of pantothenate kinase-associated neurodegeneration. *Neurology* **64**, 1810–1812.

Quinn, N.P., Rothwell, J.C., Thompson, P.D. & Marsden, C.D. (1988): Hereditary myoclonic dystonia, hereditary torsion dystonia and hereditary essential myoclonus: an area of confusion. *Adv. Neurol.* **50**, 391–401.

Risch, N., de Leon, D., Ozelius, L., Kramer, P., Almasy, L., Singer, B., Fahn, S., Breakefield, X. & Bressman, S. (1995): Genetic analysis of idiopathic torsion dystonia in Ashkenazi Jews and their recent descent from a small founder population. *Nat. Genet.* **9**, 152–159.

Saunders-Pullman, R., Shriberg, J., Heiman, G., Raymond, D., Wendt, K., Kramer, P., Schilling, K., Kurlan, R., Klein, C., Ozelius, L.J., Risch, N.J. & Bressman, S.B. (2002): Myoclonus dystonia: possible association with obsessive-compulsive disorder and alcohol dependence. *Neurology* **58**, 242–245.

Shimura, H., Hattori, N., Kubo, S., Mizuno, Y., Asakawa, S., Minoshima, S., Shimizu, N., Iwai, K., Chiba, T., Tanaka, K. & Suzuki, T. (2000): Familial Parkinson disease gene product, Parkin, is a ubiquitin-protein ligase. *Nat. Genet.* **25**, 302–305.

Slominsky, P.A., Markova, E.D., Shadrina, M.I., Illarioshkin, S.N., Miklina, N.I., Limborska, S.A. & Ivanova-Smolenskaya, I.A. (1999): A common 3-bp deletion in the DYT1 gene in Russian families with early-onset torsion dystonia. *Hum. Mutat.* **14**, 269.

Steinberger, D., Weber, Y., Korinthenberg, R., Deuschl, G., Benecke, R., Martinius, J. & Muller U. (1998): High penetrance and pronounced variation in expressivity of GCH1 mutations in five families with dopa-responsive dystonia. *Ann Neurol.* **43**, 634–639.

Tassin, J., Durr, A., Bonnet, A.M., Gil, R., Vidailhet, M., Lucking, C.B., Goas, J.Y., Durif, F., Abada, M., Echenne, B., Motte, J., Lagueny, A., Lacomblez, L., Jedynak, P., Bartholome, B., Agid, Y. & Brice, A. (2000): Levodopa-responsive dystonia. GTP cyclohydrolase I or Parkin mutations? *Brain* **123**, 1112–1121.

Thöny, B., Auerbach, G. & Blau, N. (2000): Tetrahydrobiopterin biosynthesis, regeneration and functions. *Biochem. J.* **347**, 1–16.

Torres, G.E., Sweeney, A.L., Beaulieu, J.-M., Shashidharan, P. & Caron, M.G. (2004): Effect of torsinA on membrane proteins reveals a loss of function and a dominant-negative phenotype of the dystonia-associated delta-E-torsinA mutant. *Proc. Natl. Acad. Sci. USA* **101**, 15650–15655.

Valente, E.M., Warner, T.T., Jarman, P.R., Mathen, D., Fletcher, N.A., Marsden, C.D., Bhatia, K.P. & Wood, N.W. (1998): The role of DYT1 in primary torsion dystonia in Europe. *Brain* **121**, 2335–2339.

Valente, E.M., Misbahuddin, A., Brancati, F., Placzek, M.R., Garavaglia, B., Salvi, S., Nemeth, A., Shaw-Smith, C., Nardocci, N., Bentivoglio, A.R., Berardelli, A., Eleopra, R., Dallapiccola, B. & Warner, T.T. (2003): Analysis of the epsilon-sarcoglycan gene in familial and sporadic myoclonus-dystonia: evidence for genetic heterogeneity. *Mov. Disord.* **18**, 1047–1051.

Valente, E.M., Abou-Sleiman, P.M., Caputo, V., Muqit, M.M., Harvey, K., Gispert, S., Ali, Z., Del Turco, D., Bentivoglio, A.R., Healy, D.G., Albanese, A., Nussbaum, R., Gonzalez-Maldonado, R., Deller, T., Salvi. S., Cortelli, P., Gilks, W.P., Latchman, D.S., Harvey, R.J., Dallapiccola, B., Auburger, G. & Wood, N.W. (2004): Hereditary early-onset Parkinson's disease caused by mutations in PINK1. *Science* **304**, 1158–1160.

Williams, A., Eldridge, R., Levine, R., Lovenberg, W. & Paulson, G. (1979): Low CSF hydroxylase cofactor (tetrahydrobiopterin) levels in inherited dystonia. *Lancet* ii, 410–411.

Zhou, B., Westaway, S.K., Levinson, B., Johnson, M.A., Gitschier, J. & Hayflick, S.J. (2001): A novel pantothenate kinase gene (PANK2) is defective in Hallervorden-Spatz syndrome. *Nat. Genet.* **28**, 345–349.

Zimprich, A., Grabowski, M., Asmus, F., Naumann, M., Berg, D., Bertram, M., Scheidtmann, K., Kern, P., Winkelmann, J., Muller-Myhsok, B., Riedel, L., Bauer, M., Muller, T., Castro, M., Meitinger, T., Strom, T.M. & Gasser, T. (2001): Mutations in the gene encoding epsilon-sarcoglycan cause myoclonus-dystonia syndrome. *Nat. Genet.* **29**, 66–69.

Zorzi, G., Garavaglia, B., Invernizzi, F., Girotti, F., Soliveri, P., Zeviani, M., Angelini, L. & Nardocci, N. (2002): Frequency of DYT1 mutation in early-onset primary dystonia in Italian patients. *Mov. Disord.* **17**, 407–408.

Chapter 3

Neuroradiological findings in paediatric movement disorders

Luisa Chiapparini, Marina Grisoli and Mario Savoiardo

Department of Neuroradiology, Fondazione IRCCS Istituto Neurologico 'C. Besta',
via Celoria 11, 20133 Milan, Italy
lchiapparini@istituto-besta.it

Summary

In primary dystonia, neuroradiological studies are generally normal, but they may show characteristic abnormalities in most acquired dystonias and in heredodegenerative and metabolic diseases. In cases whose diagnosis is already established by the clinical history, such as in perinatal post-anoxic or post-haemorrhagic damage to the basal ganglia, the value of magnetic resonance imaging (MRI) is limited, and it may reveal only the extent of the damage. In other delayed-onset movement disorders such as kernicterus, or in infantile bilateral striatal necrosis, MRI may help to focus attention on the possible aetiology by demonstrating the areas that are selectively affected. In other degenerative or metabolic disorders, the value of MRI in suggesting the diagnosis may be crucial, at least in cases with an atypical clinical presentation. An example of this is Wilson's disease, in which tissue changes and copper or iron deposition in the basal ganglia, thalami, and brain stem may be detected by MRI. In Hallervorden-Spatz disease (pantothenate kinase-associated neurodegeneration), specific signal intensity abnormalities in the nucleus pallidus (eye-of-the-tiger sign) caused by iron deposition and focal anterior destructive changes are observed. Selective involvement of different deep nuclei, sometimes accompanied by brain stem, cerebellar, or white matter abnormalities in different combinations, may help to restrict the differential diagnosis. Disorders in which the use of MRI may result in diagnostic benefit include mitochondrial diseases (particularly Leigh's disease) and several organic acidurias. Advanced MRI techniques for studying movement disorders (magnetic resonance spectroscopy, voxel-based morphometry, functional magnetic resonance imaging) have given valuable results in adults; their application will soon be expanded to children.

Introduction

Neuroimaging has improved our understanding of several paediatric movement disorders and aided their diagnosis and management. Accurate observation of structural imaging studies – computed tomography (CT) and magnetic resonance imaging (MRI) – looking for subtle signal abnormalities caused by neuronal loss, gliosis, changes in the water content of the nervous tissue, or deposition of paramagnetic substances – is the best way of reaching a neuroradiological diagnosis.

Advanced magnetic resonance techniques such as diffusion (Sener, 2003) and MR spectroscopy (Alanen et al., 1999; Schapiro et al., 2004) have been applied for years in children. Other techniques, such as diffusion tensor imaging (DTI) and voxel-based morphometry (VBM), have found more recent application in the younger population, either because of technical improvements (Ashburner & Friston, 2000) or because it has become clear that VBM may be capable of uncovering subtle changes in the deep nuclei or in focal cortical areas in juvenile degenerative diseases (Thieben et al., 2002; Kassubek et al., 2004). Functional MRI (fMRI) using the BOLD (blood oxygenation level-dependent) effect has also now been applied to the investigation of paediatric patients (Lehéricy et al., 2003), although its use in children may be limited by the need for a good level of cooperation. However, neither activation on fMRI (Butterworth et al., 2003) – for example, in dystonic patients in the primary sensorimotor cortex, cerebellum, or thalamus – nor demonstration of increased volume or tissue density in cortical areas on VBM (Draganski et al., 2003; Garraux et al., 2004) clarifies whether such modifications are the primary event or the consequence of malfunctioning in a different area. Thus the use of these techniques is still the subject of research.

In this chapter, we shall concentrate on MRI, describing the characteristic MRI findings in some of the paediatric movement disorders and in diseases which, while not primarily characterized as movement disorders, nevertheless affect the basal ganglia and must therefore be considered in the differential diagnosis. These include primary and secondary dystonias, heredodegenerative disorders, and metabolic diseases.

Anatomy of the basal ganglia

Movement disorders usually result from structural lesions or dysfunction of the basal ganglia (Eckert & Eidelberg, 2005). The basal ganglia are a collection of nuclei located deep in the cerebral hemispheres and in the midbrain. They include the caudate nucleus, putamen, globus pallidus, nucleus accumbens, subthalamic nucleus, and substantia nigra.

The globus pallidus, which is divided in pars externa (GPe) and pars interna (GPi), represents the paleostriatum and with the putamen forms the lenticular nucleus. The putamen and the caudate nucleus form the neostriatum, which is often referred to as the 'striatum'. The anatomy of these structures is well demonstrated on coronal and axial sections of the cerebral hemispheres (Fig. 1).

The substantia nigra, which includes the pars compacta (which produces dopamine) and the pars reticulata, is located in the midbrain. The subthalamic nucleus is located in the subthalamic area, very close to the substantia nigra, slightly cranially and laterally with respect to the latter and close to the red nucleus. All the nuclei of the basal ganglia are well demonstrated on MRI except for the subthalamic nucleus, which is clearly visible on conventional MRI studies only when it has abnormal signal intensity – for example, in Leigh's disease.

Primary and secondary dystonias

In primary dystonia the MRI appearances are normal (Rutledge et al., 1988). Secondary dystonias result from various insults to the brain (Marsden et al., 1985). The damage is usually stable and often recognizable on MRI studies, while the clinical history leaves no doubt about the aetiology. In this group, perinatal hypoxic-ischaemic or haemorrhagic cerebral injury, kernicterus, postnatal focal cerebral vascular injury, and cerebral infections are the most common causes.

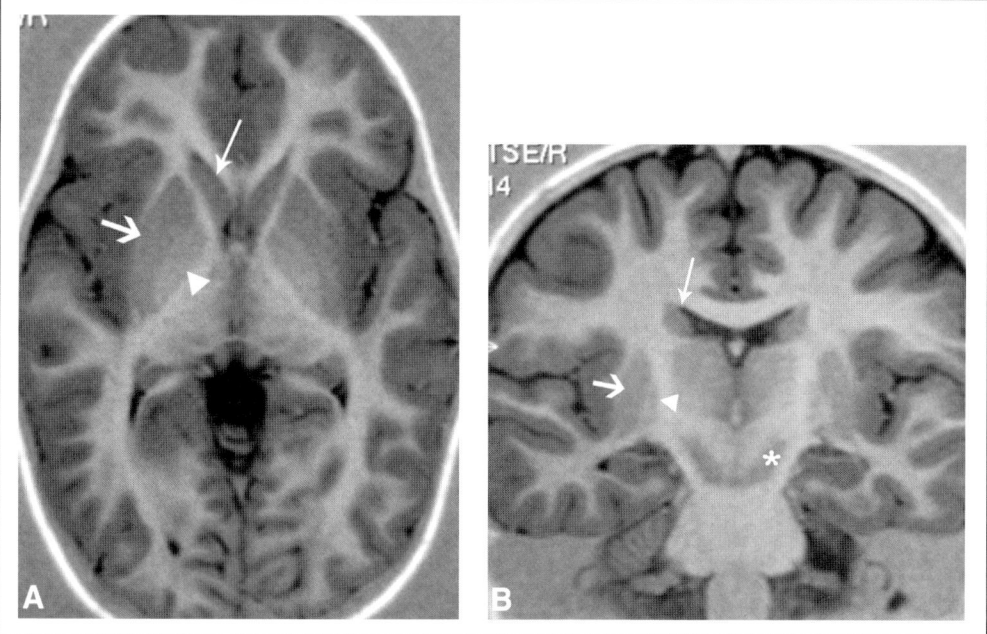

Fig. 1. (A) Axial and coronal inversion recovery images showing the putamen (short arrow), the nucleus pallidus (arrowhead), and the head of the caudate nucleus (long arrow). Asterisk is positioned on the substantia nigra (B).

Hypoxic-ischaemic brain injury

Perinatal hypoxic-ischaemic brain injury secondary to asphyxia results in the development of 'cerebral palsy', and dystonia may appear sooner or later. The lesion may predominate in the deep grey matter, where haemorrhages in the germinal matrix in the periventricular area may occur. The distribution of the lesions varies depending on the gestational age. Preterm babies usually show the periventricular leukomalacia pattern, whereas babies born at term have lesions in the ventrolateral part of the thalami, the posterolateral lentiform nuclei (Fig. 2), the hippocampi, and the rolandic and perirolandic cerebral cortex.

In early studies, MRI may show hypo- or hyperintensity in T1-weighted images and hyperintensity in T2-weighted images in these regions (Fig. 2). T1-weighted images and gradient-echo sequences may reveal signal changes consistent with presence of haemoglobin derivatives in haemorrhagic cases (Barkovich et al., 1995). Years after injury, MRI may show atrophy and only subtle hyperintensities on T2-weighted images; these can, however, still indicate the age of the stroke because of the particular distribution of the lesions (Fig. 3), as there is a selective vulnerability of particular structures at different stages of development. One of the factors underlying such selective involvement of these areas of the brain is the metabolic demands of the brain tissue involved. Active myelination of certain pathways seems to play a significant role in determining the regional susceptibility to injury of the neurons from which they originate (Barkovich, 1992; Barkovich et al., 1995).

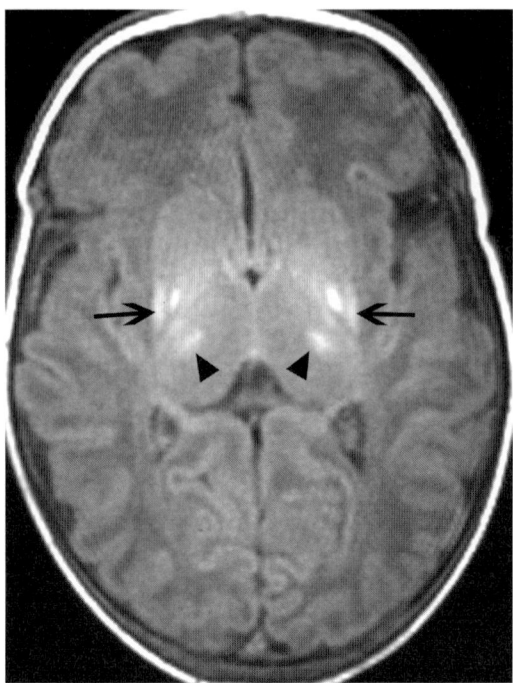

Fig. 2. Perinatal hypoxia in a neonate born at term. Axial SE T1-weighted image showing the damaged areas as spontaneous hyperintensity in the postero-lateral lentiform nuclei (arrows) and ventrolateral thalami (arrowheads), probably related to microhaemorrhages.

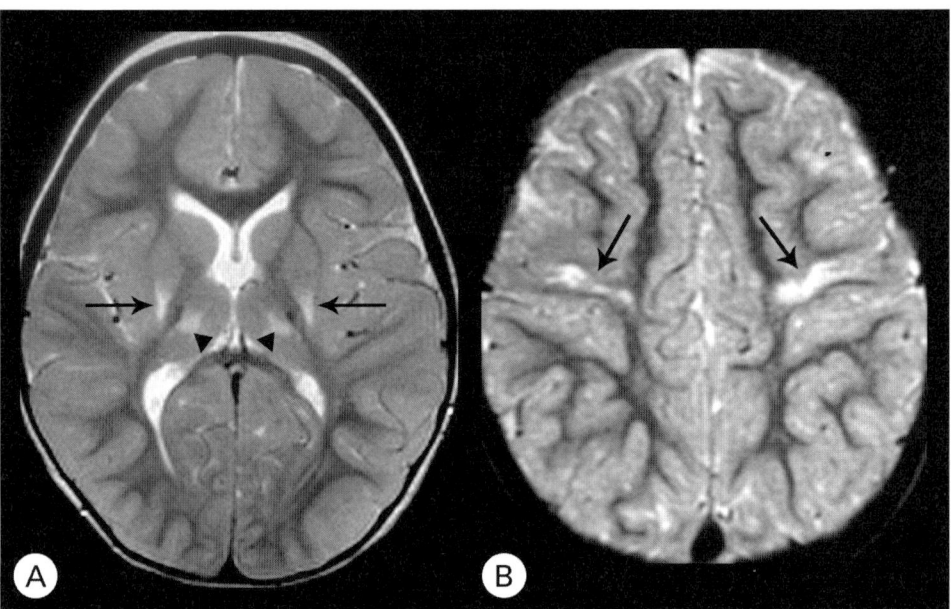

Fig. 3. Magnetic resonance imaging in a 10-year-old child with cerebral palsy. Axial SE T2-weighted images through the basal ganglia (A) and at the upper convexity level (B) show abnormal signal intensity in the lentiform nuclei (arrows) and thalami (arrowheads) and in the Rolandic regions, which also appear shrunk (arrows, B). This distribution is characteristic of perinatal hypoxia in a child born at term.

Focal cerebral vascular injury

Acute infarction of the basal ganglia, most often involving the putamen, is usually characterized by acute motor and neuropsychological dysfunction. Dystonia may occur after the resolution of the motor impairment, leading to a clinical syndrome called late-onset dystonia (Bhatia & Marsden, 1994; Nardocci *et al.*, 1996). The delayed development of dystonia is attributed to the slow development of abnormal sprouting of the surviving neurons, which may be the anatomical correlate of dystonia.

The cause may be disease of the small arteries or a dissection of the wall of the internal carotid artery, acting either directly or causing an embolus, or else a thromboembolic complication of heart disease. On MRI, T2-weighted images and diffusion-weighted sequences in the early stages of stroke show hyperintensity and swelling of the basal ganglia involved. In later stages, shrinkage of the nuclei is generally observed (Fig. 4).

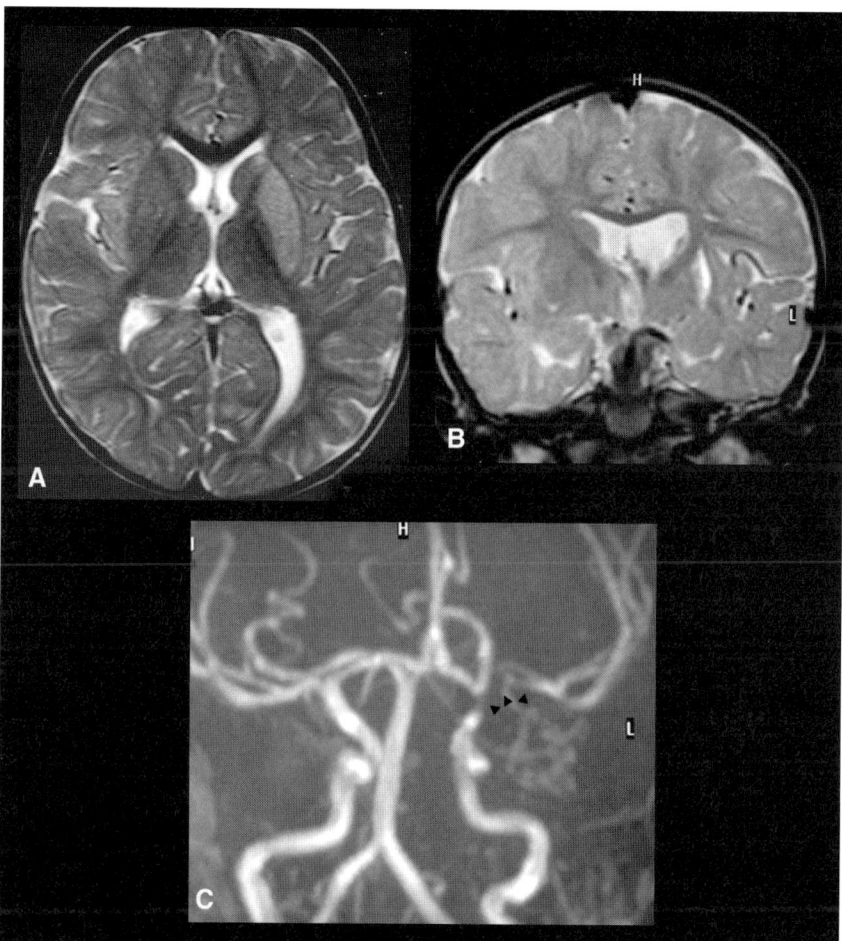

Fig. 4. Stroke in a 9-year-old-child. (A) The axial T2-weighted image 3 days after the abrupt onset of right hemiplegia shows mild hyperintensity in the left putamen and caudate nucleus. The coronal T2-weighted image obtained 4 months later (B) shows marked atrophy of the nuclei and enlargement of the frontal horn of the ipsilateral ventricle. Magnetic resonance angiography (C) shows the occlusion of the distal segment of the left internal carotid artery and the M1 segment of the middle cerebral artery (arrowheads).

Inflammatory, infectious, and toxic causes

Several agents can cause damage to the basal ganglia, with selective involvement that may mimic the distribution of an infarct in the territory of the lenticulostriate arteries, resulting in the development of dystonia. The neostriatum or the pallidum, or both, may be involved.

Carbon monoxide poisoning and possible autoimmune reactions stimulated by infections, either viral or from other agents (as we have seen in a few instances after *Mycoplasma pneumoniae* infection) or associated with presence of antiphospholipid autoantibodies (Angelini *et al.*, 1996) can result in damage to the deep grey matter, most often to the putamen. In streptococcal infections, which may lead to anterior neostriatal involvement as observed in Sydenham's chorea, it is likely that molecular mimicry explains the selective involvement of the neurons. In most cases of Sydenham's chorea, brain MRI is normal. Sometimes abnormal signal intensity in the basal ganglia is visible at the onset of the disease, rarely accompanied by abnormalities of the blood-brain barrier (Kienzle, 1991).

The onset of the lesion may go undetected in another condition – infantile bilateral striatal necrosis. This condition, of uncertain aetiology, has occasionally been associated with a mitochondrial disorder or related in a few families to genetic causes (Straussberg *et al.*, 2002; Basel-Vanagaite *et al.*, 2004). In this disorder, the development of dystonia may prompt clinical investigation. MRI may show a stable slit necrosis in the putamen, and sometimes in the head of the caudate nucleus as well, demonstrating the selective vulnerability of the neostriatum, particularly of the putamen, to an unknown agent or pathogenic mechanism (Fig. 5).

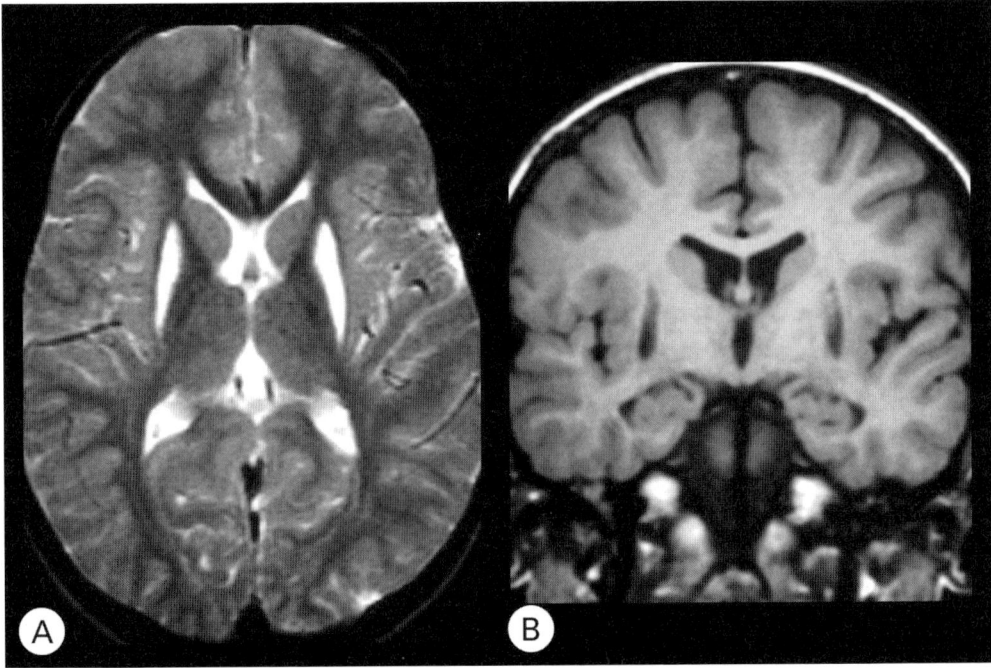

Fig. 5. Bilateral striatal necrosis. Axial T2-weighted image (A) and coronal T1-weighted image (B) showing bilateral symmetrical destructive changes in the putamina.

Kernicterus

Kernicterus or bilirubin encephalopathy is caused by deposition of toxic unconjugated bilirubin in the globi pallidi, subthalamic nuclei, and hippocampi secondary to infantile hyperbilirubinaemia when free bilirubin exceeds 20 mg/100 dL (340 µmol/L). Less marked deposition occurs in the substantia nigra, lateral nuclei of the thalamus, vestibular and dentate nuclei, and inferior olivary nuclei.

The most important cause of hyperbilirubinaemia in newborns is erythroblastosis fetalis, a haemolytic anaemia resulting from maternal-fetal incompatibility of the rhesus or, less often, the ABO blood groups. Prematurity, hypoxia, and any conditions that induce haemolysis are predisposing factors to kernicterus (Erbetta *et al.*, 1998; Rorke, 1998).

The MRI abnormalities correlate well with the gross findings in this disease, characterized by yellow staining of the selected nuclei listed above. The constant and most easily recognizable MRI feature is the presence of high signal intensity in T2-weighted images in the atrophic globi pallidi (Erbetta *et al.*, 1998) (Fig. 6). In situations where details about the perinatal history are not available, this finding should prompt further inquiry.

Huntington's disease

Huntington's disease is a hereditary neurodegenerative autosomal dominant disorder characterized by choreoathetoid movements, cognitive deterioration, and behavioural disturbances. The mean age of onset is 37 years, and childhood onset is rare (Ho *et al.*, 1995). In young patients, the rigid, akinetic variant – often accompanied by intellectual decline and cerebellar symptoms – is more often seen than the classic hyperkinetic form.

Longitudinal MRI studies (Aylward *et al.*, 1997) in Huntington's disease show progressive neostriatal atrophy which begins in the presymptomatic period. There is an inverse relation between the length of the CAG trinucleotide repeat (=40 repeats) and the age at onset of the disease. A younger age of onset and a greater number of CAG repeats correlate significantly with greater volume loss of the caudate nuclei and total basal ganglia, as shown by recent volumetric studies (Rosas *et al.*, 2001).

In the typical adult hyperkinetic patient, MRI studies show diffuse brain atrophy, most prominent in the frontal lobes, and a more marked atrophy of the head of the caudate nucleus and the putamen. Atrophy of the heads of the caudate nuclei results in a characteristic enlargement of the frontal horns of the lateral ventricles. Signal abnormalities – consisting of slight hyperintensity in proton density and T2-weighted images in the atrophic neostriatum, probably related to greater neuronal loss and gliosis – are a constant finding in the rigid variant (Savoiardo *et al.*, 1991) and are correlated with greater motor and cognitive impairment (Oliva *et al.*, 1993). In young patients with Huntington's disease, signal abnormalities in the severely atrophic neostriatum are commonly seen (Fig. 7).

Wilson's disease

Wilson's disease, or hepatolenticular degeneration, is an autosomal recessive disease of copper metabolism caused by mutations in the ATP7B gene, in which copper accumulates in several organs, primarily the liver and brain (Ferenci, 2005). The diagnosis is made on laboratory studies by demonstration of decreased serum caeruloplasmin and copper levels and raised

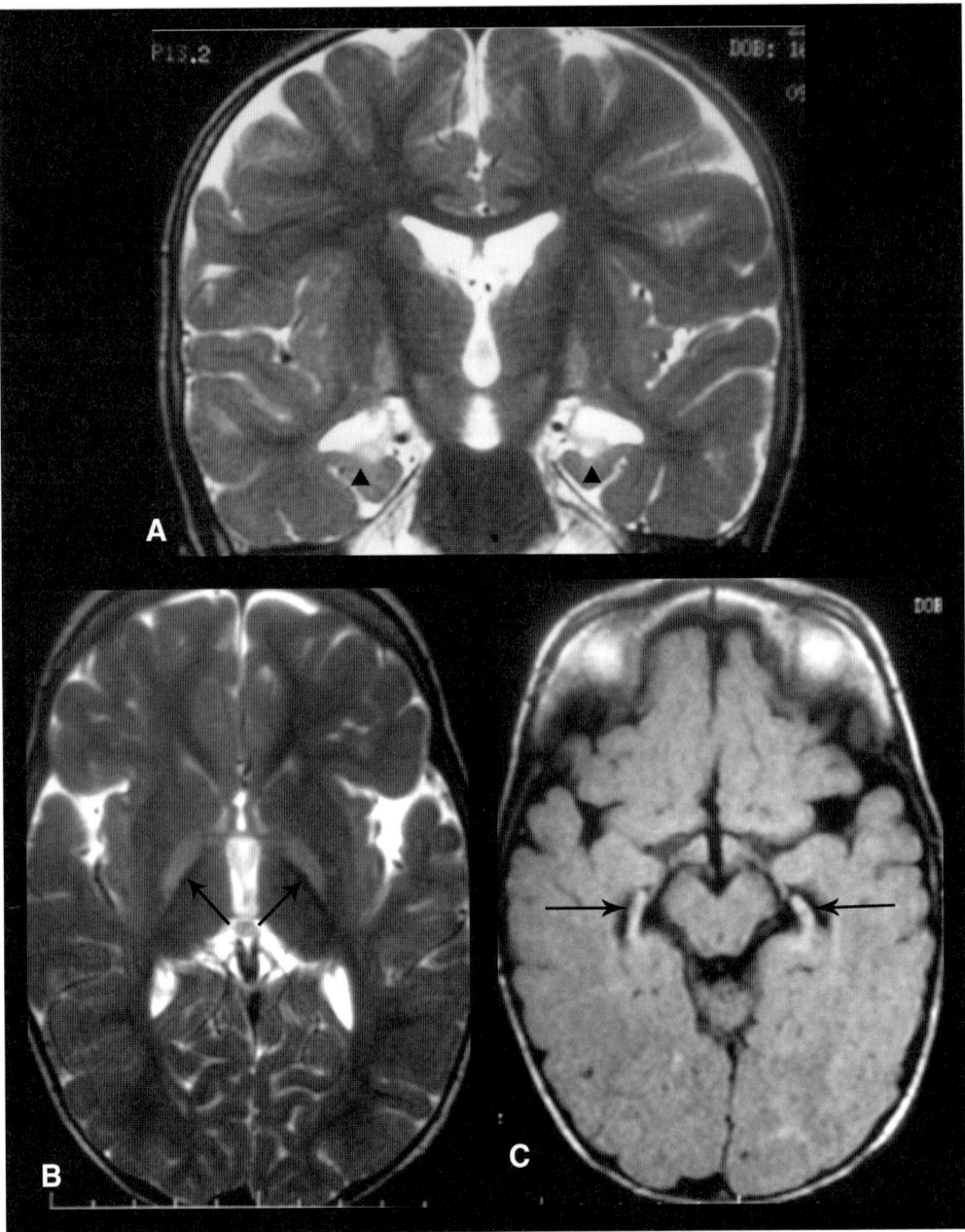

Fig. 6. Kernicterus. Coronal T2-weighted image (A), axial T2-weighted image (B), and axial FLAIR (fluid-attenuated inversion recovery) image (C), showing shrinkage and abnormal signal intensity of the pallida (A and B, arrows in B) and marked atrophy and hyperintensity of the hippocampi (A, arrowheads, and C, arrows).

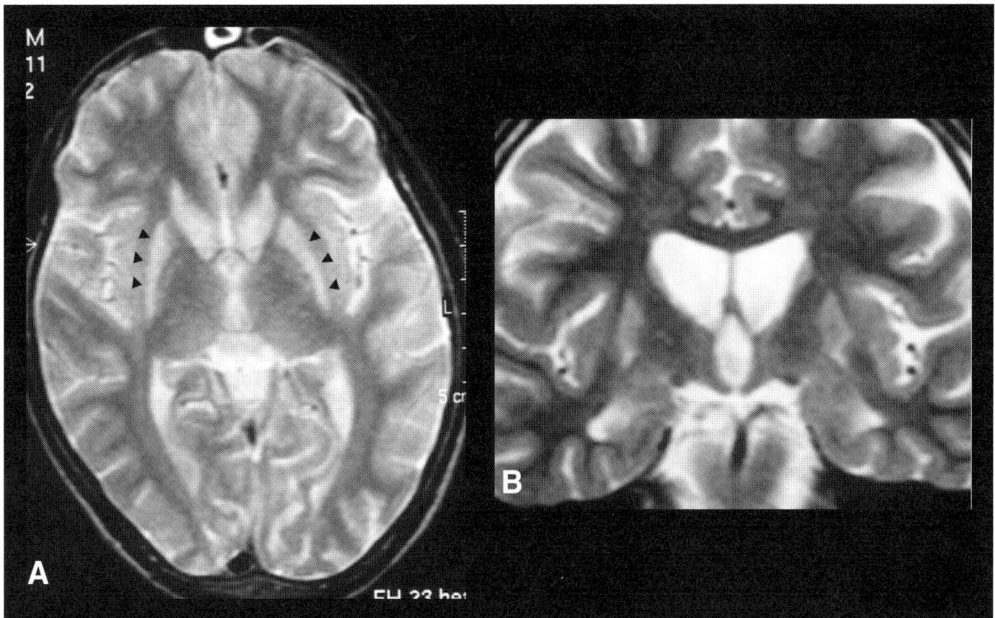

Fig. 7. Huntington's disease in a 10-year-old girl. SE axial (A) and coronal (B) T2-weighted images showing atrophy and moderate hyperintensity of the putamina (arrowheads) and heads of the caudate nuclei. Atrophy of the heads of the caudate nuclei is best appreciated in the coronal section (B).

urinary excretion of copper, and by the presence of Kayser-Fleischer rings. Neuronal loss, vacuolization, astrocytic hyperplasia, and degeneration of myelinated fibres are present in the lenticular nuclei, particularly in the putamina, and less frequently in the caudate, substantia nigra, and dentate nuclei. The lateral nuclei of the thalami are often affected. In advanced cases, cavitations may develop in the lentiform nuclei, mainly in the putamina, which can easily be demonstrated by CT. Copper deposition and microhaemorrhages may also be present in the basal ganglia. These changes account for the signal abnormalities visible on MRI studies.

Two main types of signal abnormalities are found. The most common type is high signal intensity in proton density, FLAIR (fluid-attenuated inversion recovery), and T2-weighted images in the putamen, lateral part of the thalami, midbrain (substantia nigra, red nuclei, and periaqueductal area), and pons. The involvement of the putamen is often more marked on its outer rim, which appears markedly hyperintense, and the whole nucleus may be swollen. Sometimes the claustra are markedly abnormal. In the pons, a characteristic feature is sparing of a thin rim along the cisternal surface. The cerebral white matter, corpus callosum, corticospinal tracts, middle and superior cerebellar peduncles, and the white matter of the cerebellar hemispheres are less frequently or less markedly affected (King et al., 1996; Savoiardo & Grisoli, 2002) (Fig. 8).

The second and rarer type of MRI abnormality consists of a decrease in or loss of signal intensity in T2-weighted images in the putamen, pallidum, and the head of the caudate nucleus, probably caused by deposition of copper or iron and well documented on high field intensity MRI (1.5 T), particularly with magnetic susceptibility sensitive sequences. The pattern of distribution of these low signals is often characteristic: the loss of signal intensity is located in the central part of the nucleus involved, whereas the hyperintensity tends to remain more peripheral (Savoiardo & Grisoli, 2002) (Fig. 8C).

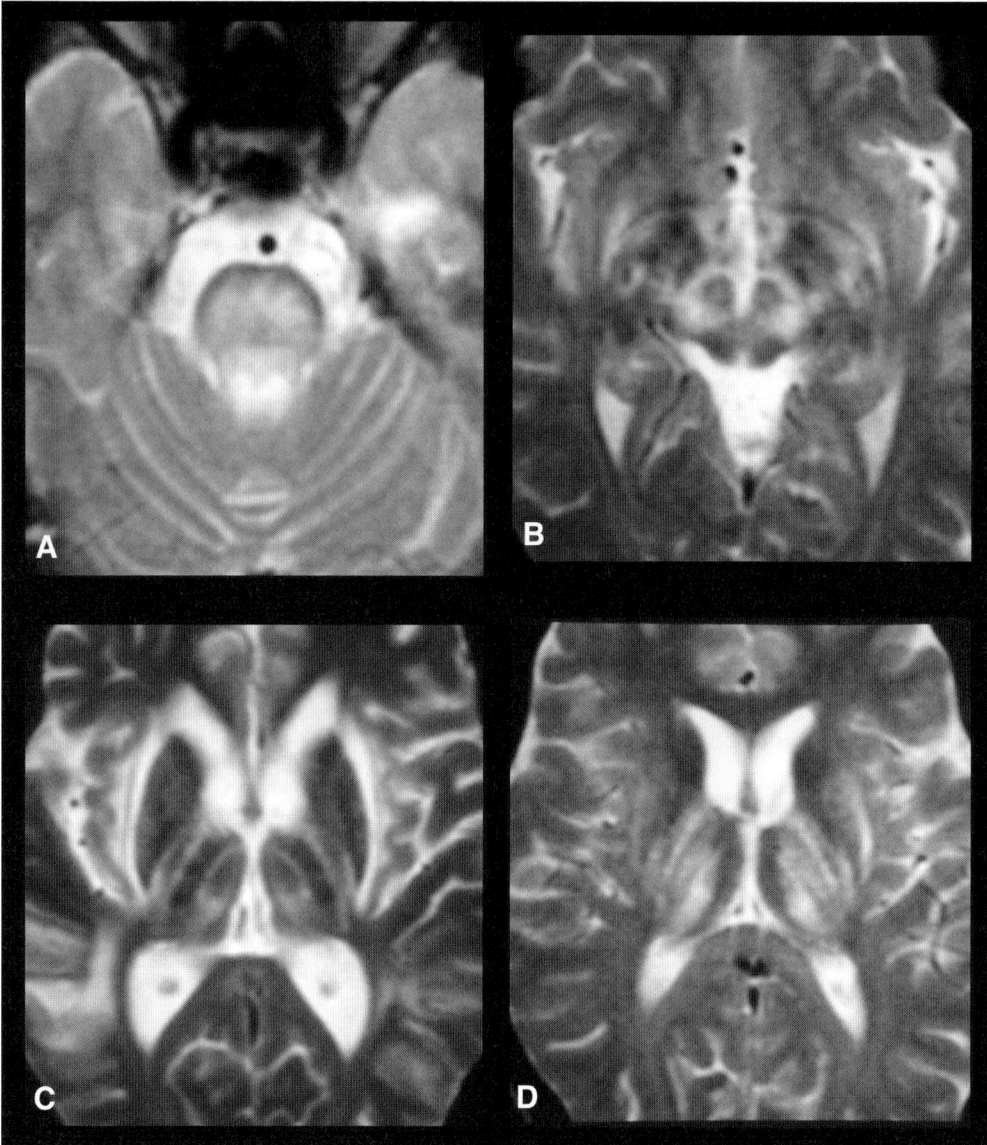

Fig. 8. Wilson's disease in a 9-year-old boy (A-C). Axial T2-weighted image sections on the brain stem (A, B) showing involvement of the pons with sparing of a thin outer rim (A), and of the midbrain ('giant panda' image, B). Axial T2-weighted image at level of the basal ganglia (C) shows hypointensity in the neostriatum and hyperintensities diffusely involving the external capsule, claustrum, and thalami. Axial T2-weighted image in another patient (D) shows abnormal signal intensity in the putamina, and a more typical involvement of the lateral part of the thalami.

A third and more subtle type of signal change observed on MRI in patients with Wilson's disease – probably associated with hepatic insufficiency – is signal hyperintensity in T1-weighted images in the pallida, usually extending toward the substantia nigra, which is attributed to a paramagnetic effect of manganese or copper (King et al., 1996; Saatci et al., 1997).

After treatment, improvement and sometimes near disappearance of the signal abnormalities (mainly the T2 hyperintensities) may occur; more marked T2 hypointensities have also been noted, tentatively attributed to deposits of iron in exchange for copper (Engelbrecht *et al.*, 1995).

Hallervorden-Spatz disease, or pantothenate kinase-associated neurodegeneration

Hallervorden-Spatz disease is the old term for an autosomal recessive disorder pathologically characterized by neuroaxonal swelling limited to the brain, and by iron deposits and destructive changes in the globi pallidi resulting in brownish pigmentation of these atrophic nuclei. In recent years the disease has been genetically defined (the gene *PANK2* maps on chromosome 20p13) (Zhou *et al.*, 2001) and metabolically characterized by the recognition of the key regulatory role of a pantothenate kinase enzyme encoded by this gene in the biosynthesis of the coenzyme A; a deficit in this enzyme may lead to neurodegeneration and iron accumulation (Gordon, 2002; Hayflick *et al.*, 2003). The main clinical findings include dystonia, parkinsonism, mental deterioration, and retinal degeneration. Brain CT may show foci of high density in the globus pallidus, probably caused by mineralization in its anteromedial part.

The most characteristic and pathognomonic findings are shown on MRI. With high field strength scanners (1.5 T or more), MRI shows hypointensity in the globi pallidi on T2-weighted images resulting from iron deposition, associated with an anteromedial focus of hyperintensity which corresponds to a loose tissue with destructive changes but devoid of iron. This pattern was named by Sethi the 'eye-of-the-tiger sign' (Sethi *et al.*, 1988; Savoiardo *et al.*, 1993; Hayflick *et al.*, 2003). In the hyperintense focus, a central spot of marked hypointensity, corresponding to the 'calcifications' seen on CT, may also be present (Fig. 9).

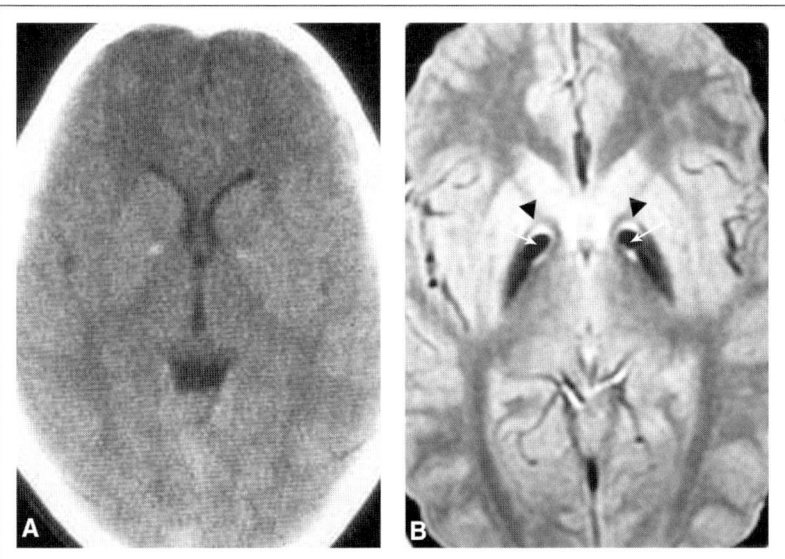

Fig. 9. Hallervorden-Spatz disease. Computed tomography (CT) (A) and magnetic resonance imaging sections (B) through the basal ganglia. CT shows bilateral foci of hyperdensity caused by mineralization in the anteromedial part of the globus pallidus. SE proton density image at 1.5 T (B) reveals marked hypointensity in the globi pallidi with high signal intensity foci in the anteromedial region ('eye-of-the-tiger'sign, arrowheads); in this patient a central spot of low signal intensity (arrows), which corresponds to the calcifications seen on CT, is also visible.

Evaluation of brain iron by MRI provides important clues for the recognition and diagnosis of patients with movement disorders. In parkinsonism, for instance, distribution of iron in the basal ganglia may be different from that observed in normal subjects. Iron is not present at birth. During life, gradual accumulation occurs, predominantly in the globus pallidus and the substantia nigra. Lesser amounts are found in the red nucleus and dentate nucleus. Only in old age does the amount of iron in the putamen reach that present in the pallidum. At younger ages, increased amounts of iron in the putamen suggest multiple system atrophy. Thus one has to take into account the age of the patient when judging T2 hypointensity on MRI. There is no doubt that the hypointensity observed in the pallidum in children with pantothenate kinase-associated neurodegeneration is grossly abnormal.

Metabolic disorders

On MRI studies the basal ganglia appear to be involved in several metabolic disorders. In many instances, however, movement disorders are not the most characteristic feature, although they may be observed. Signal abnormalities in the basal ganglia or in the brain stem and cerebellum present a pattern of distribution that may sometimes suggest a specific disorder or may limit the differential diagnosis to a group of disorders.

In this section we will refer only to mitochondrial disorders and the organic acidurias.

Mitochondrial disorders

In mitochondrial disorders the basal ganglia are often affected. In children, the most common disorder is Leigh's syndrome which is characterized by lesions in the basal ganglia, particularly the posterior part of the putamen, the brain stem (in the periaqueductal area, the pontine tegmentum, and the medulla), and in the dentate nuclei. In Leigh's disease associated with cytochrome-oxidase (COX) deficiency and *SURF1* mutation, the abnormalities in the brain stem predominate and are almost always present in the subthalamic nuclei (Farina *et al.*, 2002) (Fig. 10).

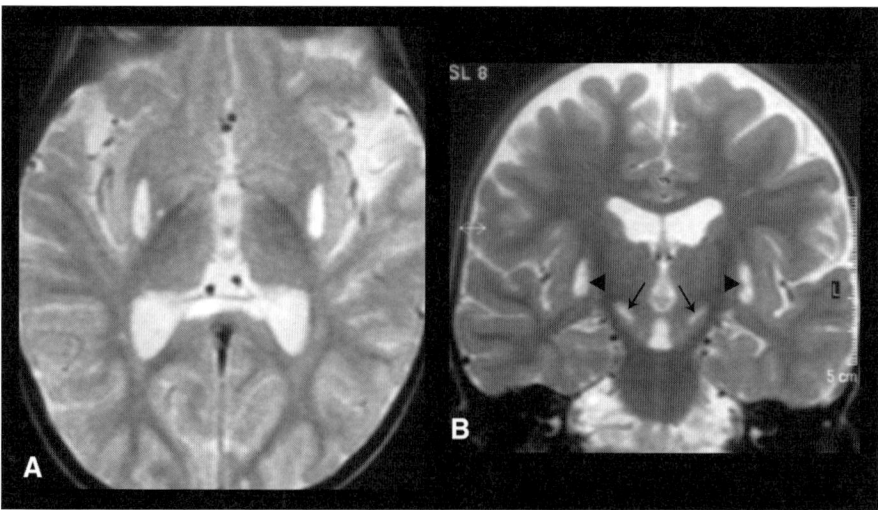

Fig. 10. Leigh syndrome in a 3-year-old boy with SURF-1 mutation. Axial (A) and coronal (B) T2-weighted image showing bilateral, symmetrical hyperintense lesions in the putamina (arrowheads) and in the subthalamic nuclei (arrows). Cerebellar and brain stem lesions (not shown) were also present.

In Kearns-Sayre syndrome, calcifications may be seen in the basal ganglia, mainly in the pallida. On MRI, mild signal hyperintensities in T2-weighted images are usually present in the pallida, in the thalami, and, diffusely, in the upper brain stem, with a pattern that may have similarities to that observed in Wilson's disease. In addition, supratentorial abnormalities in the subcortical white matter – particularly in the central regions, related to status spongiosus – are a characteristic feature.

Organic acidurias

Similar subcortical abnormalities are seen in many organic acidurias. These are sometimes very limited, being present only in the peripheral part of a cerebral gyrus (usually F1 and the temporopolar area); at other times they may be more extensive, reaching nearly to the periventricular white matter. In an acute presentation, the signal abnormalities are usually very marked and may be associated with swelling of the convolutions. A combination of this pattern with various degrees of involvement of the basal ganglia, thalami, brain stem (mostly in its upper part and in the tegmentum), and dentate nuclei is also seen in this group of metabolic disorders (D'Incerti *et al.*, 1998).

The diseases most commonly observed in a paediatric neurology department include glutaric aciduria type 1, Canavan disease, L2-hydroxy-glutaric aciduria (D'Incerti *et al.*, 1998), and methylmalonic aciduria. Without going into detail, it is worth recording that certain features may provide a clue to the correct diagnosis. For example, the MR spectroscopic finding of raised N-acetyl-aspartate indicates Canavan's disease; isolated involvement of the pallidum points to methylmalonic acidaemia; while marked peripheral subcortical abnormalities, also visible as hypointensities on T1-weighted images, combined with pallidal and dentate nucleus involvement suggest L2-OH-glutaric aciduria.

Conclusions

Magnetic resonance imaging, supported by ^{1}H-magnetic resonance spectroscopy and computed tomography to demonstrate calcifications, provides the imaging features that may suggest a specific diagnosis to the clinician. However, in recent years, it has become clear that advanced MR techniques such as functional magnetic resonance imaging, diffusion tensor imaging, and volumetric studies may supply new insights into the pathogenesis of diseases with positive MRI findings, and may also help to uncover abnormalities in disorders where conventional MRI fails to reveal any morphological abnormalities.

References

Alanen, A., Komu, M., Penttinen, M. & Leino, R. (1999): Magnetic resonance imaging and proton MR spectroscopy in Wilson's disease. *Br. J. Radiol.* **72**, 749–756.

Angelini, L., Zibordi, F., Zorzi, G., Nardocci, N., Caporali, R., Ravelli, A. & Martini, A. (1996): Neurological disorders, other than stroke, associated with antiphospholipid antibodies in childhood. *Neuropediatrics* **27**, 149–153.

Ashburner, J. & Friston, K.J. (2000): Voxel-based morphometry – the methods. *Neuroimage* **11**, 805–821.

Aylward, E.H., Li, Q., Stine, O.C., Ranen, N., Sherr, M., Barta, P.E., Bylsma, F.W., Pearlson, G.D. & Ross, C.A. (1997): Longitudinal change in basal ganglia volume in patients with Huntington's disease. *Neurology* **48**, 394–399.

Barkovich, A.J. (1992): MR and CT evaluation of profound neonatal and infantile asphyxia. *AJNR Am. J. Neuroradiol.* **13**, 959–972.

Barkovich, A.J., Westmark, K., Partridge, C., Sola, A. & Ferriero, D.M. (1995): Perinatal asphyxia: MR findings in the first 10 days. *AJNR Am. J. Neuroradiol.* **16**, 427–438.

Basel-Vanagaite, L., Straussberg, R., Ovadia, H., Kaplan, A., Magal, N., Shore, Z., Shalev, H., Walsh, C. & Shohat, M. (2004): Infantile bilateral striatal necrosis maps to chromosome 19q. *Neurology* **13**, 87–90.

Bhatia, K.P. & Marsden, C.D. (1994): The behavioural and motor consequences of focal lesions of the basal ganglia in man. *Brain* **117**, 859–876.

Butterworth, S., Francis, S., Kelly, E., McGlone, F., Bowtell, R. & Sawle, G.V. (2003): Abnormal cortical sensory activation in dystonia: an fMRI study. *Mov. Disord.* **18**, 673–682.

D'Incerti, L., Farina, L., Moroni, I., Uziel, G. & Savoiardo, M. (1998): L-2-Hydroxyglutaric aciduria: MRI in seven cases. *Neuroradiology* **40**, 727–733.

Draganski, B., Thun-Hohenstein, C., Bogdahn, U., Winkler, J. & May, A. (2003): 'Motor circuit' gray matter changes in idiopathic cervical dystonia. *Neurology* **61**, 1228–1231.

Eckert, T. & Eidelberg, D. (2005): Neuroimaging and therapeutics in movement disorders. *NeuroRx®: Journal of the American Society for Experimental Neurotherapeutics* **2**, 361–371.

Engelbrecht, V., Schlaug, G., Hefter, H., Kahn, T. & Modder, U. (1995): MRI of the brain in Wilson disease: T2 signal loss under therapy. *J. Comput. Assist. Tomogr.* **19**, 635–638.

Erbetta, A., Ciceri, E., Chiapparini, L., Botteon, G., Erba, A., Nardocci, N. & Savoiardo, M. (1998): Magnetic resonance imaging findings in bilirubin encephalopathy. *Int. J. Neuroradiol.* **4**, 161–164.

Farina, L., Chiapparini, L., Uziel, G., Bugiani, M., Zeviani, M. & Savoiardo, M. (2002): MR findings in Leigh syndrome with COX deficiency and *Surf-1* mutation. *AJNR Am. J. Neuroradiol.* **23**, 1095–1100.

Ferenci, P. (2005): Wilson's disease. *Clin. Gastroenterol. Hepatol.* **3**, 726–733.

Garraux, G., Bauer, A., Hanakawa, T., Wu, T., Kansaku, K. & Hallett, M. (2004): Changes in brain anatomy in focal hand dystonia. *Ann. Neurol.* **55**, 736–739.

Gordon, N. (2002): Pantothenate kinase-associated neurodegeneration (Hallervorden-Spatz syndrome). *Eur. J. Pediatr. Neurol.* **6**, 243–247.

Hayflick, S.J., Westaway, S.K., Levinson, B., Zhou, B., Johnson, M.A., Ching, K.H. & Gitschier, J. (2003): Genetic, clinical, and radiographic delineation of Hallervorden-Spatz syndrome. *N. Engl. J. Med.* **348**, 33–40.

Ho, V.B., Chuang, H.S., Rovira, M.J. & Koo, B. (1995): Juvenile Huntington disease: CT and MRI features. *AJNR Am. J. Neuroradiol.* **16**, 1405–1412.

Kassubek, J., Juengling, F.D., Kioschies, T., Henkel, K., Karitzky, J., Kramer, B., Ecker, D., Andrich, J., Saft, C., Kraus, P., Aschoff, A.J., Ludolph, A.C. & Landwehrmeyer, G.B. (2004): Topography of cerebral atrophy in early Huntington's disease: a voxel based morphometric MRI study. *J. Neurol. Neurosurg. Psychiatry* **75**, 213–220.

Kienzle, G.D. (1991): Sydenham chorea: MR manifestations in two cases. *AJNR Am. J. Neuroradiol.* **12**, 73–76.

King, A.D., Walshe, J.M., Kendall, B.E., Chinn, R.J., Paley, M.N., Wilkinson, I.D., Halligan, S. & Hall-Craggs, M.A. (1996): Cranial MR imaging in Wilson's disease. *AJR Am. J. Roentgenol.* **167**, 1579–1584.

Lehéricy, S., Meunier, S., Garnero, L. & Vidailhet, M. (2003): Dystonia: contributions of functional imaging and magnetoencephalography. *Rev. Neurol.* **159**, 874–879.

Marsden, C.D., Obeso, J.A., Zarranz, J.J. & Lang, A.E. (1985): The anatomical basis of symptomatic hemidystonia. *Brain* **108**, 463–483.

Mazziotta, J.C., Hutchinson, M., Fife, T.D. & Woods, R. (1998): Advanced neuroimaging methods in the study of movement disorders: dystonia and blepharospasm. *Adv. Neurol.* **78**, 153–160.

Nardocci, N., Zorzi, G., Grisoli, M., Rumi, V., Broggi, G. & Angelini, L. (1996): Acquired hemidystonia in childhood: a clinical and neuroradiological study of thirteen patients. *Pediatr. Neurol.* **15**, 108–113.

Oliva, D., Carella, F., Savoiardo, M., Strada, L., Giovannini, P., Testa, D., Filippini, G., Caraceni, T. & Girotti, F. (1993): Clinical and magnetic resonance features of the classic and akinetic-rigid variants of Huntington's disease. *Arch. Neurol.* **50**, 17–19.

Rorke, L.B. (1998): Neuropathologic findings in bilirubin encephalopathy (kernicterus). *Int. J. Neuroradiol.* **4**, 165–170.

Rosas, H.D., Goodman, J., Chen, Y.I., Jenkins, B.G., Kennedy, D.N., Makris, N., Patti, M., Seidman, L.J., Beal, M.F. & Koroshetz, W.J. (2001): Striatal volume loss in HD as measured by MRI and influence of CAG repeat. *Neurology* **57**, 1025–1028.

Rutledge, J.N., Hilal, S.K., Silver, A.J., Defendini, R. & Fahn, S. (1988): Magnetic resonance imaging of dystonic states. *Adv. Neurol.* **50**, 265–275.

Saatci, I., Topcu, M., Baltaoglu, F.F., Kose, G., Yalaz, K., Renda, Y. & Besim, A. (1997): Cranial MR findings in Wilson's disease. *Acta Radiol.* **38**, 250–258.

Savoiardo, M. & Grisoli, M. (2002): Magnetic resonance imaging of movement disorders. In: *Parkinson's disease and movement disorders*, eds. J. Jankovic & E. Tolosa, pp. 596-609. Philadelphia: William & Wilkins.

Savoiardo, M., Strada, L., Oliva, D., Girotti, F. & D'Incerti, L. (1991): Abnormal MRI signal in the rigid form of Huntington's disease. *J. Neurol. Neurosurg. Psychiatry* **54**, 888–891.

Savoiardo, M., Halliday, W.C., Nardocci, N., Strada, L., D'Incerti, L., Angelini, L., Rumi, V. & Tesoro-Tess, J.D. (1993): Hallervorden-Spatz disease: MR and pathologic findings. *AJNR Am. J. Neuroradiol.* **14**, 155–162.

Schapiro, M., Cecil, K.M., Doescher, J., Kiefer, A.M. & Jones, B.V. (2004): MR imaging and spectroscopy in juvenile Huntington's disease. *Pediatr. Radiol.* **34**, 640–643.

Sener, R.N. (2003): Diffusion MR imaging changes associated with Wilson disease. *AJNR Am. J. Neuroradiol.* **24**, 965–967.

Sethi, K.D., Adams, R.J., Loring, D.W. & el Gammal, T. (1988): Hallervorden-Spatz syndrome: clinical and magnetic resonance imaging correlations. *Ann. Neurol.* **24**, 692–694.

Straussberg, R., Shorer, Z., Weitz, R., Basel, L., Kornreich, L., Corie, C.I., Harel, L., Djaldetti, R. & Amir, J. (2002): Familial infantile bilateral striatal necrosis: clinical features and response to biotin treatment. *Neurology* **8**, 983–989.

Thieben, M.J., Duggins, A.J., Good, C.D., Gomes, L., Mahant, N., Richards, F., McCusker, E. & Frackowiak, R.S. (2002): The distribution of structural neuropathology in pre-clinical Huntington's disease. *Brain* **125**, 1815–1828.

Zhou, B., Westaway, S.R., Levinson, B., Johnson, M.A., Gitschier, J. & Hayflick, S.J. (2001): A novel pantothenate kinase gene (PANK2) is detective in Hallervorden-Spatz syndrome. *Nat. Genet.* **28**, 345–349.

Chapter 4

Neurophysiological investigations in movement disorders

Silvana Franceschetti, Laura Canafoglia, Flavia Tripaldi, Claudia Ciano and Ferruccio Panzica

Department of Neurophysiology, Epilepsy Centre, Fondazione IRCCS Istituto Neurologico 'C. Besta', via Celoria 11, 20133 Milan, Italy
franceschetti@istituto-besta.it

Summary

Neurophysiological tests should be considered as tools to support the clinical diagnosis of a specific movement disorder, to aid the differential diagnosis when there is a complex or atypical clinical presentation, and for quantitative monitoring of brain dysfunction in cases of pharmacological, surgical, or rehabilitative interventions.

Young patients may not be able to collaborate in carrying out these tests; however, within appropriate settings most neurophysiological investigations can be undertaken satisfactorily. In this chapter, we briefly summarize the types of electrophysiological techniques that can be applied to myoclonic and dystonic syndromes, two common forms of movement disorders in infancy and childhood. The electrophysiological findings are often necessary for diagnostic assessment and differential diagnosis. Neurophysiological evaluation may help to increase our knowledge of brain structures and of the dysfunctional circuitry sustaining specific types of myoclonus or dystonic movement in the heterogeneous nervous system diseases presenting with these classes of movement disorders.

Introduction

Neurophysiological tests, usually involving complex protocols, are often used in patients with movement disorders, with a variety of aims: to support a clinical diagnosis, to help in the differential diagnosis in cases of complex or atypical clinical presentation, and to monitor brain dysfunction quantitatively during therapeutic trials or rehabilitative interventions. Table 1 summarizes common applications of electrophysiological techniques in the field of movement disorders.

Neurophysiological investigations are based on techniques that are particularly suitable for following in real time events occurring in a range of milliseconds, to evaluate input-output relations (for example, the results of an afferent stimulus on a motor output), and to assess the functional state of a neural circuit. They are therefore appropriate tools to evaluate the

Table 1. Neurophysiological techniques are currently applied in order to:

- detect involuntary movements that are not easy to identify clinically (for example, movement disorders occurring during sleep or in wake-sleep transition)
- define precisely the type of movement disorder and its relation to specific conditions (such as rest/action, vigilance, stimuli)
- determine the presence/absence of synchrony activation of agonist and antagonist muscles
- determine the duration of EMG busts associated with hyperkinesias, and the frequency and consistency of rhythmic or repetitive phenomena
- aid in the differential diagnosis between different hyperkinesias and often to differentiate psychogenic from 'organic' movement disorders
- attribute an involuntary movement to a specific system (spinal cord, brain stem, basal ganglia, neocortex, and so on)
- assess the associated nervous dysfunctions (for example, evaluation of reflex responses, magnetic stimulations, evoked potentials, and so on)

characteristics of short-lasting 'phasic' events such as paroxysmal movement disorders and underlying brain dysfunction.

Complex neurophysiological protocols, including several electrophysiological techniques and sophisticated post-analyses, are also applied to gain a better understanding of the pathophysiological mechanisms sustaining a given movement disorder.

Significance and applicability of the neurophysiological tests

It is important to emphasize that young patients may not be able to collaborate fully in carrying out neurophysiological tests. Moreover, most of the electrophysiological procedures, even non-invasive ones, are time-consuming, sometimes poorly tolerated, and generally done without the support of strong sedation or anaesthesia, to avoid interference with the excitability of neural circuits. However, almost all the tests can be carried out if the investigators are sufficiently relaxed, have enough time, and if the clinical setting is appropriate and the child kindly entertained. Movement artefacts are usually recognized automatically and rejected.

Protocols aimed at evaluating movement disorders include one or more of the following electrophysiological procedures:

(1) *Polymyographic recordings often combined with EEG or video-EEG recordings.* Polymyography is considered the basic way of evaluating movement disorders and a mandatory diagnostic procedure in all uncertain or borderline conditions in which paroxysmal movement disorders may occur. Electromyographic (EMG) recordings using surface electrodes are usually well tolerated and are essential to define the following:

- the duration and time course of EMG activity associated with the pathological movement;
- the involvement of antagonist muscles;
- the pattern of muscle activation (including the order of activation and latencies between different muscles);
- the relation with voluntary movements, habituation;
- susceptibility of the EMG phenomena to multimodal stimuli delivered using appropriate devices (somatosensory, acoustic, visual, or magnetic stimuli)
- latencies between a given stimulus and the appearance of the EMG burst, allowing hypotheses about the circuitry involved.

A concomitant EEG recording allows to analyse the EEG-EMG relationship, vigilance level, and the presence of epileptic activity. Video recordings may often help in recognizing the movement disorder and in precisely evaluating the relation between the paroxysmal movement and a specific polygraphic pattern.

(2) *Study of reflex responses* including long and short loop reflexes, spinal reflexes (H-reflex and F-responses), and blink reflexes to investigate the circuitry involved in the movement disorder.

(3) *Somatosensory evoked potentials (SSEPs)* or other types of evoked potentials, which should be investigated under particular circumstances.

(4) *Transcranial magnetic stimulation (TMS) protocols*, to evaluate the excitability of the motor cortex and the conduction time of motor outputs.

Neuroimaging techniques such as positron emission tomography (PET), single photon emission computed tomography (SPECT), and functional magnetic resonance imaging (fMRI) can be applied in the specific field of movement disorders and are often complementary to the neurophysiological investigations. The main limits of imaging techniques are the slow time resolution and the high susceptibility to movement artefacts.

All the electrophysiological signals are currently analysed using 'mathematical' procedures, including simple average and spectral analysis. More sophisticated analyses of waveforms with appropriate algorithms are constantly being investigated to improve the results and abbreviate or simplify the diagnostic procedures.

In this chapter, we will try to sum up the evidence that can be acquired using electrophysiological tests in myoclonus and dystonia, two common forms of movement disorder. Myoclonus is the most extensively studied and heterogeneous type of movement disorder, occurring in a wide range of nervous diseases arising from different causes. Conversely, the origin of dystonia is assumed to be less heterogeneous, mainly involving the basal ganglia; however, dystonia probably implies the involvement of various neuronal circuits, which can be suitably investigated using electrophysiological tests. Dystonic syndromes result from a variety of diseases, either genetically determined or acquired, and it is to be expected that these will involve different circuitries.

Myoclonus

The term 'myoclonus' refers to both physiological and pathological events. Physiological myoclonus may occur on drowsiness or during rapid eye movement (REM) sleep, or as hiccups. The term can also be used to define normal fetal movements or primitive infantile reflex responses.

In pathological conditions, myoclonus occurs as a symptom of different progressive and non-progressive diseases or in isolation, as essential myoclonus. The first approach to the patient should be to verify the myoclonic nature of the movement disorder using a battery of neurophysiological tests. For example, repetitive and small myoclonic jerks are impossible to distinguish from tremor by the phenotypic appearance alone and need neurophysiological characterisation.

The presence in some neurological disorders of a 'reflex' type of myoclonus facilitates the characterisation of the circuits involved (typically opposing cortical *vs.* subcortical or 'reticular' myoclonus) (see Ugawa *et al.*, 2002; Hallett, 2002 for reviews). More recently, the extensive application of TMS (see Cantello, 2002 for a review) and the analysis of the EEG-EMG relations (Brown, 2000; Silen *et al.*, 2002; Panzica *et al.*, 2003) during repetitive myoclonic jerks have provided further information on the physiological and pathological circuitry (Grosse *et al.*, 2003) within the motor cortex. For all these reasons, the protocols used to define myoclonus electrophysiologically should be considered as a prototype of the investigations for other types of movement disorder.

Polymyographic recordings

The classification of EMG bursts using pure polymyographic criteria is in general considered essential to validate the diagnosis of myoclonus. Polymyography is commonly undertaken using pairs of surface electrodes positioned on different muscles, chosen on the basis of the clinical examination.

The concomitant activation (or inhibition) of couples of antagonist muscles is in general included in the definition of myoclonus. Myoclonic jerks are further classified as positive, positive-negative (where the EMG burst is followed by obvious inhibition of the muscle contraction), or negative (where there is pure inhibition of the EMG activity).

The positive component of a myoclonic jerk can be detected at rest as well as during muscle activation, while the negative component appears only when the patient sustains a tonic muscle contraction. The duration (Fig. 1A) of the EMG bursts and their time course may directly suggest a cortical *vs* a subcortical generator. Short duration (less than 100 ms) is common in cortical myoclonus. Likewise, short bursts recurring with a rhythmic course at a rather high frequency (usually over 10 Hz) and involving couples of antagonist muscles also strongly suggest a cortical origin (Fig. 1B and 1C). A variable EMG burst duration can be found in brain stem or spinal cord myoclonus, which may occur irregularly or with a rhythmic or quasi-periodic course. A long EMG burst duration often indicates a subcortical origin, particularly in basal ganglia diseases.

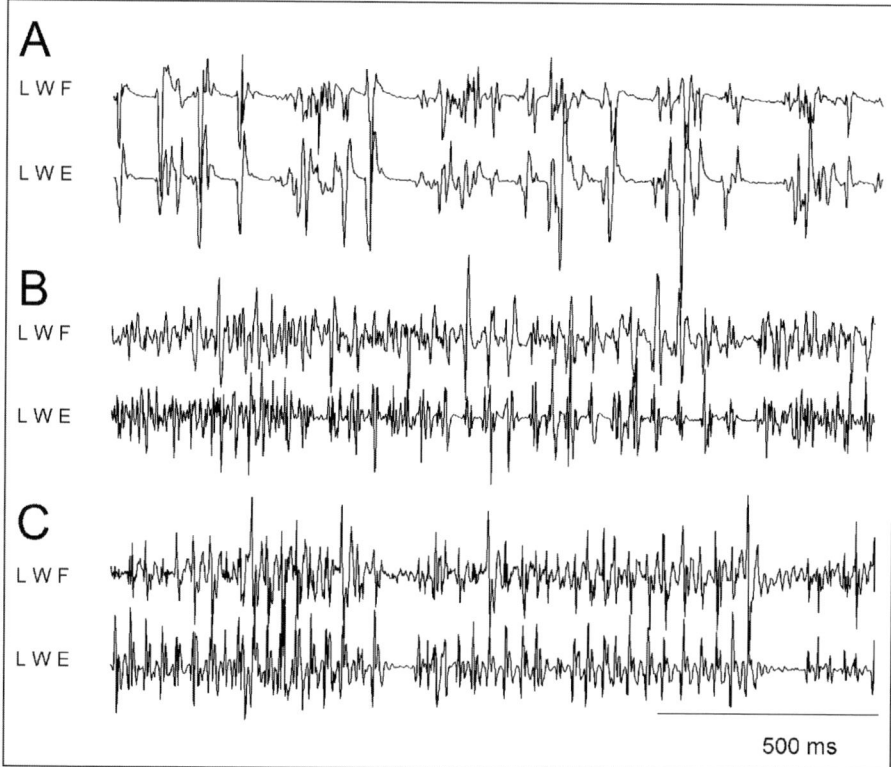

Fig. 1. (A) Cortical myoclonus: brief arrhythmic jerks occurring synchronously on antagonist muscles (L WF=left wrist flexor; L WE=left wrist extensor). (B) and (C) Rhythmic cortical myoclonus occurring at different frequencies on antagonist muscles. All the recordings were made in patients with progressive myoclonic epilepsies.

The temporal sequence of activation of different muscles is generally considered an important feature distinguishing myoclonus generated by brain stem structures from cortically generated myoclonus. In the so-called 'reticular reflex myoclonus' – a rather rare type of myoclonus resulting from a severe anoxic brain insult (post-anoxic myoclonus) or metabolic disorders – myoclonic jerks can be triggered by either a voluntary movement or an external stimulus and usually involve the whole body, with muscles on both sides being affected simultaneously. Upstream activation of the cranial muscles (with activation of sternocleidomastoid or trapezium preceding activation of masseter) plus downstream activation of skeletal muscles are considered typical features, indicating a lower brain stem generator (Hallet, 2002). In contrast, the muscle order involvement is typically downstream in cortically generated myoclonus (Ugawa et al., 2002).

The startle syndrome (startle disease) or hyperekplexia, which also probably arises from a brain stem generator, presents with well defined polymyographic characteristics. Excessive startles are linked with the appearance of prolonged EMG bursts, usually involving both sides of the body, in response to sudden stimuli. The massive myoclonic jerks can be distinguished from normal startle responses because of the lower threshold, the abnormal spread of myoclonic jerks to the axial and limb muscles, and the resistance to habituation when repeated stimuli are applied over a short interval (Brown, 2002). Moreover, the sequence of downstream muscle activation shows especially long latencies between the EMG bursts recorded on the proximal and distal limb muscles, consistent with slow propagation through slow-conducting descending pathways.

Myoclonic jerks, probably generated at a subcortical level, can sometimes be mixed with other types of movement disorders, as typically occurs in myoclonic dystonia (Obeso et al., 1983). In that case, EMG surface recordings may characterize the hyperkinesias as a mixture of involuntary 'dystonic' muscle contractions (see below) and rather long myoclonic bursts involving segmental axial and limb muscles (Fig. 2A and 2B).

EMG bursts with a generalized or segmental distribution may occur in different neurological disorders, sometimes with rhythmical or periodic repetition. The polygraphic characteristics and the time relations between the activation of different muscles may indicate a brain stem or spinal origin (as in spinal myoclonus or propriospinal myoclonus) or, coupled with EEG recordings, may help to distinguish cortically generated from subcortically generated focal myoclonic jerks.

Reflex responses

Because of the extreme variability of the generators of myoclonic jerks and their neuropathological contexts, the evaluation of reflex responses may vary depending on the segment investigated. For example, in patients with nocturnal periodic limb movements, spinal reflexes – such as the H-reflex (see below) – may show diminished inhibition occurring at spinal level (probably reflecting altered function of the descending spinal tracts), a peripheral influence, or changes in the spinal inhibitory circuitry (Rijsman et al., 2005). However, the more typically investigated reflex in cases of myoclonus is the so-called C-reflex (Shibasaki & Hallett, 2005), included in the 'long loop reflex' (LLR), the converse of the short loop (SLR) monosynaptic spinal reflex. The LLR is mediated by fast-conducting fibers from muscle spindles and cutaneous afferents and includes different components (I, II, III) reflecting the different circuits that are enhanced in the various myoclonic syndromes (Shibasaki & Hallett, 2005). The LLR reflex is present in healthy subjects during active muscle contraction (motor activation) but can also appear at rest in patients with myoclonus, when abnormally large amplitudes occur during motor activation. The LLR is commonly increased in cortical myoclonus, but one of the three components can also be

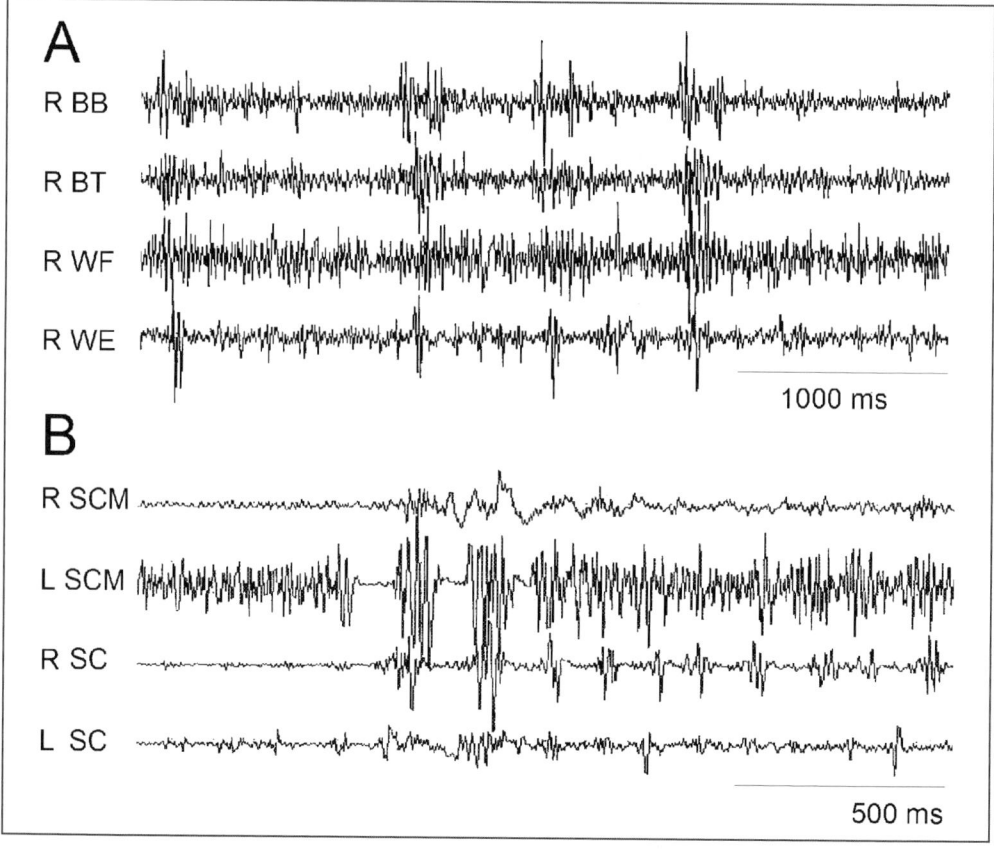

Fig. 2. Polymyographic recordings made in a patient with myoclonic dystonia. (A) Irregular tonic contraction occurring at the moment of dorsal hand flexions, overflowing on brachial biceps and triceps. Myoclonic bursts with different shapes and durations occur intermingled with the tonic contraction. (B) Long myoclonic jerks occurring spontaneously in axial muscles, superimposed on tonic muscle contraction. BB, biceps brachii; BT, triceps brachii; L, left; R, right; SCM, sternocleidomastoid; SC, splenius capitis; WE, wrist flexor; WF, wrist flexor.

enhanced in non-cortical myoclonus and in other neurological disorders involving both pyramidal and non-pyramidal systems (Deuschl & Lucking, 1990) – such as, for example, corticobasal degeneration (Carella et al., 1997) and severe epileptic syndromes (Guerrini et al., 1998).

Sensory evoked potentials

Specific changes of SSEPs have been reported in patients with cortical myoclonus caused by acquired cortical damage or progressive myoclonic epilepsies (Shibasaki & Hallett, 2005).

Enlargement of the short latency P25 and N33 components of the SSEPs evoked by electrical stimulation of the median nerve is assumed to be a characteristic of cortical reflex myoclonus (Shibasaki & Hallett, 2005). In a recent study undertaken by our group (Canafoglia et al., 2004), significant differences were found between patients with different forms of progressive myoclonic epilepsies, in particular those affected by the commonest forms of the disorder, Unverricht-Lundborg disease and Lafora body disease. Thus, while in Unverricht-Lundborg patients the 'enlarged' SEP components exactly match those characterizing 'classical' cortical reflex myoclonus, the most consistent aspect of the SSEPs in Lafora body disease was a considerably enlarged middle latency component. This suggests that the thalamo-cortical volley and the sensorimotor recipient cortex are involved in the pathological process that sustains hyperexcitability in both these subgroups of progressive myoclonic epilepsy, but that the distortion of cortical circuitry is more complex and sustained in Lafora body disease, and involves an enhanced multisynaptic elaboration of the somatosensory stimulus responsible for medium latency SSEP components.

EEG correlates

EEG correlates are typically found in myoclonic seizures or in focal motor seizures in many epileptic syndromes. In these cases, the EEG correlates are in general easily detectable by inspection of the EEG. The time relation between a specific EEG transient (or specific EEG rhythms) and the EMG jerks has been extensively studied in those conditions presenting with suspected cortical myoclonus without an obvious (that is, visually detectable) EEG correlate. Jerk-locked back averaging is a commonly applied technique aimed at clarifying the relation between muscle jerks and recorded EEG activity. It is based on the average of several EEG segments preceding and following the onset of myoclonic jerks (Shibasaki & Hallett, 2005). Averaging of the EEG signal containing both myoclonus-correlated and myoclonus-non-correlated EEG activity over a sufficient number of epochs attenuates the non-correlated EEG components and enhances the 'time-locked' transients. In cortical myoclonus, the time difference between the EEG transient and the EMG burst allows the time transfer to be calculated. This is usually consistent with fast corticospinal conduction. However, the same technique may also allow detection of EEG transients following myoclonic jerks, which can occur in cases of reticular myoclonus because of an afferent volley from the brain stem towards the cortical structures.

Alternative and sometimes more powerful techniques aimed at evaluating the cortical-EMG relations are based on the assessment of spectral EEG and EMG properties, and estimates of the coherence of the EEG-EMG relation (a high value of coherence in a certain frequency range suggests a common origin of the EEG activity in that frequency band) and phase function (related to the time transfer between EEG and EMG components) (Brown, 2000; Silen et al., 2002; Panzica et al., 2003). These techniques are especially suitable in cases of high-frequency rhythmic myoclonus, which prevents the evaluation of a one-to-one relation between EEG activities and recurrent EMG bursts. Figure 3 demonstrates the application of this analytical method on EEG-EMG traces made in our laboratory in a patient with bursts of rhythmic myoclonic jerks.

Transcranial magnetic stimulation studies

TMS allows the investigation of intracortical inhibition and facilitation and of sensorimotor integration; it can therefore be suitably applied in the evaluation of patients with known or suspected cortical myoclonus. Magnetic stimulation has been used by applying twin magnetic stimuli or a sensory stimulus delivered before the magnetic stimulus (Manganotti et al., 2001; Canafoglia et al., 2004). Sensory stimuli have been found to facilitate the conditioned motor evoked potentials (MEPs) abnormally at short interstimulus intervals in comparison with healthy controls.

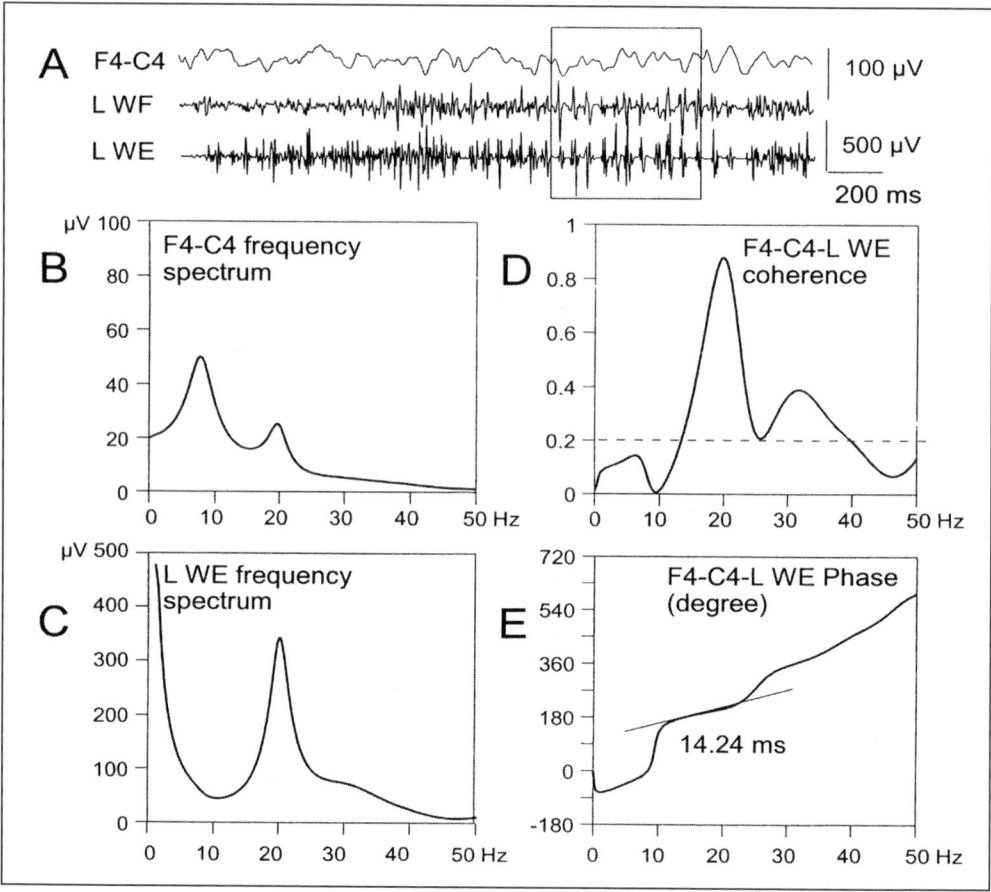

Fig. 3. (A) EEG-EMG recording in a patient with sequences of rhythmic cortical myoclonus (L WF, left wrist flexor; L WE, left wrist extensor). (B) and (C) Amplitude spectrum of EEG and EMG traces. (D) and (E) Coherence and phase analyses which allow the detection of a common generator and a cortex-muscle time difference consistent with cortico-spinal transfer.

Dystonia

Dystonia is commonly defined as the presence of sustained contraction of one or more muscle groups, which causes a twisting/distortion of that part of the body, resulting in an abnormal posturing or positioning. It can be generalized or focal, as in blepharospasm, torticollis, Meige's syndrome, spasmodic dysphonia, and writer's cramp.

Clinical assessment of dystonia does not need the support of electrophysiological tests when the presentation is obvious, but they may be of diagnostic value in cases of mild or atypical presentation. Electrophysiological investigations can also help in distinguishing between the different dystonic syndromes, the genetic basis of which is under extensive investigation, and in quantitatively assessing the results of therapeutic (pharmacological or surgical) interventions. Recent studies based on neurophysiological investigation have shown that dystonia involves cortical circuits and that the motor dysfunction results from a complex disturbance of sensori-motor integration. This suggests that extensive neurophysiological diagnostic procedures should be applied to obtain a better understanding of the different forms of nervous system dysfunction that result in dystonic syndromes.

Polymyographic recordings

Polymyographic recordings are usually undertaken on the basis of the characteristics and distribution of dystonic movements. After applying surface disk electrodes on selected muscles, the patient is stimulated to perform simple movements that elicit dystonic posturing. The EMG pattern associated with dystonia can vary, with isolated or recurrent EMG bursts of variable duration. One of the most important characteristics revealed by polymyographic evaluation is the failure of reciprocal inhibition. Thus antagonist muscles contract simultaneously (co-contraction); furthermore, the contraction unintentionally 'overflows' to muscle groups that are not needed for the motor task. Figure 4 shows the concurrent activation of sternocleiodomastoid and splenii capitis muscles on both sides during mild and clumsy right head deviation in a patient with spasmodic torticollis.

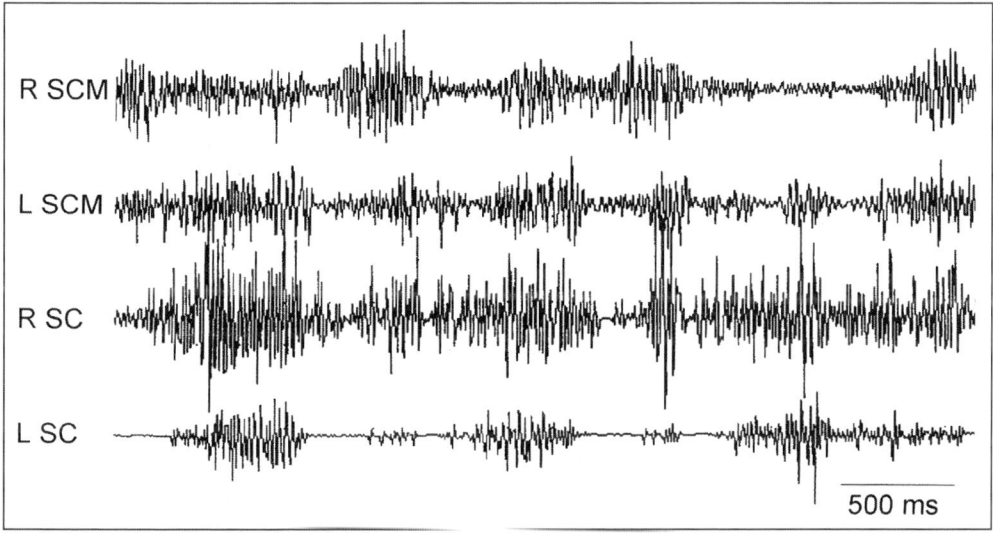

Fig. 4. EMG recording made in a patient with spasmodic torticollis showing the abnormal co-contraction of both sternocleidomastoid muscles (SCM) and the concurrent activation of the splenius capitis (SC) muscle when the patient tried to rotate his head slightly to the right.

Reflex responses

Segmental inhibitory circuits in the brain stem and spinal cord are impaired in dystonic patients owing to the defective influence of suprasegmental brain structures. Various neurophysiological tests are capable of revealing this dysfunctional circuitry. Reduced reciprocal inhibition should be demonstrated by paired stimulation of nerves innervating antagonist muscles in focal and generalized dystonia (for review, see Berardelli et al., 1998; Mavroudakis, 2005). Evaluation of the spinal H-reflex cycle is also often carried out, using paired pulse protocols. This procedure shows enhanced recovery in patients with generalized dystonia, as well as in those with focal dystonia (spasmodic torticollis and writer's cramp). Moreover, the recovery cycle of the blink reflex (elicited by paired trigeminal stimuli) is enhanced in patients with cranial, cervical, and generalized dystonia, with reduced inhibition of the conditioned multisynaptic response

(R2) which can be recorded bilaterally from the orbicular muscles, and marked enhancement of the recovery curve. Figure 5 shows the enhancement of the multisynaptic late component of the blink reflex occurring contralateral to a dystonic disturbance, leading to spasmodic torticollis, as observed in our laboratory. Interestingly, the blink reflex recovery cycle also shows reduced inhibition in patients with DOPA-responsive dystonia, recovering towards normal values after effective treatment with dopamine (Huang et al., 2006). This may suggest that in selected patients with dystonic syndromes the evaluation of reflex responses may be an objective way of evaluating the patient under basal conditions and of testing the effectiveness of pharmacological treatment.

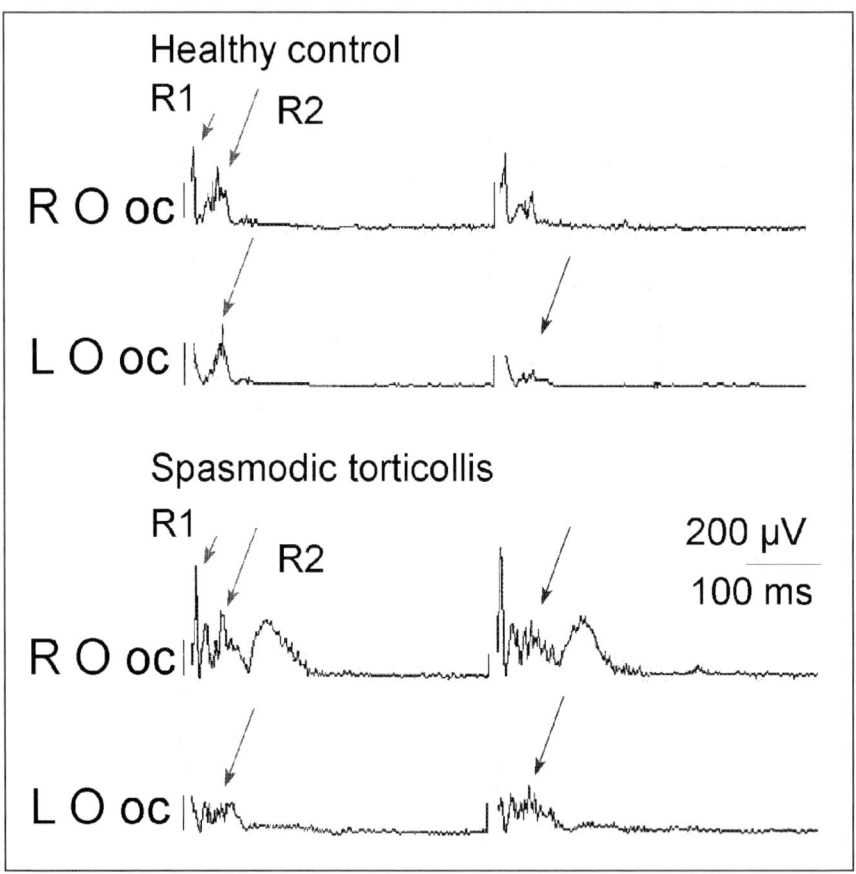

Fig. 5. Blink reflex evaluation using paired pulse protocol (stimuli are delivered to the right trigeminal nerve). R1 (arrow head) is the oligosynaptic response recorded on the stimulated side; R2 (arrows) is the multisynaptic response recorded on both sides. In the patient with spasmodic torticollis, note the large multi-synaptic response (arrows) occurring in the orbicularis oculi (OOc) ipsilateral and contralateral with respect to the stimulated trigeminal nerve, and the early recovery of the conditioned stimulus delivered 400 ms after the conditioning one. By contrast, at the same time R2 is obviously inhibited in the healthy control.

Electrophysiological evaluation of sensorimotor cortical integration

Various electrophysiological investigations have provided evidence that the abnormality in the central nervous system in dystonic syndromes is located not only at the subcortical level but also at the cortical level – specifically, cortical excitability and intracortical inhibition have been shown to be abnormal. From this evidence, dystonic movements appear to involve abnormal function of somatosensory pathways and sensorimotor integration.

Two movement-related cortical events, reflecting the preparation or anticipation of movement – the so-called Bereitschaftspotential (readiness potential, appearing with self-paced, 'voluntary' movements) and the contingent-negative variation (CNV, occurring between a warning stimulus and a 'go' stimulus) – reflect dynamic changes in motor cortical activity taking place during the 1.5 seconds preceding the onset of the movement. These two components (the Bereitschaftspotential and the CNV) have been found to be depressed and abnormally distributed in focal hand dystonia (Deuschl *et al.*, 1995; Ikeda *et al.*, 1996; Hamano *et al.*, 1999) and in jaw deviation dystonia (Yoshida & Iizuka, 2003), indicating that abnormalities of the motor programme involve neocortical function directly in patients with focal dystonias.

More recently, the functional state of the motor cortex has been extensively evaluated by means of TMS protocols aimed at examining cortical excitability and the effect of sensory stimuli on the motor cortex.

Many studies, mainly on focal dystonias, have revealed dysfunctional conditions of the motor cortex and of sensorimotor integration. These include a shortening of the refractory period (following individual magnetic stimuli), decreased short interval intracortical inhibition (evaluated by paired magnetic pulse protocols), distorted projection of the motor cortex to the muscles (evaluated by MEP mapping), and a pathological facilitation of MEPs by peripheral sensory stimuli (see Cantello, 2002 for a review). Interestingly, some of these changes can be attenuated after local botulinum toxin injections with a time course corresponding to the clinical effectiveness of this agent, suggesting that the peripheral input resulting from dystonic movements may significantly influence the function and excitability of the motor cortex, probably by modifying afferent inputs from muscle spindles.

Conclusions and prospectives

The evidence briefly summarized here is only a small sample of what can be obtained by neurophysiological procedures in the field of movement disorders. In general, these procedures are useful and sometimes necessary to support the clinical diagnosis in cases of doubtful presentation (for example, psychogenic disorders) or to clarify the differential diagnosis between the various types of movement disorders, which are sometimes difficult to distinguish on the basis of purely phenotypical manifestations. Moreover, the evidence obtained by neurophysiological investigation plays a fundamental role in clarifying the generators and the pathological circuits sustaining a given movement disorder.

Polygraphic recordings represent the primary tool in evaluating abnormal movements or posturing, and are generally suitable for use in infants and children. However, the increasing accuracy and power of other techniques – including reflex responses analysis, TMS protocols, and analytical algorithms capable of better characterisation of the recorded signal – are additional important ways to illuminate the pathophysiological mechanisms underlying movement disorders. The detection and characterization of abnormal sensorimotor integration in various myoclonic and dystonic syndromes (as well in other movement disorders) is an example of the special contribution of neurophysiological procedures in understanding the pathophysiology of movement disorders.

The application of neurophysiological tests to monitor and follow up patients submitted to therapeutic deep brain stimulation needs further research, but they may be considered promising tools for identifying specific features that are predictive of outcome. Moreover, intraoperative recordings from implanted electrodes (Zhuang *et al.*, 2004; Starr *et al.*, 2006) as well as concomitant intraoperative EMG monitoring (Liu *et al.*, 2005) may support surgical procedures and supply direct information about the mechanisms sustaining movement disorders.

Acknowledgments: We thank the technicians Alessandra Peirano, Laura Grigoletti, Angela Napolitano and Paola Anversa for their skilful technical assistance in the neurophysiological recordings.

References

Berardelli, A., Rothwell, J.C., Hallett, M., Thompson, P.D., Manfredi, M. & Marsden, C.D. (1988): The pathophysiology of primary dystonia. *Brain* **121**, 1195–1212.

Brown, P. (2000): Cortical drives to human muscle: the Piper and related rhythms. *Prog. Neurobiol.* **60**, 97–108.

Brown, P. (2002): Neurophysiology of the startle syndrome and hyperekplexia. *Adv. Neurol.* **89**, 153–159.

Canafoglia, L., Ciano, C., Panzica, F., Scaioli, V., Zucca, C., Agazzi, P., Visani, E., Avanzini, G. & Franceschetti, S. (2004): Sensorimotor cortex excitability in Unverricht-Lundborg disease and Lafora body disease. *Neurology* **63**, 2309–2315.

Cantello, R. (2002): Applications of transcranial magnetic stimulation in movement disorders. *J. Clin. Neurophysiol.* **19**, 272–293.

Carella, F., Ciano, C., Panzica, F. & Scaioli, V. (1997): Myoclonus in corticobasal degeneration. *Mov. Disord.* **12**, 598–603.

Deuschl, G. & Lucking, C.H. (1990): Physiology and clinical applications of hand muscle reflexes. *Electroencephalogr. Clin. Neurophysiol. Suppl.* **41**, 84–101.

Deuschl, G., Toro, C., Matsumoto, J. & Hallett, M. (1995): Movement-related cortical potentials in writer's cramp. *Ann. Neurol.* **38**, 862–868.

Grosse, P., Guerrini, R., Parmeggiani, L., Bonanni, P., Pogosyan, A. & Brown, P. (2003): Abnormal corticomuscular and intermuscular coupling in high-frequency rhythmic myoclonus. *Brain* **126**, 326–342.

Guerrini, R., Bonanni, P., Parmeggiani, L., Santucci, M., Parmeggiani, A. & Sartucci, F. (1998): Cortical reflex myoclonus in Rett syndrome. *Ann. Neurol.* **43**, 472–479.

Hallett, M. (2002): Neurophysiology of brainstem myoclonus. *Adv. Neurol.* **89**, 99–102.

Hamano, T., Kaji, R., Katayama, M., Kubori, T., Ikeda, A., Shibasaki, H. & Kimura, J. (1999): Abnormal contingent negative variation in writer's cramp. *Clin. Neurophysiol.* **110**, 508–515.

Huang, Y.Z., Trender-Gerhard, I., Edwards, M.J., Mir, P., Rothwell, J.C. & Bhatia, K.P. (2006): Motor system inhibition in dopa-responsive dystonia and its modulation by treatment. *Neurology* **66**, 1088–1090.

Ikeda, A., Shibasaki, H., Kaji, R., Terada, K., Nagamine, T., Honda, M., Hamano, T. & Kimura, J. (1996): Abnormal sensorimotor integration in writer's cramp: study of contingent negative variation. *Mov. Disord.* **11**, 683–690.

Liu, X., Aziz, T.Z. & Bain, P.G. (2005): Intraoperative monitoring of motor symptoms using surface electromyography during stereotactic surgery for movement disorders. *J. Clin. Neurophysiol.* **22**, 183–191.

Manganotti, P., Tamburin, S., Zanette, G. & Fiaschi, A. (2001): Hyperexcitable cortical responses in progressive myoclonic epilepsy: a TMS study. *Neurology* **57**, 1793–1799.

Mavroudakis, N. (2005): Clinical neurophysiology of dystonia. *Acta Neurol. Belg.* **105**, 23–29.

Obeso, J.A., Rothwell, J.C., Lang, A.E. & Marsden, C.D. (1983): Myoclonic dystonia. *Neurology* **33**, 825–830.

Panzica, F., Canafoglia, L., Franceschetti, S., Binelli, S., Ciano, C., Visani, E. & Avanzini, G. (2003): Movement-activated myoclonus in genetically defined progressive myoclonic epilepsies: EEG-EMG relationship estimated using autoregressive models. *Clin. Neurophysiol.* **114**, 1041–1052.

Rijsman, R.M., Stam, C.J. & de Weerd, A.W. (2005): Abnormal H-reflexes in periodic limb movement disorder; impact on understanding the pathophysiology of the disorder. *Clin. Neurophysiol.* **116**, 204–210.

Shibasaki, H. & Hallett, M. (2005): Electrophysiological studies of myoclonus. *Muscle Nerve* **31**, 157–174.

Silen, T., Forss, N., Salenius, S., Karjalainen, T. & Hari, R. (2002): Oscillatory cortical drive to isometrically contracting muscle in Unverricht-Lundborg type progressive myoclonus epilepsy (ULD). *Clin. Neurophysiol.* **113**, 1973–1979.

Starr, P.A., Turner, R.S., Rau, G., Lindsey, N., Heath, S., Volz, M., Ostrem, J.L. & Marks, W.J. (2006): Microelectrode-guided implantation of deep brain stimulators into the globus pallidus internus for dystonia: techniques, electrode locations, and outcomes. *J. Neurosurg.* **104**, 488–501.

Ugawa, Y., Hanajima, R., Okabe, S. & Yuasa, K. (2002): Neurophysiology of cortical positive myoclonus. *Adv. Neurol.* **89**, 89–97.

Yoshida, K. & Iizuka, T. (2003): Jaw deviation dystonia evaluated by movement-related cortical potentials and treated with muscle afferent block. *Cranio* **21**, 295–300.

Zhuang, P., Li, Y. & Hallett, M. (2004): Neuronal activity in the basal ganglia and thalamus in patients with dystonia. *Clin. Neurophysiol.* **115**, 2542–2557.

Chapter 5

Quantitative assessment of paediatric movement disorders

Renata Bono, Emanuela Pagliano, Elena Andreucci, Simona Malinverni and Alice Corlatti

Department of Developmental Neurology, Fondazione IRCCS Istituto Neurologico 'C. Besta', via Celoria 11, 20133 Milan, Italy
renatabono@libero.it
Video 1

Summary

The functional evaluation of paediatric movement disorders depends on several internationally validated instruments, which have been developed for each disorder. These tools allow an objective and standardized assessment sufficient to provide a diagnostic definition of each disorder, to characterize its clinical course, and to evaluate the effectiveness of medical and surgical therapeutic interventions.

In this chapter, we summarize the developmental scales that are most suited to assessing motor impairment in static encephalopathies, including the Gross Motor Function Measure (GFMF) and the Gross Motor Performance Measure (GMPM). We then provide an overview of the tools that specifically evaluate the motor function of the hand (the Melbourne scale) and foot (the Boyd test), and of the complex battery of five different tests developed by Fedrizzi et al. for a detailed assessment of dystonic-dyskinetic syndromes. Next, we illustrate the scale used clinically to assess the severity and functional disability of torsion dystonia, as well as the computerized instruments available to define sitting, standing, and walking patterns (gait analysis). Finally, for assessing treatments that result in the greatest self-sufficiency in activities of daily living, we review the Wee FIM scale of functional independence, the Paediatric Evaluation of Disability Inventory (PEDI), and a simple tool developed to evaluate disability in torsion dystonia. These tools supply the clinician all the information necessary to select the therapeutic strategy most suited to the individual patient.

Introduction

Tools for the functional assessment of paediatric movement disorders must first of all be objective. To satisfy the requirements of evidence-based medicine, a given tool must be reliable – that is, consistently give the same result in different evaluations; valid – that is, be sensitive to change but stable under fixed conditions; and produce reproducible results. Reliability and validity are achieved when a tool is successfully tested on a large population of patients fulfilling the criteria for statistical applicability. Different functional scales are available that meet these requirements. Nevertheless, the choice between one scale and another must be made according to the clinical features of the particular patient. For the evaluation of paediatric movement disorders, these tools are necessary to reach a diagnosis, to follow the clinical course of the disease, and to assess the effectiveness of treatment.

The diagnostic work-up of paediatric movement disorders involves several different steps. These include a detailed history, a thorough neurological examination, and an initial overview of the child (gestalt) sufficient to provide a working diagnosis of the possible underlying disease. This first analysis involves the collection of a great deal of information about the semiology of the movement disorder, the co-occurrence of systemic signs, the duration of the disease, the constancy or variability of a given symptom, the degree of functional impairment, the ability of the child to cope with or compensate for the symptoms, and the patterns that are typical or pathognomonic of each movement disorder. While laboratory investigations make a substantial contribution to the diagnostic process, a sound knowledge of the natural history of the main childhood neurological disorders is the basis for the correct identification of the signs and symptoms that are useful in making a diagnosis.

The use of standardized scales must therefore be integrated into the clinical practice, making it possible to quantify a disorder, to compare different case series, and to evaluate the outcome of different treatment regimens. However, only clinicians can interpret and make best use of the information derived from these scales, in accordance with their own experience and competence.

Functional evaluation

There are various functional evaluation scales, each addressing a different aspect of movement disorders. Discriminative measures allow to identify a disorder and provide information on the neuromotor features, including their pattern repertoire, their scarcity or stereotypy, their symmetry, the quality of motor sequences, the type of abnormal movement involved, and so on. Predictive scales – such as the Assessment of General Movements in neonates with cerebral palsy (Prechtl & Hopkins, 1986) – specifically provide prognostic indexes. Finally, quantitative and qualitative scales monitor the magnitude of change, whether spontaneous or following interventions, that occurs over time.

There are several functional scales available for a reliable and valid assessment of changes in the clinical picture of children with cerebral palsy. One of the most commonly used is the Gross Motor Function Measure (GMFM), developed by Russell *et al.* (1989, 1994) at McMaster University (Ontario, Canada), which allow the prompt evaluation of quantitative changes in different motor functions. The GMFM is composed of 88 items grouped into five dimensions: (1) lying and rolling; (2) crawling and kneeling; (3) sitting; (4) standing; and (5) walking, running, and jumping. Generally, normal children are able to complete all items. Items are scored on a 4-point ordinal scale:

0 = the child does not initiate the item;
1 = the child initiates the item (< 10 per cent of the maximum score);
2 = the child partially completes the item (> 10, but < 100 per cent of the maximum score);
3 = the child completes the item.

Each dimension contributes equally to the total score. Scores for each dimension are expressed as a percentage of the maximum score for that dimension. The total score is obtained by adding the scores for all dimensions and dividing by the total number of dimensions. The GMFM was created to measure gross motor function quantitatively, not taking into account the quality of movements. It takes approximately 45 to 60 minutes to administer and the examiners must be

Table 1. Gross Motor Function Measure (GMFM), fifth domain: walking, running, and jumping

1.	From standing, can walk 5 steps on the right while holding on a bench
2.	From standing, can walk 5 steps on the left while holding on a bench
3.	From standing, can walk 10 steps with both hands held
4.	From standing, can walk 10 steps with one hand held
5.	From standing, can walk 10 steps with arms free
6.	From standing, can walk 10 steps backward
7.	From standing, can walk 10 steps while holding a ball with two hands
8.	From standing, can walk 10 consecutive steps between 2 lines 20 cm apart
9.	From standing, can walk 10 consecutive steps on a line 2 cm wide
10.	Can get over a stick placed at the knee level with the right foot
11.	Can get over a stick placed at the knee level with the left foot
12.	Can run 5 metres, stop and run back
13.	Can kick a ball with the right foot
14.	Can kick a ball with the left foot
15.	Can jump 30 cm high with both feet simultaneously
16.	Can jump forward 30 cm with both feet simultaneously
17.	Can jump 10 times on the right foot, within a circle of 35 cm in diameter
18.	Can jump 10 times on the left foot, within a circle of 35 cm in diameter
19.	Can walk up 4 steps, alternating feet, while holding one rail
20.	Can walk down 4 steps, alternating feet, while holding one rail
21.	Can walk up 4 steps, alternating feet, with arms free
22.	Can walk down 4 steps, alternating feet, with arms free
23.	Can jump down a 10 cm step with both feet simultaneously

paediatric therapists. The level of agreement improves significantly when therapists are trained to administer and score the GMFM using videotaped simulations.

An example of functional evaluation within the GMFM fifth dimension (walking, running, and jumping) is given in the accompanying DVD, video 1, track 1 (see also Table 1).

When assessing the severity of paediatric motor disorders, it is most useful to define the child's degree of independence. In this respect, the classification of severity developed by Palisano *et al.* (1997) is internationally recognized as the primary reference. It is a five-level classification system assessing gross motor function, ranging from complete self-sufficiency (level I) to severe disability (level V) (Table 2).

The Gross Motor Performance Measure (GMPM) (Boyce *et al.*, 1995) is a qualitative evaluation tool employing 20 items derived from the GMFM. It focuses on the child's posture and locomotor functions, which are assessed using five performance attributes: (1) postural alignment; (2) coordination (considering the direction, speed, strength, and amplitude of each motor sequence); (3) dissociated movements (isolated and independent movements); (4) postural

Table 2. Gross motor function classification system (from Palisano *et al.*, 1997)

Level	Mobility	Outdoor independence
I	Walks without restriction	Limited by more advanced motor skills (running, jumping)
II	Walks indoor without assistive devices	Limitations when walking outdoor or in the community
III	Walks with assistive devices, both indoor and outdoor	Needs transportation when travelling for long distances
IV	Cannot walk, even with assistive devices	Needs assistance to move from sitting to standing
V	Self-mobility severely limited even with assistive devices	Unable to maintain antigravity of head and trunk

stability; (5) weight transfer. This scale provides information on the structure of movements and is therefore sensitive enough to evaluate small changes in even severely disabled children.

Functional evaluation of upper limb movements can be carried out using the Melbourne scale for assessing upper limb function (Johnson *et al.*, 1994). This scale was developed in the early 1990s and was validated definitively in 1997. It is composed of 16 items exploring different functional tasks, including reaching the mouth to eat, or grasping objects in different spatial directions. The Melbourne scale is particularly useful for evaluating selected actions, such as reaching for an object, grasping, releasing, manipulating, and reaching the mouth with the hand. Two operators are needed to administer the scale, one instructing the child and the other videotaping. It takes approximately 30 minutes to administer, plus 30 minutes to score. The items are scored on a four-point scale, following predefined criteria. They are intended to evaluate different aspects of upper limb function: some focus on the quality of movements, including their range, precision, fluidity, and speed, while others focus on the developmental level. The total score is expressed as a percentage, obtained by summing the scores for all the items, then dividing by the maximum score, and finally multiplying by 100. The Melbourne scale is most useful for evaluating the magnitude of change after medical, surgical, or physiotherapeutic interventions. It is worth remembering that this tool focuses on motor activity, and takes no account of other aspects such as cognition, language, or perception.

The administration of the first four items of the Melbourne scale to a 5-year-old child with mixed-type quadriparesis is illustrated in the accompanying DVD (video 1, track 2).

Hand function may also be evaluated using the assessment protocol for upper limb function (Protocollo di Valutazione Arto Superiore) devised by Fedrizzi (1989). This scale was developed specifically to assess hemiparetic children. It is administered every six months and is composed of two different instruments: first, evaluation of grasping with the paretic hand, using standardized material (three cubes of 0.5, 2, and 4 cm each); this allows a four-point quantification of hand function (0 = no grasping; 1 = hand grasping; 2 = tri-digital grasping; 3 = pincer grasping); second, a qualitative evaluation of bimanual manipulation, either during spontaneous play activity or using material selected according to the child's age.

The quality of the motor patterns is scored according to its variability (a score of 3) or stereotypy (a score of 1):

0 = the child does not use the paretic upper limb;

1 = the child uses the paretic limb only as a support, and with a stereotypic pattern (supports objects with the wrist);

2 = the paretic hand cooperates in manipulation as a support (holds objects), although with simple plain patterns;
3 = the paretic hand cooperates in manipulation, carrying out simultaneous movements (both supporting and manipulating), and with a variable repertoire of motor patterns.

The administration of these two instruments allows an extensive and detailed assessment from both a quantitative and a qualitative standpoint. The evaluation of grasping provides qualitative information in relation to 'best performance', while evaluation of use provides information on the child's spontaneous capacity to employ the paretic hand in play activities and in other activities of daily living, thus providing a reliable tool for assessing his real functional ability. The evaluation of grasping on demand is not sufficient on its own to assess disability in a child with hemiplegia, but the integration of the data derived from both these instruments allows a much more precise and reliable form of evaluation.

The accompanying DVD (video 1, track 3) illustrates an example of how the protocol devised by Fedrizzi et al. is employed in the evaluation of a 5-year-old child with a right hemiparesis, showing the child's use of the paretic hand in grasping standardized material.

The Boyd test (Boyd & Graham, 1999) is a useful tool for assessing the selective control of motor function in the foot. While the test is administered, the child must be sitting with the lower limbs loose. The test is scored on a four-point scale, and the maximum score is given when the child is able to dorsiflex the foot actively.

A brief example of this test is illustrated in the accompanying DVD (video 1, track 4).

The Service for the Diagnosis and Treatment of Motor Development Disorders in our Institute has developed a qualitative-quantitative protocol to assess children with dystonic-dyskinetic disorders (Broggi & Fedrizzi, 1978; Broggi et al., 1983). This protocol allows global neuro-functional balance to be defined, the variety and variability of dyskinetic movements to be evaluated, and useful data on function in relation to treatment to be obtained. The protocol involves five videotaped tests (Bono et al., 1978):

1. *The Bobath test chart of ability* (Bobath & Bobath, 1958). This test is composed of 20 items assessing postural control in different positions, from lying to standing; each item is scored from 0 to 5 (total score = 100);
2. *Upper limb movements test*. This is composed of 11 items assessing movement sequences and quantifies the motor performance; every item is scored from 0 to 5, each side of the body being evaluated separately (total score = 55 per side);
3. *Grasping*. The patient is asked to grasp and release three objects of different size; the test is scored on a three-point scale according to difficulty, and each side of the body is evaluated separately;
4. *Independence in feeding and dressing*. This test comprises 26 items assessing gross and fine motor abilities with respect to the activities of daily living. It is a yes/no test, irrespective of the time needed and how the task is performed (total score = 26);
5. *Precision and speed of upper limb movements*. The patient is asked to follow with a pencil a simplified version of the trace proposed by Siegfried & Perret (Siegfried et al., 1970); the performance is scored on a six-point scale, according to the number of squares touched in a definite time (the test was normalized on 10 age-matched healthy subjects).

The protocol is entirely videotaped. It takes approximately 90 minutes to administer to quadriplegic children, and 40 minutes to hemiplegic children.

The accompanying DVD (video 1, track 5) illustrates a quadriparetic dystonic child carrying out the Siegfried & Perret trace test (test number 5).

Evaluation of dystonia

In the mid 1980s, Fahn & Marsden (1987) proposed the clinical rating of torsion dystonia and developed different scales to assess overall dystonia severity and to quantify disability (Tables 3, 4, and 5).

More recently, different groups of investigators have developed and compared other scales and rating systems (Comella et al., 2003). The administration of these scales allows precise and detailed documentation of dystonia. The sessions are always videotaped. Burke et al. (1985) proposed a video recording protocol lasting about 4 minutes in which the following postures and movements are examined: lying position at rest; sitting position; speech (name, date, days of the week, months of the year); upper limbs suspended in front of the body; finger-nose test; rapid succession movements (hands and feet); standing up and sitting down, turning four times by 90°; walking; and handwriting (name, date, drawing a spiral). The overall time for video-taping is 4 minutes, 15 seconds.

Other investigations

Various devices are available for assessing selected and specific aspects of movement. Using equipment of varying technological complexity, it is possible to study the different neurophysiological parameters of standing, sitting, and walking.

Table 3. Staging of torsion dystonia (from Marsden & Schachter, 1981)

STAGE I	Focal: a single segment (e.g., one limb, torticollis, blepharospasm, dysphonia, both arms or both legs)
STAGE II	Segmental: 2–3 continuous segments (i.e., Meige syndrome, torticollis plus shoulder)
STAGE III	Unilateral arm and leg
STAGE IV	Bilateral generalized

Table 4. Dystonia severity evaluation scale (from Marsden & Schachter, 1981)

Segments	Provoking factor	Severity factor	Product
Eyes	0-4	0-4	
Mouth	0-4	0-4	
Speech and swallowing	1-4	1-4	
Neck	0-4	0-4	
Right arm	0-4	0-4	
Left arm	0-4	0-4	
Trunk	0-4	0-4	
Right leg	0-4	0-4	
Left leg	0-4	0-4	
Total			

Provoking factors: (0) no dystonia at rest or action; (1) dystonia on particular action; (2) dystonia on many actions; (3) dystonia on action of distant part of body; (4) dystonia present at rest.
Speech and swallowing: (1) occasional either or both; (2) frequent either; (3) frequent one and occasional other; (4) frequent both.
Severity factor: (0) no dystonia present; (1) slight dystonia, but not causing impairment: clinically insignificant; (2) mild: impairment, but not disabling; (3) moderate: disabling, but not eliminating basic function; (4) severe: preventing basic function.

Table 5. Functional disability scale for torsion dystonia (from Marsden & Schachter, 1981)

A. *Language*		E. *Hygiene*	
0	Normal	0	Normal
1	Slightly involved, easily understood	1	Clumsy, independent
2	Some difficulty to understand	2	Needs help with some activities
3	Marked difficulty to understand	3	Needs help with most activities
4	Completely or almost completely aphonic or anarthric activities	4	Needs help with all
B. *Handwriting*		F. *Dressing*	
0	Normal	0	Normal
1	Slight difficulty, legible	1	Clumsy, independent
2	Almost illegible	2	Needs help with some
3	Illegible	3	Needs help with most
4	Unable to grasp or maintain hold on pen	4	Helpless
C. *Feeding*		G. *Walking*	
0	Normal	0	Normal
1	Uses 'tricks', independent	1	Slightly abnormal, hardly noticeable
2	Can feed, but not cut	2	Moderately abnormal, obvious to observer
3	Finger food only	3	Considerably abnormal
4	Completely dependent	4	Wheel-chair bound
D. *Eating*			
0	Normal		
1	Occasionally choking		
2	Chokes frequently, difficult swallowing		
3	Unable to swallow firm foods		
4	Marked difficulty swallowing soft foods and liquid		

To assess the sitting position, the patient is asked to sit on a membrane connected to a computer, which can measure the degree of pressure at different points of the membrane. This allows a correctly balanced sitting position to be obtained through the use of special pillows.

Stabilometry is a technique for evaluating, in the standing position, shifts of the baricentre projected to the ground; different variables are analysed, including the mean load and the speed and amplitude of the shift in different perceptive modalities. A single platform with three or four collecting points may be used, or separate platforms, which can be placed in different positions with respect to the anterior or posterior segment of the foot (Riach & Starkes, 1993).

Finally, computerized gait analysis is an opto-electronic 3D instrument for measuring the cinematic (joint angles), dynamic (moment and power at joint), and electromyographic aspects of movement during walking. It is widely used in clinical practice, and is most useful for assessing patients before and after medical or surgical interventions (Gage, 1991). Gait analysis has many advantages: it provides simultaneous tridimensional information; it allows the differentiation of pathological from compensatory mechanisms; it can monitor the efficacy of medical or surgical treatment objectively; and it is widely validated and internationally accepted.

Evaluation of independence and functionality

The disability scales are intended to assess the limitations of the activities of daily living as the result of a movement disorder. These scales are widely used in chronic diseases, and were created on populations of normal subjects.

The functional independence measure for children (WeeFIM) (Msall *et al.*, 1994) is composed of 19 items exploring six different developmental domains, including self-care, sphincter control, mobility, locomotion, communication, and social relationships. It is intended for children aged 6 months to 7 years. The items are scored on a seven-point scale, reflecting an increasing degree of independence and with respect to the need for assistance and assistive devices. Being focused on the impact of disability in daily living, this scale is most useful in assessing disability, and does not quantify impairment.

Another internationally adopted tool for evaluating disability is the Paediatric Evaluation of Disability Inventory (PEDI) (Haley *et al.*, 1992). This scale is intended for children aged 6 months to 7.6 years and is composed of two different subscales: capability (exploring acquired functions), and performance (assessing the degree of disability through the measure of the level of assistance and the environmental modifications needed). The inventory, carried out with the collaboration of the family, takes about 45 minutes to administer.

Finally, Burke *et al.* (1985) developed a scale especially intended to assess disability in dystonic children (the torsion dystonia disability scale). This scale explores different functional domains, including speech, handwriting, feeding, hygiene, dressing, and walking. Each item is scored 0 to 4 or 0 to 6 according to increasing severity (maximum score = 30).

An example of the training of a severely affected quadriparetic anarthric patient in the use of a modified keyboard for communication is illustrated in the accompanying DVD (video 1, track 6).

The last track in the DVD (video 1, track 7) addresses the underlying importance of a videotape-documented follow-up in an early-onset movement disorder (choreoathetosis), showing an improving course during the first 5 years of life.

Conclusions

The tools described here may help in assessing and quantifying very severe and disabling clinical syndromes. They are useful, but not definitive, in the diagnostic work-up and the therapeutic strategies necessary to reveal adaptive abilities and competences that often go unrecognized or underestimated in children with movement disorders.

References

Bobath, K. & Bobath, R.(1958): An assessment of children with cerebral palsy and of their response to treatment. *Ann. J. Occup. Ther.* **21**, 19–25.

Bono, R., Broggi, G., Fedrizzi, E., Fugolin, A. & Oleari, G. (1978): Metodica di valutazione neurofunzionale di soggetti discinetici sottoposti ad interventi stereotassici. *Saggi* **1**, 33–42.

Boyce, W., Gowland, C., Rosembaum, P., Lane, M., Plews, N., Goldsmith, C., Russell, D., Wright, V., Zdrobov, S. & Harding, D. (1995): The gross motor performance measure: validity and responsiveness of a measure of quality of movement. *Phys. Ther.* **75**, 603–613.

Boyd, R.N. & Graham, H.K. (1999): Objective measurement of clinical findings in the use of botulinum toxin type A for the management of children with cerebral palsy. *Eur. J. Neurol.* **6**, S23–S35.

Broggi, G. & Fedrizzi, E. (1978): Méthodes d'évaluation des mouvements anormaux dans l'infirmité motrice cérébrale. *Med. Hyg.* **39**, 2046–2050.

Broggi, G., Angelini, L., Bono, R., Giorgi, C., Nardocci, N. & Franzini, A. (1983): Long-term results of stereotactic thalamotomy for cerebral palsy. *Neurosurgery* **12**, 195–202.

Burke, R.E., Fahn, S., Marsden, C.D., Bressman, S.B., Moskowitz, C. & Friedman, J. (1985): Validity and reliability of a rating scale for the primary torsion dystonias. *Neurology* **35**, 73–77.

Comella, C.L., Leurgans, S., Wuu, J., Stebbins, G.T., Chmura, T. & The Dystonia Study Group (2003): Rating scales for dystonia: a multicenter assessment. *Mov. Disord.* **18**, 303–312.

Fahn, S. & Marsden, C.D. (1987): Classification and investigation of dystonia. In: *Movement disorders*, eds. C.D. Marsden & S. Fahn, pp. 332–358. London: Butterworth and Co.

Fedrizzi, E. (1989): Emiplegia spastica: aspetti metodologici e implicazioni riabilitative. *Gior. Neuropsich. Età Evol.* **4**, 56–72.

Gage, J.R. (1991): Gait analysis in cerebral palsy. In: *Clinics in Developmental Medicine*, vol. 121. London: MacKeith Press.

Haley, S.M., Coster, W.J., Ludlow, L.H., Haltiwanger, J.T. & Andrellos, P.J. (1992): Pediatric evaluation of disability inventory (PEDI). *Development standardization and administration manual.* Boston: Boston University Press.

Johnson, L.M., Randall, M.J., Oke, L.E., Byrt, T.A. & Bach, T.M. (1994): Development of a clinical assessment of quality of movement for unilateral upper limb function. *Dev. Med. Child Neurol.* **36**, 965–973.

Marsden, C.D. & Schachter, M. (1981): Assessment of extrapyramidal disorders. *Br. J. Clin. Pharmacol.* **11**, 129–151.

Msall, M.E., DiGaudio, K., Rogers, B.T., LaForest, S., Catanzaro, N.L., Campbell, J., Wilczenski, F. & Duffy, L.C. (1994): The functional independence measure for children (WeeFIM): conceptual basis and pilot use in children with developmental disabilities. *Clin. Pediatr.* **33**, 421–430.

Palisano, R.J., Rosenbaum, P.L., Walter, S., Russell. D., Wood, E. & Galluppi, B. (1997): Development and reliability of a system to classify gross motor function in children with cerebral palsy. *Dev. Med. Child Neurol.* **39**, 214–223.

Prechtl, H.F. & Hopkins, B. (1986): Developmental transformations of spontaneous movements in early infancy. *Early Hum. Dev.* **14**, 233–238.

Riach, C.L. & Starkes, J.L. (1993): Stability limits of quiet standing postural control in children and adults. *Gait Posture* **1**, 105–111.

Russell, D.J., Rosenbaum, P.L., Cadman, D.T., Gowland, C., Hardy, S. & Jarvis, S. (1989): The gross motor function measure: a means to evaluate the effects of physical therapy. *Dev. Med. Child Neurol.* **31**, 341–352.

Russell, D.J., Rosenbaum, P.L., Lane, M., Gowland, C., Goldsmith, C.H., Boyce, W.F. & Plews, N. (1994): Training users in the gross motor function measure: methodological and practical issues. *Phys. Ther.* **74**, 630–636.

Siegfried, J., Esslen, E., Gretener, V., Ketz, E. & Perret, E. (1970): Functional anatomy of the dentate nucleus in the light of stereotaxic operations. *Confin. Neurol.* **32**, 1–10.

Chapter 6

Primary dystonia

Nardo Nardocci, Federica Zibordi, Caterina Costa and Giovanna Zorzi

Unit of Child Neuropsychiatry, Fondazione IRCCS Istituto Neurologico 'C. Besta',
via Celoria 11, 20133 Milan, Italy
nnardocci@istituto-besta.it
Video 2

Summary

Dystonia is a syndrome characterized by sustained muscle contractions, frequently causing twisting and repetitive movements or abnormal postures. It is classified in three ways: by age at onset, by distribution, and by aetiology. The aetiological classification distinguishes four main categories: primary, dystonia plus, secondary, and heredodegenerative dystonia. Primary dystonia and dystonia plus are thought to be the result of neurochemical disorders, while secondary and heredodegenerative dystonia are the consequence of neuronal cell death.

Primary dystonia is defined as clinical condition characterized by dystonia as the only neurological abnormality apart from tremor. Different genetic alterations and gene loci have been mapped in familial and sporadic patients. DYT1 dystonia is transmitted as an autosomal dominant trait with reduced penetrance. The underlying mutation is a GAG deletion in the coding region of the *DYT1* gene, located at chromosome 9q34. In patients not carrying the *DYT1* mutation other genetic loci have been mapped: DYT2, DYT4, DYT6, and DYT13.

Definition and classification of dystonia

Dystonia is a syndrome characterized by sustained muscle contractions, frequently causing twisting and repetitive movements or abnormal postures (Marsden *et al.*, 1976). It is classified in three ways: by age at onset, by distribution, and by aetiology.

Classification by *age at onset* distinguishes childhood onset (0–12 years), adolescent onset (13–20), and adult onset (> 20). Age at onset is an important factor related to prognosis: the younger the age, the more likely it is that the dystonia will become generalized (Marsden *et al.*, 1976; Fahn *et al.*, 1987).

Classified by *distribution*, dystonia is defined as focal (affecting a single part of the body), segmental (two or more contiguous parts of the body), multifocal (two or more non-contiguous parts of the body), unilateral (one half of the body), or generalized (involvement of leg plus any other area of the body). Hemidystonia usually suggests a symptomatic cause. The distribution of dystonia can also be considered an indicator of its severity and is useful for planning therapeutic strategies.

Identification of the cause is the main goal in the clinical evaluation of patients with dystonia. The *aetiological classification* distinguishes four main categories: primary, dystonia plus, secondary, and heredodegenerative dystonia. Primary dystonia and dystonia plus are thought to be the result of neurochemical disorders; secondary and heredodegenerative dystonias are the consequence of neuronal cell death.

Primary torsion dystonia (PTD) is characterized by dystonia as the only neurological abnormality apart from tremor (Marsden *et al.*, 1976) and is a clinically and genetically heterogeneous disorder (Table 1). *Dystonia plus* syndromes are characterized by dystonia associated with parkinsonism and myoclonus [see: 'Dopa-responsive syndromes' for a detailed clinical description (this volume, chapter 11)]. *Secondary or symptomatic dystonia* is defined as a dystonic syndrome caused by environmental insults resulting in structural brain damage. Damage to the spinal cord or peripheral nerves has been reported to contribute to dystonia. A list of the conditions causing secondary dystonia is given in Table 2. Patients with secondary dystonia usually have dystonia plus other neurological signs and symptoms, but in some instances – for example, in tardive dystonia – dystonia may be the only neurological abnormality and can thus mimic a primary condition (Fahn *et al.*, 1998).

Heredodegenerative dystonia is associated with a wide range of neurodegenerative CNS disorders (Table 3) and the diagnosis requires a complex multistep process. Dystonia is usually found in combination with other neurological signs and symptoms (pyramidal tract signs, parkinsonism, dementia, epilepsy, visual disturbances); it may be a prominent feature or it may occur at late stages of the disease or even fail to appear at all (Jancovic *et al.*, 2002).

Primary torsion dystonia

Early-onset PTD (EO-PTD) represents the most severe form of primary dystonia and can be transmitted as an autosomal dominant trait with reduced penetrance (Marsden *et al.*, 1976; Bressmann *et al.*, 1989). The most common underlying mutation of autosomal dominant EO-PTD is a GAG deletion in the coding region of the *DYT1* gene, located at chromosome

Table 1. Classification of primary dystonia

Dystonia type	**Inheritance**	**Locus**	**Chromosomal location**	**Gene product and mutation**
Dystonia 1; early-onset	AD	DYT1	9q34	ATP-binding protein
Dystonia 7; late-onset focal dystonia, adult onset	AD	DYT7	18p	Unknown
Dystonia 6; adolescent and early adult onset of mixed phenotype	AD	DYT6	8p21-8p22	Unknown
Dystonia 12; rapid-onset dystonia-parkinsonism	AD	DYT12	19q13	Unknown
Dystonia 4	AD	DYT4	Unknown	Unknown
Dystonia 2	AR	DYT2	Unknown	Unknown
Dystonia 13; early and adult onset; cranial cervical brachial	AD	DYT13	1p36	Unknown

AD, autosomal dominant; AR, autosomal recessive.

Table 2. Secondary dystonia

Cerebral palsy
Encephalitis
Head trauma
Cervical cord injury
Peripheral injury
Focal vascular lesion
Brain tumours
Multiple sclerosis
Drug-induced (levodopa, D2-receptor blockade, anticonvulsant)
Psychogenic

Modified from Fahn *et al.*, 1998.

Table 3. Heredodegenerative dystonia

Autosomal recessive	**Autosomal dominant**
Wilson disease	Rapid onset dystonia-parkinsonism
Niemann-Pick type C	Juvenile parkinsonism
GM1 gangliosidosis	Huntington disease
GM2 gangliosidosis	Machado-Joseph disease (SCA3)
Metachromatic leukodystrophy	Dentato-rubral-pallidoluysian atrophy
Lesch-Nyan	
Glutaric acidaemia	
Methylmalonic acidaemia	**Mitochondrial**
Hartnup disease	Leigh disease
Ataxia-telangiectasia	Other mitochondrial encephalopathies
PANK2 deficiency	
Juvenile neuronal lipofuscinoses	
Neuroacanthocytosis	
Intranuclear hyaline inclusion disease	
MECP2 deficiency	

Modified from Fahn *et al.*, 1998.

9q34, causing expression of an abnormal protein named torsinA (Ozelius *et al.*, 1989; 1997; Walker & Shashidharan, 2003). TorsinA, a protein of unclear function, interacts with endocellular membranes and may regulate vesicular exocytosis (Misbahuddin *et al.*, 2005). The most frequent presentation of DYT1 dystonia is with onset in a limb and progression to a generalized distribution, sparing the cranial muscles; however, DYT1 PTD is clinically heterogeneous with variable phenotypic expression (Opal *et al.*, 2002). The clinical presentation may vary widely, even in members of the same family. Since the early reports on dystonia, it has been observed that cases with childhood onset have a worse prognosis than those with adult onset (Fahn et al., 1987).

The *DYT1* gene is responsible for a large proportion of EO-PTD, mainly in North American series. However, there remains a large group of EO-PTD cases, especially among non-Jewish patients, in whom there is no linkage to this gene (Jarman et al., 1999; Bressmann et al., 2000; Zorzi et al., 2002).

Four phenotypes of EO-PTD have been described in patients not carrying the *DYT1* mutations: DYT2, DYT4, DYT6, and DYT13. DYT2 and DYT4 are two genetically unclassified family phenotypes characterized by onset of dystonia in childhood with subsequent generalization. DYT2 was described as an autosomal recessive form of EO-PTD in Spanish gypsies. Two other similar phenotypes with autosomal recessive transmission have been named DYT2, based on clinical similarities with the original families (Gimenez-Roldan et al., 1988; Khan et al., 2003; Moretti et al., 2005). A large Australian pedigree containing cases across more than four generations was named DYT4. Dystonia was inherited as an autosomal dominant trait; involvement of the larynx and generalization were common (Parker, 1985; Ahmad et al., 1993). DYT6 and DYT13 patients belong to families linking to chromosomes 8p21-q22 and 1p36.13-36.32 (Almasy et al., 1997; Valente et al., 2001). The DYT6 phenotype, described in two related Mennonite families with autosomal dominant transmission, is characterized by frequent cranial-cervical involvement and occasional generalization. Onset is early (on average 18.9 years) and the disease is progressive, some generalized cases being indistinguishable from those with generalized DYT1 dystonia (Almasy et al., 1997). The DYT13 phenotype has autosomal dominant transmission, with prevalent involvement of the upper body and frequent early-onset. There are similarities in body prevalence with DYT6 dystonia, but the clinical course is more benign; generalization is uncommon and usually only mildly disabling (Bentivoglio et al., 2004a).

Other sporadic or familial patients with EO-PTD have been reported apart from these well characterized familial cases. Their phenotype partially overlaps with the descriptions of DYT1 EO-PTD cases, raising the question as to whether specific clinical genetic correlates can be identified in EO-PTD (Bressman et al., 2000; Edwards et al., 2003). All these families encompass subjects with EO-PTD as well as others with onset in adult life. EO-PTD cases can be included in two main phenotypes with autosomal dominant transmission and incomplete penetrance: a focal type with upper limb, cervical, or cranial involvement; and a so-called 'mixed phenotype' (Almasy et al., 1997; Nemeth, 2002; Bentivoglio et al., 2004b). The latter phenotype is more severe and clinically heterogeneous, with onset often in childhood; the site of onset is commonly cervical or in one upper limb, and there is constant involvement of the cranial-cervical region (including the larynx); progression to generalization is not uncommon. Examples of the first phenotype are two large non-Jewish families; the affected members presented with dystonia of early or adult onset which was confined to the cervical region or to the upper limbs (Uitti et al., 1993; Bressman et al., 1996). Other examples of the first phenotype are families with onset in childhood, in which dystonia was manifested as blepharospasm, cervical dystonia, or writer's cramp (Kamm et al., 2000; Munchau et al., 2000; Wunderlick et al., 2001; Brancati et al., 2002; Defazio et al., 2003; Maniak et al., 2003). Examples of the second phenotype encompass a Swedish family with age at onset varying from the second to the fifth decade, prominent cranial-cervical involvement, upper limb tremor, and occasional generalization (Holmgren et al., 1995). Another Italian family from South Tyrol had a variable phenotype – cervical or upper limb dystonia with onset in adulthood was the most common presentation, but some patients suffered from typical early-onset generalized dystonia (Klein et *al.*, 1998). A member of this family had unusually slow progression with eventual generalization resembling the index case of the DYT13 family (Bentivoglio *et al.*, 2004b).

From these data it appears that cervical involvement is a distinct clinical feature of non-DYT1 early-onset cases; in keeping with this observation, it has been hinted that cranial or cervical onset is a specific feature of non-DYT1 cases (Bressman *et al.*, 1994a; Bressman *et al.*, 1994b; Kamm *et al.*, 1999; Munchau *et al.*, 2000; Wunderlick *et al.*, 2001; Bentivoglio *et al.*, 2004a). However, cervical or laryngeal onset has also been observed in DYT1 patients (Bressman *et al.*, 2000). The phenotypic overlap observed in DYT1 and non-DYT1 dystonias raises questions about the specificity and sensitivity of the observed clinical features.

Video – Illustrative cases

Primary DYT1 dystonia (video 2, track 1) – Patient with primary DYT1 dystonia with onset at age 6 years. At the age of 9 he shows generalized dystonia, with dystonic movements of legs and arms, evident at rest and during action.

Primary non-DYT1 dystonia (video 2, track 2) :

– Patient 1

A 5-year-old patient, after 6 months from the onset of the disease. The neurological picture is characterized by action dystonia involving neck and upper limbs. The neck dystonia can be reduced by a sensory trick. The same patient at the age of 7, after 2.5 years from the onset: dystonia has worsened causing a more severe retrocollis, involving also the trunk.

– Patient 2

A 7-year-old patient, after 1 year from the onset of the disease. He shows dystonic posturing of hands, dystonic tremor of the left hand and bilateral leg dystonia during walking.

After 3 years from the onset, dystonia has worsened, with oro-mandibular involvement and a more evident limb dystonia.

References

Ahmad, F., Davis, M.B., Waddy, H.M., Oley, C.A., Marsden, C.D. & Harding, A.E. (1993): Evidence for locus heterogeneity in autosomal dominant torsion dystonia. *Genomics* **15**, 9–12.

Almasy, L., Bressman, S.B., Raymond, D., Kramer, P.L., Greene, P.E. & Heiman, G.A. (1997): Idiopathic torsion dystonia linked to chromosome 8 in two Mennonite families. *Ann. Neurol.* **42**, 670–673.

Bentivoglio, A.R., Ialongo, T., Contarino, M.F., Valente, E.M. & Albanese, A. (2004a): Phenotypic characterization of DYT13 primary torsion dystonia. *Mov. Disord.* **19**, 200–206.

Bentivoglio, A.R., Elia, A.E., Filippini, G., Valente, E.M., Fasano, A. & Albanese, A. (2004b): Clinical presentation and progression of sporadic and familial primary torsion dystonia in Italy. *Adv. Neurol.* **94**, 171–178.

Brancati, F., Defazio, G., Caputo, V., Valente, E.M., Pizzuti, A., Livrea, P., Berardelli, A. & Dallapiccola, B. (2002): Novel Italian family supports clinical and genetic heterogeneity of primary adult-onset torsion dystonia. *Mov. Disord.* **17**, 392–397.

Bressman, S.B., de Leon, D., Brin, M.F., Risch, N., Burke, R.E., Greene, P.E., Shale, H. & Fahn, S. (1989): Idiopathic dystonia among Ashkenazi Jews: evidence for autosomal dominant inheritance. *Ann. Neurol.* **26**, 612–620.

Bressman, S.B., de Leon, D., Kramer, P.L., Ozelius, L.J., Brin, M.F., Greene, P.E., Fahn, S., Breakefield, X.O. & Risch, N.J. (1994a): Dystonia in Ashkenazi Jews: clinical characterization of a founder mutation. *Ann. Neurol.* **36**, 771–777.

Bressman, S.B., Hunt, A.L., Heiman, G.A., Brin, M.F., Burke, R.E., Fahn, S., Trugman, J.M., de Leon, D., Kramer, P.L., Wilhelmsen, K.C. *et al.* (1994b): Exclusion of the DYT1 locus in a non-Jewish family with early-onset dystonia. *Mov. Disord.* **9**, 626–632.

Bressman, S.B., Warner, T.T., Almasy, L., Uitti, R.J., Greene, P.E., Heiman, G.A., Raymond, D., Ford, B., de Leon, D., Fahn, S., Kramer, P.L., Risch, N.J., Maraganore, D.M., Nygaard, T.G. & Harding, A.E. (1996): Exclusion of the DYT1 locus in familial torticollis. *Ann. Neurol.* **40**, 681–684.

Bressman, S.B., Sabatti, C., Raymond, D., deLeon, D., Klein, C. & Kramer, P.L. (2000): The DYT1 phenotype and guidelines for diagnostic testing. *Neurology* **54**, 1746–1752.

Defazio, G., Brancati, F., Valente, E.M., Caputo, V., Pizzuti, A., Martino, D., Abbruzzese, G., Livrea, P., Berardelli, A. & Dallapiccola, B. (2003): Familial blepharospasm is inherited as an autosomal dominant trait and relates to a novel unassigned gene. *Mov. Disord.* **18**, 207–212.

Edwards, M., Wood, N. & Bhatia, K. (2003): Unusual phenotypes in DYT1 dystonia: a report of five cases and a review of the literature. *Mov. Disord.* **18**, 706–711.

Fahn, S., Marsden, C.D. & Calne, D.B. (1987): Classification and investigation of dystonia. In: *Movement disorders 2*, eds. C.D. Marsden & S. Fahn, pp. 332–358. London: Butterworths.

Fahn, S., Bressman, S. & Marsden, C.D. (1998): Classification of dystonia. *Adv. Neurol.* **78**, 1–10.

Gimenez-Roldan, S., Delgado, G., Marin, M., Villanueva, J.A. & Mateo, D. (1988): Hereditary torsion dystonia in gypsies. *Adv. Neurol.* **50**, 73–81.

Holmgren, G., Ozelius, L., Forsgren, L., Almay, B.G., Holmberg, M., Kramer, P., Fahn, S. & Breakefield, X.O. (1995): Adult onset idiopathic torsion dystonia is excluded from the DYT1 region (9q34) in a Swedish family. *J. Neurol. Neurosurg. Psychiatry* **59**, 178–181.

Jankovic, J. & Fahn, S. (2002): Dystonic disorders. In: *Parkinson's disease and movement disorders*, 4th ed., eds. J. Jankovic & E. Tolosa, pp. 331–357. Baltimore: Williams and Wilkins.

Jarman, P.R., Del Grosso, N., Valente, E.M., Leube, B., Cassetta, E. & Bentivoglio, A.R. (1999): Primary torsion dystonia: the search for genes is not over. *J. Neurol. Neurosurg. Psychiatry* **67**, 395–397.

Kamm, C., Castelon-Konkiewitz, E., Naumann, M., Heinen, F., Brack, M., Nebe, A., Ceballos-Baumann, A. & Gasser, T. (1999): GAG deletion in the DYT1 gene in early limb-onset idiopathic torsion dystonia in Germany. *Mov. Disord.* **14**, 681–683.

Kamm, C., Naumann, M., Mueller, J., Mai, N., Riedel, L., Wissel, J. & Gasser, T. (2000): The DYT1 GAG deletion is infrequent in sporadic and familial writer's cramp. *Mov. Disord.* **15**, 1238–1241.

Khan, N.L., Wood, N.W. & Bhatia, K.P. (2003): Autosomal recessive, DYT2-like primary torsion dystonia: a new family. *Neurology* **61**, 1801–1803.

Klein, C., Pramstaller, P.P., Castellan, C.C., Breakefield, X.O., Kramer, P.L. & Ozelius, L.J. (1998): Clinical and genetic evaluation of a family with a mixed dystonia phenotype from South Tyrol. *Ann. Neurol.* **44**, 394–398.

Maniak, S., Sieberer, M., Hagenah, J., Klein, C. & Vieregge, P. (2003): Focal and segmental primary dystonia in north-western Germany – a clinico-genetic study. *Acta Neurol. Scand.* **107**, 228–232.

Marsden, C.D., Harrison, M.J. & Bundey, S. (1976): Natural history of idiopathic torsion dystonia. *Adv. Neurol.* **14**, 177–187.

Misbahuddin, A., Placzek, M.R., Taanman, J.W., Gschmeissner, S., Schiavo, G., Cooper, J.M. & Warner, T.T. (2005): Mutant torsinA, which causes early-onset primary torsion dystonia, is redistributed to membranous structures enriched in vesicular monoamine transporter in cultured human SH-SY5Y cells. *Mov. Disord.* **20**, 432–440.

Moretti, P., Hedera, P., Wald, J. & Fink, J. (2005): Autosomal recessive primary generalized dystonia in two siblings from a consanguineous family. *Mov. Disord.* **20**, 245–247.

Munchau, A., Valente, E.M., Davis, M.B., Stinton, V., Wood, N.W., Quinn, N.P. & Bhatia, K.P. (2000): A Yorkshire family with adult-onset cranio-cervical primary torsion dystonia. *Mov. Disord.* **15**, 954–959.

Nemeth, A.H. (2002): The genetics of primary dystonias and related disorders. *Brain* **125**, 695–721.

Opal, P., Tintner, R., Jankovic, J., Leung, J., Breakefield, X.O. & Friedman. J. (2002): Intrafamilial phenotypic variability of the DYT1 dystonia: from asymptomatic TOR1A gene carrier status to dystonic storm. *Mov. Disord.* **17**, 339–345.

Ozelius, L., Kramer, P.L., Moskowitz, C.B., Kwiatkowski, D.J., Brin, M.F., Bressman, S.B., Shuback, D.E., Falk, C.T., Risch, N. & deLeon, D. (1989): Human gene for torsion dystonia located on chromosome 9q32-q34. *Neuron* **2**, 1427–1434.

Ozelius, L.J, Hewett, J.W., Page, C.E., Bressman, S.B., Kramer, P.L. & Shalish, C. (1997): The early-onset torsion dystonia gene (DYT1) encodes an ATP-binding protein. *Nat. Genet.* **17**, 40–48.

Parker, N. (1985): Hereditary whispering dysphonia. *J. Neurol. Neurosurg. Psychiatry* **48**, 218–224.

Uitti, R.J. & Maraganore, D.M. (1993): Adult onset familial cervical dystonia: report of a family including monozygotic twins. *Mov. Disord.* **8**, 489–494.

Valente, E.M., Bentivoglio, A.R., Cassetta, E., Dixon, P.H., Davis, M.B., Ferraris, A., Ialongo, T., Frontali, M., Wood, N.W. & Albanese, A. (2001): DYT13, a novel primary torsion dystonia locus, maps to chromosome 1p36.13-36.32 in an Italian family with cranial-cervical or upper limb onset. *Ann. Neurol.* **49**, 362–366.

Walker, R.H. & Shashidharan, P. (2003): Developments in the molecular biology of DYT1 dystonia. *Mov. Disord.* **18**, 1102–1107.

Wunderlich, S., Reiners, K., Gasser, T. & Naumann, M. (2001): Cervical dystonia in monozygotic twins: case report and review of the literature. *Mov. Disord.* **16**, 714–718.

Zorzi, G., Garavaglia, B., Invernizzi, F., Girotti, F., Soliveri, P., Zeviani, M., Angelini, L. & Nardocci, N. (2002): Frequency of DYT1 mutation in early-onset primary dystonia in Italian patients. *Mov. Disord.* **17**, 407–408.

Chapter 7

Update on myoclonus-dystonia

Enza Maria Valente[*][§] and Bruno Dallapiccola[*][#]

[*] *Neurogenetics Unit, CSS-Mendel Institute, viale Regina Margherita 261, 00198 Rome, Italy;*
[§] *Department of Medical and Surgical Paediatric Sciences, University of Messina, via Consolare Valeria 1, 98100 Messina, Italy;*
[#] *Department of Experimental Medicine and Pathology, University 'La Sapienza', viale Regina Elena 324, 00161 Rome, Italy*
e.valente@css-mendel.it

Summary

Myoclonus-dystonia is an autosomal dominant condition characterized by myoclonus mainly in the upper body, which can be accompanied by focal or segmental dystonia of the neck, arms, and face (mostly spasmodic torticollis and writer's cramp). The onset of the disorder is typically in childhood or the teenage years and progression is slow, with a benign course and limited disability. Additional clinical features are psychiatric disturbances and a positive response to alcohol ingestion, with temporary amelioration of symptoms. Although this condition is genetically heterogeneous, a proportion of cases (about 25 per cent) are caused by mutations in the *SGCE* gene on chromosome 7q21, encoding ε-sarcoglycan. This protein is highly expressed in the central nervous system and it is thought to play a role in regulating synaptic transmission of aminergic neurons. The reduced penetrance of the disease is largely explained by the maternal imprinting of the *SGCE* gene. Therefore, patients are more likely to have inherited the pathogenic mutations from their father, while unaffected carriers have more often inherited the mutation from their mother. Most mutations are loss-of-function and there are no mutational hotspots, making it difficult to carry out genotype-phenotype correlations.

A second locus for myoclonus-dystonia has recently been mapped to chromosome 18, but the responsible gene has not yet been cloned. No specific treatments for myoclonus-dystonia are currently available, although chronic bilateral stimulation of the globus pallidus internus may represent a valid strategy in selected cases with severe phenotypes.

Introduction

Dystonia is a movement disorder characterized by involuntary sustained muscle contractions causing twisting movements and abnormal postures (Fahn *et al.*, 1987). According to the latest classification, the dystonias can be divided into four groups:

• primary torsion dystonia (PTD) where the phenotype is of dystonia alone, which may be accompanied by tremor;

- dystonia-plus syndromes, where dystonia is associated to another movement disorder, such as parkinsonism (dopa-responsive dystonia and rapid onset dystonia-parkinsonism) or myoclonus (myoclonus-dystonia);
- heredodegenerative diseases, where dystonia is part of a more complex neurodegenerative phenotype, such as pantothenate kinase-associated neurodegeneration (PKAN) syndromes, Huntington's disease, and Wilson's disease;
- secondary dystonias resulting from environmental factors (Fahn et al., 1998).

Myoclonus is a clinical sign defined as sudden very rapid, shock-like involuntary jerks caused by muscle contraction or relaxation. It can present at rest, with action, or in response to a specific stimulus, and can be classified as positive myoclonus, characterised by sudden muscle activation, or negative myoclonus, where the lightning jerk is due to sudden muscle relaxation. The aetiological classification of myoclonus distinguishes four major categories: *physiological myoclonus*, normally observed in healthy individuals; *essential myoclonus*, where the myoclonus is the most prominent or the only clinical finding and is either idiopathic or inherited; *epileptic myoclonus*, where the myoclonus is part of a more complex chronic seizure disorder which usually dominates the clinical picture (such as the Uverricht-Lundborg syndrome, Lennox-Gastaut syndrome, and others); and *symptomatic myoclonus*, manifesting in the setting of a specific underlying disorder, which can be neurological or non-neurological (for example, metabolic disorders, toxic and drug-induced syndromes, neurodegenerative conditions, focal nervous system damage, and so on) (Marsden et al., 1982).

The nosology of conditions incorporating both myoclonic jerks and torsion dystonia has been the subject of considerable debate over the years (Quinn et al., 1988). Such patients have been classified as having myoclonus or myoclonus-dystonia, benign essential myoclonus (despite dystonic features being present on examination), or myoclonus-dystonia with 'lightning jerks' responsive to alcohol (Quinn, 1996). Recent advances in the genetics of these conditions, with the identification of one major disease gene *(SGCE*, see below), has brought some welcome order to this area, providing a unifying link between different phenotypes which have now been grouped under the term 'myoclonus-dystonia'.

Clinical features of myoclonus-dystonia

Classical myoclonus-dystonia is characterized by myoclonus usually involving the arms and axial muscles, which can be accompanied by focal or segmental dystonia of the neck, arms, and face (mainly spasmodic torticollis and writer's cramp). The upper body is most often involved, although myoclonus can occasionally involve the legs as well. Onset of the disorder is typically in childhood or the teenage years, and progression is slow, with a benign course and limited disability. However, onset in adult life and severe phenotypes interfering with daily life activities have been reported. Many patients find that their symptoms improve transiently with alcohol, and this is responsible for alcohol dependence in a subset of patients with myoclonus-dystonia (Quinn, 1996; Asmus & Gasser, 2004). Obsessive-compulsive behaviour and panic attacks have also been reported in some families (Saunders-Pullman et al., 2002). The identification of one major gene responsible for myoclonus-dystonia *(SGCE* – see below) and subsequent mutation screening of large cohorts of patients has broadened the clinical spectrum of this movement disorder. For instance, two families have been reported with an association of myoclonus-dystonia and seizures or EEG abnormalities, previously thought to be an exclusion criterion for the clinical diagnosis of this syndrome (Foncke et al., 2003; O'Riordan et al., 2004).

Representative video recordings of patients with myoclonus-dystonia can be found within selected references cited in this chapter (Liu *et al.*, 2002; Hjermind *et al.*, 2003; Cif *et al.*, 2004; Kock *et al.*, 2004; O'Riordan *et al.*, 2004).

Genetics of myoclonus-dystonia

The *SGCE* gene

Myoclonus-dystonia is inherited as an autosomal dominant trait with incomplete penetrance, although sporadic cases have often been reported. In 1999, Nygaard and collaborators mapped a major myoclonus-dystonia locus (DYT11) on chromosome 7q21-q31 in a large family (Nygaard *et al.*, 1999). Subsequently, linkage was confirmed in several other myoclonus-dystonia families, allowing refinement of the DYT11 candidate interval to a 7 cM region (Klein *et al.*, 2000a; Asmus *et al.*, 2001; Vidailhet *et al.*, 2001). The phenotype was not homogeneous, with variable age of onset (up to 38 years) and with different combinations of myoclonic jerks and dystonic movements and postures, usually confined to the upper body but occasionally involving the lower limbs as well. Alcohol responsiveness and psychiatric disturbances were observed only in a subset of patients. Subsequently, mutations within the ε-sarcoglycan *(SGCE)* gene have been identified in families linked to the DYT11 locus (Zimprich *et al.*, 2001).

Epsilon-sarcoglycan was initially discovered because of its 50 per cent sequence homology to α-sarcoglycan, a major constituent of the dystrophin-glycoprotein complex in striated muscle, along with β, γ, and δ sarcoglycans (Ettinger *et al.*, 1997). Mutations in these four genes cause autosomal recessive limb girdle muscular dystrophies. Epsilon-sarcoglycan forms part of the dystrophin-glycoprotein complex in smooth muscle, and is part of the sarcoglycan complex in the Schwann cell membrane (Straub *et al.*, 1999; Imamura *et al.*, 2000). *SGCE* is also widely expressed in several areas of the brain (Zimprich *et al.*, 2001). Mouse embryonic studies showed that *SGCE* expression can be detected in a wide distribution early in development (Straub *et al.*, 1999; Imamura *et al.*, 2000). A recent study showed that ε-sarcoglycan exists in two distinct isoforms, of which one (εSG1) has ubiquitous expression, while the other (εSG2) is selectively expressed in the central nervous system. Both isoforms were found to be highly expressed in mouse brain, especially within aminergic neuronal groups in the substantia nigra, olfactory bulb, dentate gyrus, pons, and cerebellar cortex. Subcellular fractionation experiments showed that the εSG1 isoform is mostly found in post-synaptic membranes, while εSG2 is concentrated within presynaptic membranes. Although the significance of this finding is still unclear, the investigators have suggested that the two isoforms may play distinct roles in regulating aminergic synaptic function across the central nervous system (Nishiyama *et al.*, 2004; Chan *et al.*, 2005).

In the original report, families with *SGCE* mutations presented a uniform phenotype, with onset in the first two decades of life, more marked myoclonus than dystonia, upper body involvement, and in most cases a good response to alcohol consumption (Zimprich *et al.*, 2001). Mutations in the *SGCE* gene were subsequently found in all families previously linked to the chromosome 7 locus and in several additional cases worldwide (Asmus *et al.*, 2002; DeBerardinis *et al.*, 2003; Foncke *et al.*, 2003; Han *et al.*, 2003; Hjermind *et al.*, 2003; Marechal *et al.*, 2003; Hedrich *et al.*, 2004; Kock *et al.*, 2004; O'Riordan *et al.*, 2004; Schule *et al.*, 2004; Asmus *et al.*, 2005; Tezenas du Montcel *et al.*, 2006). Several distinct truncating, splice-site, and missense mutations, exon deletions, and whole gene deletion have been identified, allowing the definition of a broader clinical spectrum of the myoclonus-dystonia syndrome. Although the vast majority of patients presented a typical phenotype with early-onset and upper body myoclonus as the sole or the most relevant feature, atypical presentations with late onset, dystonia alone (mostly writer's cramp), or prominent leg involvement have been reported among mutation positive cases. Moreover, *SGCE* mutations were found in two families with myoclonus-dystonia and epilepsy. In these families, some family members had pure myoclonus-dystonia while others had an association of movement disorder and epilepsy – either complex partial seizures with occasional secondary generalization or febrile seizures, responsive to antiepileptic drugs. These findings suggest that epilepsy can indeed be part of the phenotypic spectrum of myoclonus-dystonia and must not be considered an exclusion criterion (Foncke *et al.*, 2003; O'Riordan *et al.*, 2004).

To assess whether the same genetic aetiology underlies both neurological and psychiatric signs in patients with myoclonus-dystonia, Saunders-Pullman and collaborators (2002) studied the occurrence of psychiatric symptoms in affected individuals, healthy carriers, and non-carriers from three large families linked to the DYT11 locus. Alcohol dependence was observed in 43 per cent of the patients and none of the healthy subjects, and may be explained by self-medication with alcohol to improve motor symptoms of myoclonus-dystonia. Obsessive-compulsive behaviour was detected in 25 per cent of patients and in 9 per cent of healthy carriers, with an overall rate among carriers of 20 per cent, while none of the non-carriers manifested psychiatric problems. This study was the first to show a significantly higher incidence of psychiatric disturbances among mutation carriers.

Because of the frequent occurrence of obsessive-compulsive disorders among myoclonus-dystonia patients, de Carvalho Aguiar and coworkers (2004) looked for *SGCE* mutations in a cohort of patients with either obsessive-compulsive disorder alone or Gilles de la Tourette syndrome, a psychiatric condition also characterised by obsessive-compulsive behaviour. However, both the complete mutation screening of the *SGCE* gene in these patients and an association study of a *SGCE* polymorphism in patients *vs* matched controls failed to identify a role for this gene in the pathogenesis of these two psychiatric conditions. Additionally, mutations in the *SGCE* gene were not found in patients with different subtypes of primary torsion dystonia (including 'jerky' dystonia), benign hereditary chorea, or Ramsay-Hunt syndrome – all conditions that must be considered in the differential diagnosis of myoclonus-dystonia (Grundmann *et al.*, 2004; Valente *et al.*, 2005; Tezenas du Montcel *et al.*, 2006), allowing the definition of a well defined phenotypic spectrum associated with *SGCE* mutations.

In the light of these results, *SGCE* testing appears appropriate in individuals with myoclonus affecting the arms or neck, or both, with or without dystonia, in whom clinical history and initial investigations suggest a primary rather than a secondary (neurodegenerative) cause. The most important additional factor that predicts *SGCE* positivity is autosomal dominant paternal inheritance, although this is also seen in negative cases and sporadic *SGCE* disease occurs. Predominant myoclonus, upper body distribution of symptoms, young age at onset, and alcohol responsiveness are all helpful clinical features but are not exclusive to *SGCE* positive cases, and no clinical criteria can clearly differentiate between mutation-positive and mutation-negative patients (Valente *et al.*, 2005). As with all genetic testing, genetic counselling should be given before and after testing. Patients should be counselled that *SGCE* mutation testing is more often negative than positive, and that the absence of an *SGCE* mutation does not imply a non-genetic cause for their movement disorder but other, as yet unknown, genetic defects are likely to be responsible (see below).

Most identified *SGCE* mutations produce a loss of function of the ε-sarcoglycan protein; therefore genotype-phenotype correlations are difficult to perform. Nevertheless, the complete gene deletion and truncating mutations abolishing protein expression have been associated with a more severe phenotype (DeBerardinis *et al.*, 2003; Marechal *et al.*, 2003). Intrafamilial clinical variability has often been reported, further complicating genotype-phenotype correlations and suggesting that other genetic or environmental factors may play a role in modulating the phenotype.

The reduced penetrance of *SGCE* mutations is largely caused by maternal imprinting of the gene, which consists in the inactivation of the maternal allele through a mechanism of hypermethylation, with consequent selective expression of the paternally inherited gene. The promoter region of the *SGCE* gene contains several regions prone to methylation processes – a characteristic feature of imprinted genes (Muller *et al.*, 2002; Grabowski *et al.*, 2003). Because of this, clinically affected individuals are more likely to have inherited the pathogenic mutation from their father, while unaffected, non-penetrant mutation carriers have more often inherited the mutation from their mother. This also explains the lack of family history in some patients with myoclonus-dystonia and *SGCE* mutations, although screening large cohorts of patients has shown that the mutation rate is much higher in familial than in sporadic cases (Valente *et al.*, 2003; Valente *et al.*, 2005; Tezenas du Montcel *et al.*, 2006). *De novo* mutations have also been described (Hedrich *et al.*, 2004).

Other genes and loci implicated in myoclonus-dystonia

Overall, *SGCE* is responsible for about 20 to 25 per cent of patients with myoclonus-dystonia, including familial and (apparently) sporadic cases. These results, emerging from large mutation screenings, confirm that myoclonus-dystonia is a genetically heterogeneous condition.

Before the discovery of *SGCE* mutations, two other genes had been implicated in the pathogenesis of myoclonus-dystonia: the *DRD2* gene on chromosome 11, encoding the dopamine D2 receptor, and the *DYT1* gene on chromosome 9q, mutated in primary torsion dystonia. Linkage analysis of candidate regions in one large family with eight individuals affected by myoclonus-dystonia generated positive – although not fully significant – LOD score values in the genetic region containing the *DRD2* gene. Sequencing of the coding region of this gene identified a missense mutation (V154I) segregating with the phenotype (Klein *et al.*, 1999). However, the pathogenicity of this missense mutation was never demonstrated by functional experiments and several further studies failed to identify mutations in this gene in other myoclonus-dystonia families (Dürr *et al.*, 2000; Klein *et al.*, 2000b; Grimes *et al.*, 2001).

A unique 3 bp deletion (GAG) in exon 5 of the *DYT1* gene is responsible for a large proportion of patients with early-onset, generalised primary torsion dystonia (Ozelius *et al.*, 1997; Valente *et al.*, 1998). In the course of a large mutation screening of the DYT1 gene in patients with variable dystonic phenotypes, a novel 18bp in-frame deletion in the same exon 5 was identified in one sporadic case with dystonia and myoclonic features. This deletion causes the loss of six amino-acids towards the C-terminus end of the TorsinA protein, but functional studies on the effect of the mutation on the protein activity have not been undertaken. As with the *DRD2* gene, mutations in the *DYT1* gene have never been found again in patients with myoclonus-dystonia, despite extensive screening (Kabakci *et al.*, 2004; Schule *et al.*, 2004; Tezenas du Montcel *et al.*, 2006). Further doubts about the role of these two genes in the pathogenesis of myoclonus-dystonia have arisen after the identification of *SGCE* as the major gene responsible for this condition. In fact, both the affected individuals in the original *DRD2* family and the sporadic patient with the *DYT1* 18bp deletion were found to carry a pathogenic mutation in the *SGCE* gene. Although a digenic inheritance has been postulated as a possible pathogenic mechanism in these cases (Doheny *et al.*, 2002a; Doheny *et al.*, 2002b; Klein *et al.*, 2002), it must be noted that the identified *SGCE* mutations are sufficient *per se* to explain the phenotype in both cases, and the *DRD2* and *DYT1* mutations could indeed represent harmless variants unrelated to the phenotype. Yet it is interesting to note that Tezenas du Montcel and colleagues have recently described an Ashkenazi Jewish patient with clinical features of alcohol-responsive myoclonus-dystonia who carried the classical GAG deletion in the *DYT1* gene (2006). This patient had the onset of writer's cramp at age 18, and developed myoclonus some years later with involvement of both upper and lower limbs, while his mother suffered from writer's cramp only. However, the occurrence of myoclonus-dystonia features in carriers of the *DYT1* GAG deletion is extremely rare and up to now the role of *DRD2* and *DYT1* genes in myoclonus-dystonia remains unconvincing.

A novel locus for myoclonus-dystonia has recently been mapped to a 16.9 cM region on chromosome 18p11 in a large Canadian family with 13 affected members (Grimes *et al.*, 2002). The phenotype was typical, with onset in the first two decades and prominent upper body involvement; however, some intrafamilial clinical variability could be observed with respect to the presence or absence of dystonia, the distribution of myoclonus, and alcohol responsiveness (Grimes *et al.*, 2001). The responsible gene has not yet been identified and other families linked to this novel locus have not been reported.

Treatment options in myoclonus-dystonia

No specific treatments for myoclonus-dystonia are currently available, and standard antiepileptic treatments are ineffective or only mildly effective in controlling abnormal movements. A single case has been reported with excellent therapeutic response to γ-hydroxybutyric acid (GHB), a drug commonly used in the treatment of alcohol withdrawal. The patient presented a typical alcohol responsive myoclonus-dystonia, which was severe and interfered with several daily life activities such as writing, drinking, and eating. GHB at a dosage of 6.125 g/day produced an 80 per cent improvement in symptoms with no appreciable side effects (Priori *et al.*, 2000). However, further studies are needed to confirm the potential beneficial effects of this drug in the treatment of myoclonus-dystonia.

In two severe cases, chronic bilateral stimulation of the globus pallidus internus has produced excellent results, with marked amelioration of symptoms and improvement in the quality of life (Cif *et al.*, 2004; Liu *et al.*, 2002). The patient described by Cif and coworkers was an 8-year-old boy who was a carrier of an *SGCE* mutation. He developed myoclonus-dystonia at age 1 year and was severely disabled. After surgery, involuntary movements completely disappeared at rest, and action myoclonus also improved consistently. Benefits were still present after a 20 month follow-up, with no side effects. Similarly, in the patient reported by Liu and collaborators, bilateral medial pallidal stimulation abrogated the myoclonic muscle activity, with results persisting at a 20 month follow-up. Thus deep brain stimulation of the globi pallidi could represent a valid treatment option in patients with severe and handicapping myoclonus-dystonia, for whom no other treatment strategies are currently available.

References

Asmus, F. & Gasser, T. (2004): Inherited myoclonus-dystonia. In: *Dystonia 4*, eds. S. Fahn, M. Hallett & M.R. DeLong. *Adv. Neurol.* **94**, 113–119.

Asmus, F., Zimprich, A., Naumann, M., Berg, D., Bertram, M., Ceballos-Baumann, A., Pruszak-Seel, R., Kabus, C., Dichgans, M., Fuchs, S., Muller-Myhsok, B. & Gasser, T. (2001): Inherited myoclonus-dystonia syndrome: narrowing the 7q21-q31 locus in German families. *Ann. Neurol.* **49**, 121–124.

Asmus, F., Zimprich, A., Tezenas Du Montcel, S., Kabus, C., Deuschl, G., Kupsch, A., Ziemann, U., Castro, M., Kuhn, A.A., Strom, T.M., Vidailhet, M., Bhatia, K.P., Dürr, A., Wood, N.W., Brice, A. & Gasser, T. (2002): Myoclonus-dystonia syndrome: epsilon-sarcoglycan mutations and phenotype. *Ann. Neurol.* **52**, 489–492.

Asmus, F., Salih, F., Hjermind, L.E., Ostergaard, K., Munz, M., Kuhn, A.A., Dupont, E., Kupsch, A. & Gasser, T. (2005): Myoclonus-dystonia due to genomic deletions in the epsilon-sarcoglycan gene. *Ann. Neurol.* **58**, 792–797.

Chan, P., Gonzalez-Maeso, J., Ruf, F., Bishop, D.F., Hof, P.R. & Sealfon, S.C. (2005): Epsilon-sarcoglycan immunoreactivity and mRNA expression in mouse brain. *J. Comp. Neurol.* **482**, 50–73.

Cif, L., Valente, E.M., Hemm, S., Coubes, C., Vayssiere, N., Serrat, S., Di Giorgio, A. & Coubes, P. (2004): Deep brain stimulation in myoclonus-dystonia syndrome. *Mov. Disord.* **19**, 724–727.

DeBerardinis, R.J., Conforto, D., Russell, K., Kaplan, J., Kollros, P.R., Zackai, E.H. & Emanuel, B.S. (2003): Myoclonus in a patient with a deletion of the epsilon-sarcoglycan locus on chromosome 7q21. *Am. J. Med. Genet. A.* **121**, 31–36.

de Carvalho Aguiar, P., Fazzari, M., Jankovic, J. & Ozelius, L.J. (2004): Examination of the SGCE gene in Tourette syndrome patients with obsessive-compulsive disorder. *Mov. Disord.* **19**, 1237–1238.

Doheny, D.O., Brin, M.F., Morrison, C.E., Smith, C.J., Walker, R.H., Abbasi, S., Muller, B., Garrels, J., Liu, L., De Carvalho Aguiar, P., Schilling, K., Kramer, P., De Leon, D., Raymond, D., Saunders-Pullman, R., Klein, C., Bressman, S.B., Schmand, B., Tijssen, M.A., Ozelius, L.J. & Silverman, J.M. (2002a): Phenotypic features of myoclonus-dystonia in three kindreds. *Neurology* **59**, 1187–1196.

Doheny, D., Danisi, F., Smith, C., Morrison, C., Velickovic, M., De Leon, D., Bressman, S.B., Leung, J., Ozelius, L., Klein, C., Breakefield, X.O., Brin, M.F. & Silverman, J.M. (2002b): Clinical findings of a myoclonus-dystonia family with two distinct mutations. *Neurology* **59**, 1244–1246.

Dürr, A., Tassin, J., Vidailhet, M., Durif, F., Jedynak, P., Agid, Y. & Brice, A. (2000): D2 dopamine receptor gene in myoclonic dystonia and essential myoclonus. *Ann. Neurol.* **48**, 127–128.

Ettinger, A.J., Feng, G. & Sanes, J.R. (1997): (-Sarcoglycan, a broadly expressed homologue of the gene mutated in limb-girdle muscular dystrophy 2D. *J. Biol. Chem.* **272**, 32534–32538.

Fahn, S., Marsden, C.D. & Calne, D.B. (1987): Classification and investigation of dystonia. In: *Movement disorders 2*, eds. C.D. Marden & S. Fahn, pp. 332–358. London: Butterworth.

Fahn, S., Bressman, S.B. & Marsden, C.D. (1998): Classification of dystonia. In: *Dystonia 3*, eds. C.D. Marden, S. Fahn & M.R. DeLong. *Adv. Neurol.* **78**, 1–10.

Foncke, E.M., Klein, C., Koelman, J.H., Kramer, P.L., Schilling, K., Muller, B., Garrels, J., de Carvalho Aguiar, P., Liu, L., de Froe, A., Speelman, J.D., Ozelius, L.J. & Tijssen, M.A. (2003): Hereditary myoclonus-dystonia associated with epilepsy. *Neurology* **60**, 1988–1990.

Grabowski, M., Zimprich, A., Lorenz-Depiereux, B., Kalscheuer, V., Asmus, F., Gasser, T., Meitinger, T. & Strom, T.M. (2003): The epsilon-sarcoglycan gene (SGCE), mutated in myoclonus-dystonia syndrome, is maternally imprinted. *Eur. J. Hum. Genet.* **11**, 138–144.

Grimes, D.A., Bulman, D., St George-Hyslop, P. & Lang, A.E. (2001): Inherited myoclonus-dystonia: evidence supporting genetic heterogeneity. *Mov. Disord.* **16**, 106–110.

Grimes, D.A., Han, F., Lang, A.E., St George-Hyslop, P., Racacho, L. & Bulman, D.E. (2002): A novel locus for inherited myoclonus-dystonia on 18p11. *Neurology* **59**, 1183–1186.

Grundmann, K., Laubis-Herrmann, U., Dressler, D., Vollmer-Haase, J., Bauer, P., Stuhrmann, M., Schulte, T., Schols, L., Topka, H. & Riess, O. (2004): Lack of mutations in the epsilon-sarcoglycan gene in patients with different subtypes of primary dystonias. *Mov. Disord.* **19**, 1294–1297.

Han, F., Lang, A.E., Racacho, L., Bulman, D.E. & Grimes, D.A. (2003): Mutations in the epsilon-sarcoglycan gene found to be uncommon in seven myoclonus-dystonia families. *Neurology* **61**, 244–246.

Hedrich, K., Meyer, E.M., Schule, B., Kock, N., de Carvalho Aguiar, P., Wiegers, K., Koelman, J.H., Garrels, J., Dürr, R., Liu, L., Schwinger, E., Ozelius, L.J., Landwehrmeyer, B., Stoessl, A.J., Tijssen, M.A. & Klein, C. (2004): Myoclonus-dystonia: detection of novel, recurrent, and de novo SGCE mutations. *Neurology* **62**, 1229–1231.

Hjermind, L.E., Werdelin, L.M., Eiberg, H., Krag-Olsen, B., Dupont, E. & Sorensen, S.A. (2003): A novel mutation in the epsilon-sarcoglycan gene causing myoclonus-dystonia syndrome. *Neurology* **60**, 1536–1539.

Imamura, M., Araishi, K., Noguchi, S. & Ozawa, E. (2000): A sarcoglycan-dystroglycan complex anchors Dp116 and utrophin in the peripheral nervous system. *Hum. Mol. Genet.* **9**, 3091–3100.

Kabakci, K., Hedrich, K., Leung, J.C., Mitterer, M., Vieregge, P., Lencer, R., Hagenah, J., Garrels, J., Witt, K., Klostermann, F., Svetel, M., Friedman, J., Kostic, V., Bressman, S.B., Breakefield, X.O., Ozelius, L.J., Pramstaller, P.P. & Klein, C. (2004): Mutations in DYT1: extension of the phenotypic and mutational spectrum. *Neurology* **62**, 395–400.

Klein, C., Brin, M.F., Kramer, P., Sena-Esteves, M., de Leon, D., Doheny, D., Bressman, S., Fahn, S., Breakefield, X.O. & Ozelius, L.J. (1999): Association of a missense change in the D2 dopamine receptor with myoclonus-dystonia. *Proc. Natl. Acad. Sci. USA* **96**, 5173–5176.

Klein, C., Schilling, K., Saunders-Pullman, R.J., Garrels, J., Breakefield, X.O., Brin, M.F., deLeon, D., Doheny, D., Fahn, S., Fink, J.S., Forsgren, L., Friedman, J., Frucht, S., Harris, J., Holmgren, G., Kis, B., Kurlan, R., Kyllerman, M., Lang, A.E., Leung, J., Raymond, D., Robishaw, J.D., Sanner, G., Schwinger, E., Tabamo, R.E. & Tagliati, M. (2000a): A major locus for myoclonus-dystonia maps to chromosome 7q in eight families. *Am. J. Hum. Genet.* **67**, 1314–1319.

Klein, C., Gurvich, N., Sena-Esteves, M., Bressman, S., Brin, M.F., Ebersole, B.J., Fink, S., Forsgren, L., Friedman, J., Grimes, D., Holmgren, G., Kyllerman, M., Lang, A.E., de Leon, D., Leung, J., Prioleau, C., Raymond, D., Sanner, G., Saunders-Pullman, R., Vieregge, P., Wahlstrom, J., Breakefield, X.O., Kramer, P.L., Ozelius, L.J. & Sealfon, S.C. (2000b): Evaluation of the role of the D2 dopamine receptor in myoclonus-dystonia. *Ann. Neurol.* **47**, 369–373.

Klein, C., Liu, L., Doheny, D., Kock, N., Muller, B., de Carvalho Aguiar, P., Leung, J., de Leon, D., Bressman, S.B., Silverman, J., Smith, C., Danisi, F., Morrison, C., Walker, R.H., Velickovic, M., Schwinger, E., Kramer, P.L., Breakefield, X.O., Brin, M.F. & Ozelius, L.J. (2002): Epsilon-sarcoglycan mutations found in combination with other dystonia gene mutations. *Ann. Neurol.* **52**, 675–679.

Kock, N., Kasten, M., Schule, B., Hedrich, K., Wiegers, K., Kabakci, K., Hagenah, J., Pramstaller, P.P., Nitschke, M.F., Munchau, A., Sperner, J. & Klein, C. (2004): Clinical and genetic features of myoclonus-dystonia in 3 cases: a video presentation. *Mov. Disord.* **19**, 231–234.

Liu, X., Griffin, I.C., Parkin, S.G., Miall, R.C., Rowe, J.G., Gregory, R.P., Scott, R.B., Aziz, T.Z. & Stein, J.F. (2002): Involvement of the medial pallidum in focal myoclonic dystonia: a clinical and neurophysiological case study. *Mov. Disord.* **17**, 346–353.

Marechal, L., Raux, G., Dumanchin, C., Lefebvre, G., Deslandre, E., Girard, C., Campion, D., Parain, D., Frebourg, T. & Hannequin, D. (2003): Severe myoclonus-dystonia syndrome associated with a novel epsilon-sarcoglycan gene truncating mutation. *Am. J. Med. Genet. B Neuropsychiatr. Genet.* **119**, 114–117.

Marsden, C.D., Hallett, M. & Fahn, S. (1982): The nosology and pathophysiology of myoclonus. In: *Movement disorders*, eds. C.D. Marsden & S. Fahn, pp. 196–248. London: Butterworth.

Muller, B., Hedrich, K., Kock, N., Dragasevic, N., Svetel, M., Garrels, J., Landt, O., Nitschke, M., Pramstaller, P.P., Reik, W., Schwinger, E., Sperner, J., Ozelius, L., Kostic, V. & Klein, C. (2002): Evidence that paternal expression of the epsilon-sarcoglycan gene accounts for reduced penetrance in myoclonus-dystonia. *Am. J. Hum. Genet.* **71**, 1303–1311.

Nishiyama, A., Endo, T., Takeda, S. & Imamura, M. (2004): Identification and characterization of epsilon-sarcoglycans in the central nervous system. *Mol. Brain Res.* **125**, 1–12.

Nygaard, T.G., Raymond, D., Chen, C., Nishino, I., Greene, P.E., Jennings, D., Heiman, G.A., Klein, C., Saunders-Pullman, R.J., Kramer, P., Ozelius, L.J. & Bressman, S.B. (1999): Localization of a gene for myoclonus-dystonia to chromosome 7q21-q31. *Ann. Neurol.* **46**, 794–798.

O'Riordan, S., Ozelius, L.J., de Carvalho Aguiar, P., Hutchinson, M., King, M. & Lynch, T. (2004): Inherited myoclonus-dystonia and epilepsy: further evidence of an association? *Mov. Disord.* **19**, 1456–1459.

Ozelius, L.J., Hewett, J.W., Page, C.E., Bressman, S.B., Kramer, P.L., Shalish, C., de Leon, D., Brin, M.F., Raymond, D., Corey, D.P., Fahn, S., Risch, N.J., Buckler, A.J., Gusella, J.F. & Breakefield, X.O. (1997): The early-onset torsion dystonia gene (DYT1) encodes an ATP-binding protein. *Nature Genet.* **17**, 40–48.

Priori, A., Bertolasi, L., Pesenti, A., Cappellari, A. & Barbieri, S. (2000): Gamma-hydroxybutyric acid for alcohol-sensitive myoclonus with dystonia. *Neurology* **54**, 1706.

Quinn, N.P. (1996): Essential myoclonus and myoclonic dystonia. *Mov. Disord.* **11**, 119–124.

Quinn, N.P., Rothwell, J.C., Thompson, P.D. & Marsden, C.D. (1988): Hereditary myoclonic dystonia, hereditary torsion dystonia and hereditary essential myoclonus: an area of confusion. *Adv. Neurol.* **50**, 391–401.

Saunders-Pullman, R., Shriberg, J., Heiman, G., Raymond, D., Wendt, K., Kramer, P., Schilling, K., Kurlan, R., Klein, C., Ozelius, L.J., Risch, N.J. & Bressman, S.B. (2002): Myoclonus-dystonia: possible association with obsessive-compulsive disorder and alcohol dependence. *Neurology* **58**, 242–245.

Schule, B., Kock, N., Svetel, M., Dragasevic, N., Hedrich, K., De Carvalho Aguiar, P., Liu, L., Kabakci, K., Garrels, J., Meyer, E.M., Berisavac, I., Schwinger, E., Kramer, P.L., Ozelius, L.J., Klein, C. & Kostic, V. (2004): Genetic heterogeneity in ten families with myoclonus-dystonia. *J. Neurol. Neurosurg. Psychiatry* **75**, 1181–1185.

Straub, V., Ettinger, A.J., Durbeej, M., Venzke, D.P., Cutshall, S., Sanes, J.R. & Campbell, K.P. (1999): ε-sarcoglycan replaces α-sarcoglycan in smooth muscle to form a unique dystrophin-glycoprotein complex. *J. Biol. Chem.* **274**, 27989–27996.

Tezenas du Montcel, S., Clot, F., Vidailhet, M., Roze, E., Damier, P., Jedynak, C.P., Camuzat, A., Lagueny, A., Vercueil, L., Doummar, D., Guyant-Marechal, L., Houeto, J.L., Ponsot, G., Thobois, S., Cournelle, M.A., Dürr, A.,

Durif, F., Echenne, B., Hannequin, D., Tranchant, C. & Brice, A. (2006): Epsilon sarcoglycan mutations and phenotype in French patients with myoclonic syndromes. *J. Med. Genet.* **43**, 394–499.

Valente, E.M., Warner, T.T., Jarman, P.R., Mathen, D., Fletcher, N.A., Marsden, C.D., Bhatia, K.P. & Wood, N.W. (1998): The role of DYT1 in primary torsion dystonia in Europe. *Brain* **121**, 2335–2339.

Valente, E.M., Misbahuddin, A., Brancati, F., Placzek, M.R., Garavaglia, B., Salvi, S., Nemeth, A., Shaw-Smith, C., Nardocci, N., Bentivoglio, A.R., Berardelli, A., Eleopra, R., Dallapiccola, B. & Warner, T.T. (2003): Analysis of the epsilon-sarcoglycan gene in familial and sporadic myoclonus-dystonia: evidence for genetic heterogeneity. *Mov. Disord.* **18**, 1047–1051.

Valente, E.M., Edwards, M.J., Mir, P., DiGiorgio, A., Salvi, S., Davis, M., Russo, N., Bozi, M., Kim, H.T., Pennisi, G., Quinn, N., Dallapiccola, B. & Bhatia, K.P. (2005): The epsilon-sarcoglycan gene in myoclonic syndromes. *Neurology* **64**, 737–739.

Vidailhet, M., Tassin, J., Durif, F., Nivelon-Chevallier, A., Agid, Y., Brice, A. & Dürr, A. (2001): A major locus for several phenotypes of myoclonus-dystonia on chromosome 7q. *Neurology* **56**, 1213–1216.

Zimprich, A., Grabowski, M., Asmus, F., Naumann, M., Berg, D., Bertram, M., Scheidtmann, K., Kern, P., Winkelmann, J., Muller-Myhsok, B., Riedel, L., Bauer, M., Muller, T., Castro, M., Meitinger, T., Strom, T.M. & Gasser, T. (2001): Mutations in the gene encoding ε-sarcoglycan cause myoclonus-dystonia syndrome. *Nat. Genet.* **29**, 66–69.

Chapter 8

Pharmacological treatment of childhood dystonia

Agathe Roubertie, Julie Leydet, Nathalie Demonceau and Bernard Echenne

Neuropaediatric Service, Hospital Gui de Chauliac, 80 Avenue Augustin Fliche, 34295 Montpellier, France
a-roubertie@chu-montpellier.fr

Summary

Dystonia often leads to disabling conditions in childhood. The aetiology of the dystonic symptoms, the age of the patient, the anatomical distribution, and the potential risk of adverse effects are important determinants of the choice of the treatment. The wide range of available pharmacological molecules is reviewed and discussed in the light of recently published data.

Introduction and general considerations

Dystonia has been defined as a syndrome of sustained muscle contractions, frequently causing twisting and repetitive movements or abnormal postures. It is characterized by great variability in its topography, aetiology (genetic causes, metabolic disorders, brain lesion), and related functional consequences. Accurate clinical and paraclinical evaluation is the first step leading to a therapeutic strategy. It is essential to identify situations which do not need treatment – for example, localized dystonia with little functional impairment may not require pharmacological therapy, and transitory benign dystonia, which will improve spontaneously and which does not need treatment, should be distinguished from disabling disorders.

On the other hand some situations will require specific treatment. Dopa-responsive dystonia (DRD) can be classified within this category, as patients improve dramatically on even low doses of levodopa. A therapeutic trial of dopa over a three-month period should be undertaken in any child with dystonic symptoms without identified aetiology. If DRD is ruled out by this trial, as dopaminergic therapy has little effect in the other forms of dystonia, this treatment can be discontinued (Jankovic, 1998). Dopa therapy is discussed in elsewhere in this volume (chapter 11). Other metabolic disorders which require specific treatment are rare but must be recognized early, as the treatment of the underlying disease will improve the abnormal movements; example are creatine supplementation for guanidinoacetate methyltransferase deficiency (Stöckler *et al.*, 1994), and biotin supplementation for encephalopathy with biotin deficiency (Ozand *et al.*, 1998).

In many patients with dystonia, the dystonic symptoms will be so disabling that pharmacological treatment is necessary. In such cases the aim of treatment is to improve the symptoms. Its theoretical purpose is to decrease the abnormal movements, improve functional ability, and relieve pain associated with dystonic contractions.

The evaluation of medical treatment for dystonia is difficult for the following reasons:

- dystonia and its functional consequences are sometimes difficult to quantitate; many studies report crude clinical data, although validated rating scales should be used;
- dystonic symptoms can be associated with various neurological disorders with diverse aetiologies; thus groups of patients with dystonia may be very heterogeneous;
- dystonia is characterized by waxing and waning of symptoms, and given such spontaneous and transient fluctuations, assessment of the response to treatment may be difficult;
- many pharmacological trials have been carried out in small groups of patients, or even as single case reports; unless the sample size is statistically valid for the assessment of a new drug, the significance of any studies done must be interpreted carefully;
- few trials are well enough designed to determine the efficacy of a new drug unequivocally, and prospective, double-blind studies with placebo controls are rare.

For all these reasons, the assessment of various therapeutic intervention in dystonia of childhood is problematic. Table 1 illustrates the list of the pharmacological treatments given to a group of 19 patients with early-onset generalized dystonia. These patients were referred to our department from different French cities for evaluation before deep brain stimulation. During a follow-up ranging from 18 months to 21 years, 15 different classes of drugs were used by the patients' physicians, representing 31 different molecules. The patients each received between two and 11 different drugs, with a mean duration of treatment of 7 months. Table 1 highlights the variety of drugs used by physicians in France, and also suggests the limited efficacy of the available pharmacological treatments for dystonia in childhood.

Table 1. Drugs used in the treatment of dystonia in 19 children by physicians in France

Pharmacological treatment	Number of patients (total number of patients = 19)
L-dopa	19
Benzodiazepine	16
Anticholinergic	19
Baclofen	13
Tetrabenazine	7
Piracetam	4
Dopa agonist	4
Vigabatrin	2
Classical neuroleptics	4
Atypical neuroleptics	2
Carbamazepine	5
Myorelaxant	3
Sodium valproate	1
Gabapentin	1
Phenytoin	1

Retrospective analysis of the pharmacologial treatment of 19 patients with childhood-onset primary generalized dystonia. Multicentric referal for evaluation before deep brain stimulation. 12 DYT1 patients, 7 non-DYT1 patients. Mean age at onset of the disease: 7y 2m; mean age at generalization: 9y; mean follow-up: 6y (18m-21y). Fifteen different pharmacological classes have been used.

Anticholinergic treatment

Anticholinergic drugs block the action of acetylcholine on the central muscarinic receptors. Anticholinergic drugs – especially trihexiphenidyl – have long been the mainstay of treatment for dystonia, and a blinded clinical trial carried out two decades ago confirmed their efficacy in children with focal, segmental, or generalized dystonia (Burke et al., 1986). The treatment should be started at a dose of 1 mg a day, with a 2 mg/week increase up to the maximum tolerated dosage (up to 15–30 mg a day). Side effects can be controlled by slow titration but may limit the use of these agents (dry mouth, blurred vision, central adverse events with drowsiness, forgetfulness, hallucinations). Efficacy is observed in more than one-third of the patients with dystonia; the beneficial effects are seen not only in primary generalized dystonia but also in dopa-responsive dystonia and especially in cases with secondary dystonic symptoms or dystonic cerebral palsy. The best clinical effect is achieved when treatment is initiated early (Hoon et al., 2001). According to a recent meta-analysis, trihexiphenidyl was the only pharmacological treatment shown to be effective in childhood dystonia (Balash & Giladi, 2004).

Baclofen

Baclofen is a presynaptic γ-aminobutyric acid (GABA) agonist. In a retrospective study, efficacy in dystonia has been reported in about one-third of patients with primary dystonia when given at dosages ranging from 40 to 180 mg/day (Greene, 1992). High dosage is often limited by side effects (sleepiness, increased axial hypotonia). Intrathecal baclofen has been used successfully to treat dystonia, especially in patients with dystonic cerebral palsy. Albright reported a large series of patients (71 per cent with cerebral palsy); improvement in dystonia scores and quality of life was significant, especially in dystonic patients with pyramidal tract signs (Albright et al., 2001). Surgical complications occurred in 26 per cent of the patients (infection, CSF leaks).

Dopamine depleting agents

Tetrabenazine is an anti-dopaminergic agent that depletes presynaptic storage of monoamines and blocks postsynaptic dopamine receptors. A recent study analysed its efficacy on abnormal movements among 150 adult patients and reported an excellent effect in a subgroup with chorea and facial dystonia/dyskinesia (Paleacu et al., 2004). It is also effective in adult ballism and tardive dystonia. No study is available in childhood; nevertheless, this drug is considered to be effective in childhood dystonia. The usual dose ranges between 25 and 100 mg/day. Side effects, mainly drowsiness, are dose-dependent.

Dopamine blocking agents: classical and new neurolepetics

Dopamine blocking agents have classically been used to treat dystonia. Tiapride might be useful in secondary dystonia or dystonic cerebral palsy. Pimozide has been reported as useful, especially in status dystonicus (Nardocci et al., 2005). Otherwise, given their side effects (sedation, parkinsonism, tardive dyskinesia) and their limited efficacy, D2 blocking agents must be avoided or restricted to selected cases (Jankovic, 1995).

Grassi et al. (2000) reported the efficacy of risperidone (2–6 mg/day) in adult patients with idiopathic and symptomatic dystonia. Published data on the use of new antipsychotic drugs in dystonia are limited, concern adult patients, and are confined to single case reports (Balash & Giladi, 2004).

Dopamine agonists

Dopamine agonists have also been used in patients with dystonia. An improvement in dystonia has been reported with high dosage of bromocriptine (50–80 mg/day) in uncontrolled studies (Obeso & Luquin, 1984). In two randomized placebo-controlled trials, lisuride has been found to have inconclusive effects (Quinn et al., 1985). Finally, these drugs are of limited use, except in particular metabolic conditions – for example, patients with amino-acid decarboxylase deficiency can be improved by bromocriptine and the monoamine oxidase inhibitor tranylcypromine (Pons et al., 2004).

Benzodiazepines

Benzodiazepines bind to GABAa receptor and enhance GABA-mediated inhibition. Although no controlled trial has explored the clinical efficacy of benzodiazepines, these drugs are commonly used to treat dystonia (Jankovic, 1998; Edgar, 2003). High doses are often necessary to obtain a clinical response but are associated with side effects, especially sleepiness.

Botulinum toxin

Botulinum toxin has been used for more than 15 years for the treatment of adult focal dystonia. It provides obvious benefits for cervical dystonia, or blepharospasm, and is also used for writer's cramp. This neurotoxin blocks the release of acetylcholine at the neuromuscular junction, thereby inducing a progressive weakness of the muscles with subsequent improvement of the focal dystonic symptoms. Beneficial effects are temporary, and injection must be repeated every three to four months (Graham et al., 2003). In children. botulinum toxin injections can be given under general anaesthesia or using entonox.

Treatment strategy

Dystonia is only a symptom; treatment will be symptomatic and designed to improve the patient's posture and function and to relieve any associated pain. The therapeutic strategy will be determined by the aetiology of the dystonic symptoms, the age of the patient, the anatomical distribution, and the potential risk of adverse effects.

After failure of a trial of dopa (which rules out DRD), anticholinergic drugs will be the first therapeutic choice. Patients with primary focal dystonia who are old enough might benefit from botulinum toxin injections. Those with secondary focal dystonia may also benefit, and two of our patients with focal dystonia after a stoke were dramatically improved by this treatment. Botulinum toxin is useless in multifocal or generalized dystonia (Graham et al., 2003).

Many patients with multifocal or generalized primary dystonia will require a combination of several drugs – for example, tetrabenazine or baclofen can be combined with anticholinergic treatment (Jankovic, 1998; Roubertie et al., 2000). In patients with dystonic cerebral palsy or secondary dystonia, benzodiazepines may also be useful in reducing the associated spasticity. Pimozide may improve the dystonic symptoms associated with pyramidal tract signs.

Conclusions

Various pharmacological agents are available for treating dystonic manifestations but only trihexiphenidyl has scientifically proven efficacy. For these reasons, the selection of a particular choice of treatment is largely guided by empirical trials and by personal clinical experience (Jankovic, 1998).

The treatment of severe dystonia is characterized by a variable response and frequent failure of the drugs to relieve the symptoms. Despite pharmacological indications, alleviation of symptoms is often mild and the cognitive side effects of the drugs (drowsiness, sleepiness, and the related disruption of learning) aggravate the functional impairment caused by the abnormal movements. In ensuing years the challenge of this pharmacological treatment may be renewed by advances in the neurochemistry and neuropharmacology of dystonia, and a more pertinent neurobiological approach may emerge. At present, however, when drug treatment cannot prevent clinical deterioration in the dystonic patient, other treatment needs to be considered early in the course of the disease – especially functional surgical management.

References

Albright, A.L., Barry, M.J., Shafton, D.H. & Ferson, S.S. (2001): Intrathecal baclofen for generalized dystonia. *Dev. Med. Child Neurol.* **43**, 652–657.

Balash, Y. & Giladi, N. (2004): Efficacy of pharmacological treatment of dystonia: evidence-based review including meta-analysis of the effect of botulinum toxin and other cure options. *Eur. J. Neurol.* **11**, 361–370.

Burke, R.E., Fahn, S. & Marsden, C.D. (1986): Torsion dystonia: a double-blind, prospective trial of high-dosage trihexiphenidyl. *Neurology* **36**, 160–164.

Edgar, T.S. (2003): Oral pharmacotherapy of childhood movement disorders. *J. Child Neurol.* **18**, S40–S49.

Graham, H.K., Boyd, R.N. & Fehlings, D. (2003): Does intramuscular botulinum toxin A injection improve upper-limb function in children with hemiplegic cerebral palsy? *Med. J. Aust.* **178**, 95–96.

Grassi, E., Latorraca, S., Piacentini, S., Marini, P. & Sorbi, S. (2000) : Risperodone in idiopathic and symptomatic dystonia; preliminary experience. *Neurol. Sci.* **21**, 121–123.

Greene, P. (1992): Baclofen in the treatment of dystonia. *Clin. Neuropharmacol.* **15**, 276–288.

Hoon, A.H., Freese, P.O., Reinhardt, E.M., Wilson, M.A., Lawrie, W.T., Harryman, S.E., Pidcock, F.S. & Johnston, M.V. (2001): Age-dependent effects of trihexyphenidyl in extrapyramidal cerebral palsy. *Pediatr. Neurol.* **25**, 55–58.

Jankovic, J. (1995): Tardive syndromes and other drug-induced movement disorders. *Clin. Neuropharmacol.* **18**, 197–214.

Jankovic, J. (1998): Medical therapy and botulinum toxin in dystonia. In: *Advances in neurology: dystonia 3*, eds. S. Fahn, C.D. Marsden & M.R. Delong, pp. 169–183. Philadelphia: Lippincott-Raven.

Nardocci, N., Temudo, T., Echenne, B. & Roubertie, A. (2005): Status dystonicus in children. In: *Pediatric movement disorders*, eds. E. Fernandez-Alvarez, A. Arzimanoglou & E. Tolosa, pp. 71–76. London: John Libbey.

Obeso, J.A. & Luquin, M.R. (1984): Bromocriptine and lisuride in dystonias. *Neurology* **43**, 135–136.

Ozand, P.T., Gascon, G.G., Al Essa, M., Joshi, S., Al Jishi, E., Bakheet, S., Al Watban, J., Al-Kawi, M.Z. & Dabbagh, O. (1998): Biotin-responsive basal ganglia disease: a novel entity. *Brain* **121**, 1267–1279.

Paleacu, D., Giladi, N., Moore, O., Stern, A., Honigman, S. & Badarny, S. (2004): Tetrabenazine treatment in movement disorders. *Clin. Neuropharmacol.* **27**, 230–233.

Pons, R., Ford, B., Chiriboga, C.A., Clayton, P.T., Hinton, V., Hyland, K., Sharma, R. & De Vivo, D.C. (2004): Aromatic L-amino-acid decarboxylase deficiency: clinical features, treatment, and prognosis. *Neurology* **62**, 1058–1065.

Quinn, N.P., Lang, L.E., Sheehy, M.P. & Marseden, C.D. (1985): Lisuride in dystonia. *Neurology* **35**, 766–769.

Roubertie, A., Echenne, B., Cif, L., Vayssiere, N., Hemm, S. & Coubes, P. (2000): Treatment of early-onset dystonia: update and new perspective. *Childs Nerv. Syst.* **16**, 334–340.

Stöckler, S., Holzbach, U., Hanefeld, F., Marquardt, I., Helms, G., Requart, M., Hanicke, W. & Frahm, J. (1994): Creatine deficiency in the brain: a new, treatable inborn error of metabolism. *Pediatr. Res.* **36**, 409–413.

Chapter 9

Deep brain stimulation of the globus pallidus internus for the treatment of childhood-onset dystonia

Giovanni Broggi, Carlo Marras, Angelo Franzini, Giovanna Zorzi[*],
Luigi Romito[#], Dario Caldiroli[§], Luisa Chiapparini[°] and Nardo Nardocci[*]

*Unit of Neurosurgery, [*]Child Neuropsychiatry, [#]Neurology, [°]Neuroradiology, and [§]Neurointensive care,
Fondazione IRCCS Istituto Neurologico 'C. Besta',
via Celoria 11, 20133 Milan, Italy
neurochirurgia@istituto-besta.it
Video 3*

Summary

Pharmacological treatment of dystonia is generally disappointing. Surgical procedures such as thalamotomy and pallidotomy usually result in slight improvement but sometimes cause persistent side effects. In contrast, deep brain stimulation (DBS) causes few side effects and allows adjustment of the strength of stimulation according to clinical requirements.

Our study included 23 patients with childhood-onset dystonia affected by DYT1-negative primary dystonia (n = 17), DYT1-positive primary dystonia (n = 2), and symptomatic dystonia (n = 4), who underwent surgery by bilateral (n = 22) or unilateral (n = 1) globus pallidus internus (GPi) stimulation. Age at onset of symptoms ranged between 2 and 14 years. The duration of the disease at the time of surgery ranged between 4 and 30 years. Dystonia was generalized in 22 patients and unilateral in one. Five of the patients developed status dystonicus during the course of their disease. Preoperative and postoperative evaluation included video recordings and assessment of dystonia with the Burke-Fahn-Marsden dystonia rating scale (BFMRS). The mean follow-up after surgery in this series was 1.5 years and ranged between 9 months and 4.5 years. The greatest benefit was obtained in patients with primary dystonia and tardive dystonia, but significant improvement was also observed in patients with symptomatic dystonia. This technique was particularly effective on axial and limb dystonic movements and postures, while oromandibular dystonia and fixed dystonic postures were modified to a lesser extent. Our findings provide further evidence of the efficacy of pallidal DBS in childhood-onset intractable dystonia, including status dystonicus.

Introduction

Dystonia is a clinical syndrome characterized by sustained muscle contractions, frequently causing twisting repetitive movements and abnormal postures. Dystonia can be the result of acquired lesions (secondary dystonia) and neurodegenerative processes in the CNS (heterodegenerative dystonia), or it can occur in the absence of any identifiable cause (primary dystonia) (Fahn et al., 1998). Patients with dystonia of different aetiologies may develop a severe worsening of symptoms called status dystonicus (Manji et al., 1998). Although rare, this potentially life-threatening condition needs management on an intensive care unit for sedation and ventilation. In status dystonicus, metabolic complications are the rule and death is not infrequent. Pharmacological treatment of dystonia entails different drugs such as anticholinergic agents, dopamine agonists, dopamine antagonists, and benzodiazepines, often given in combination, but usually with limited efficacy.

In the last decade, deep brain stimulation (DBS) of the globus pallidus internus (GPi) has been used for the treatment of dystonia with good results in both adults and children.

Since early in the last century, neurosurgery has been applied to movement disorders such as dystonia. Horsley is considered a pioneer. He proposed selective resection of the motor cortex to control focal dystonia and parkinsonian tremor (Vilensky et al., 2005). Following Horsley's experience, stereotactic systems allowed more precise and selective procedures, consisting of small lesions of the basal ganglia and thalamic nuclei (Abosch & Lozano, 2003). In the 1960s and 1970s, a revolutionary therapeutic approach to movement disorders was proposed, based on selective electric stimulation of the neuronal networks involved in the disorder. In that period, the so-called 'brain stimulation era' was born. In the USA, Cooper undertook electrical stimulation of the cerebellar cortex to treat primary dystonia (Rosenow et al., 2002), while in the USSR, Bekhtereva treated dystonia and Parkinson's disease by electrodes implanted in the basal ganglia. Only 20 years later was this innovative approach universally accepted and routinely undertaken in the treatment of drug-resistant dystonia. However, this period of time was necessary to solve various different problems, including the choice of target and the size, biocompatibility, and longevity of the pacemaker's battery. In the current era of DBS, implantable systems composed of four contact electrodes, an extension cable, and a pulse generator with a battery duration of 4 years are available. This system is capable of supplying stimulation parameters that can be varied in the intensity of current, frequency (usually high frequency, 130–185 Hz), and pulse width according to the clinical needs of the patient. The effect is similar to a selective lesional procedure, but more stable and reversible. In this field, a group from the University of Grenoble made a major contribution by defining the target (the subthalamic nucleus; STN) and the stimulation parameters for the treatment of Parkinson's disease (Benabid et al., 2002). STN was initially used for the treatment of dystonia, with disappointing results, but the GPi – initially proposed by Laitinen for lesional procedures – was then successfully targeted (Laitinen, 2004). The first surgical series involving deep brain stimulation of the GPi for the treatment of dystonia was undertaken by Coubes. The cases included in this series mostly had primary generalized DYT1-positive dystonia (Coubes et al., 2000). Many other surgical groups then started using deep brain stimulation of the GPi and new indications were proposed. Although all investigators are in agreement about the long-term efficacy of GPi stimulation for treating dystonia, there are only incomplete guidelines for patient selection and eligibility.

Patients and methods

During the past 6 years, 38 patients affected by dystonia underwent surgery at our Institute. Twenty-three had childhood-onset dystonia and are included in this study: 17 of these had DYT1-negative primary dystonia, two had DYT1-positive primary dystonia, and the remaining four had symptomatic dystonia (tardive dystonia in two, bilateral basal ganglia calcification in one, and hemidystonia from head trauma in the remaining patient). The age at onset of symptoms ranged between 2 and 14 years. The duration of the disease at the time of surgery ranged between

4 and 30 years. Dystonia was generalized in 22 patients and unilateral in one. Five patients developed status dystonicus during the course of their disease. Four of these had primary dystonia and the remaining patient had symptomatic dystonia. Status dystonicus occurred after a duration of dystonia ranging between 6.4 and 12.6 years (mean 8.6). Status dystonicus developed progressively over months in three patients and within 2 weeks in the remaining two cases. In one case, an intercurrent infection was suggested as the precipitating factor.

The mean follow-up after surgery in this series was 1.5 years (range 3 months to 4 years). Preoperative clinical evaluation in all patients included assessment of dystonia using videotape recordings and administration of the Burke-Fahn-Marsden dystonia rating scale (BFMRS) for the disability and severity of dystonia. After surgery all the patients are evaluated monthly and their clinical status is being assessed by videotape recordings and the BMFRS.

Surgical technique

The bilateral ventroposterolateral portion of GPi was the target for surgery in all patients except the one affected by hemidystonia (who had unilateral DBS). In each patient, preoperative magnetic resonance imaging (MRI) on a 0.5 T or 1.5 T unit was carried out to determine the intercommissural plane, the mid-commissural point, and the anatomical location of the GPi. MRI axial studies included inversion recovery (IR) images passing through the anterior-posterior commissure (AC–PC) line with the following parameters: slice thickness = 2 mm, gap = 0, repetition time (TR) = 2000 ms, echo time (TE) = 13 ms, inversion time (TI) = 350 ms, Turbo factor = 9, field of view (FOV) = 260, rectangular FOV = 100 per cent, matrix size = 256×256 (scan percentage 100 per cent), and scan time = 15.36 minutes for 80 slices.

General anaesthesia was used in all patients and is strongly recommended by our group. Under general anaesthesia and the suspension of curare administration, it is possible to monitor the motor response induced by macrostimulation. Macrostimulation was carried out and when side effects could be detected this suggested an incorrect placement of the electrode. An induced motor response at low amplitude (< 5 mA) showed an overly mesial electrode placement (very close to or within the internal capsule). Under general anaesthesia, it was also possible to carry out microrecording, which allowed analysis of the neuronal discharge of the GPi and permitted better definition of the cranio-caudal and latero-mesial borders of the nucleus.

Software was developed in our department, that allowed precise definition of the distance between the electrode and the internal capsule (Fig. 1). This measurement was made possible by assessing the correlation between the motor response and the amplitude necessary to induce it. A preliminary version of the program is available on-line (www.angelofranzini.com/tardive.html).

The stereotactic frame (Leksell G, CRW) was tilted in the sagittal plane to approximate the AC–PC plane. Presurgery computed tomography (CT) was done, using a volumetric technique with a slice thickness of 2 mm. The gantry angle was 0°. MR images were fused with CT images obtained under stereotactic conditions through an *ad hoc* workstation and software (Sofamor Danek Stealth Station, Frame-link 4.0, Medtronic Inc, Minneapolis, Minnesota, USA), providing stereotactic coordinates of the three-dimensional, virtually built space. Targeting of the GPi was done using the coordinates from the midpoint of AC–PC plane. Anatomical localization was also carried out. In all cases, this corresponded to the AC–PC midpoint coordinates. The stereotactic coordinates of the GPi were also determined by the virtual ventriculography system (program available on-line). The target was 2 mm anterior to the AC–PC midpoint, 19-21 mm lateral to the midline, and at a depth of 5–6 mm below the intercommissural plane.

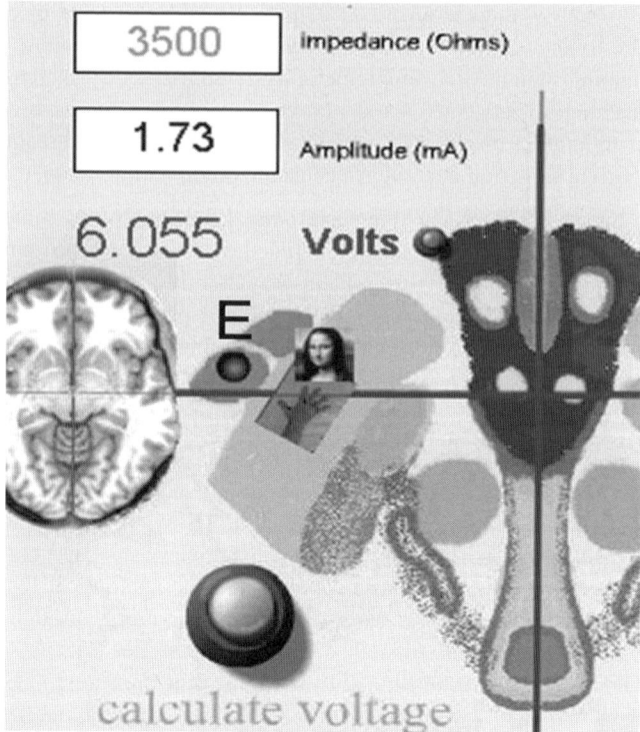

Fig. 1. Relation between the electrode (E), placed in the globus pallidus internus (GPi), and motor fibres of the internal capsule as they look on screen in a neurophysiological electrode placement program.

Through a precoronary paramedian burr hole, a rigid cannula was inserted up to 10 mm from the target. A quadripolar DBS electrode (DBS-3389, Medtronic Inc) was inserted in the ventroposterolateral part of the GPi and secured in the burr hole by a flange. The burr hole was then filled with a biological glue to obtain initial fixation of the electrode and to reduce the risk of CSF leakage. Early postoperative CT was undertaken to exclude surgical complications and to define the electrode placement by merging with the preoperative MRI (Fig. 2) (Ferroli et al., 2004). In the same surgical session, the electrodes were connected to a pulse generator (Itrel II, Soletra, Medtronic Inc) placed subcutaneously in the subclavicular or paraumbilical area.

Stimulation was started the day after surgery. In accordance with the standard practice of our group, unipolar stimulation was used in each patient, the active contact being the more distal one. The initial setting of the stimulation parameters was as follows: amplitude 1.0 V, pulse width 90 µs, frequency 130–185 Hz. These parameters were subsequently adjusted individually according to the clinical response at each follow-up visit.

Results

The postoperative BFMRS showed a mean improvement ranging between 0 and 90 per cent (mean 48 per cent) (Fig. 3). The response was delayed and appeared after a period ranging between 1 week and 2 months. Amelioration of symptoms increased progressively with time. Significant clinical improvement was observed in the first month in 70 per cent of the cases, and in the whole group within the first year. Two patients also continued to improve in the

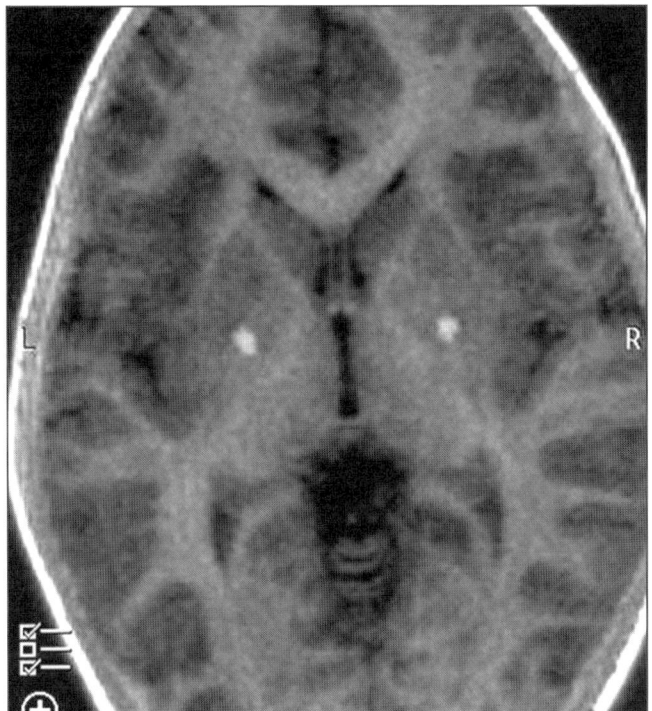

Fig. 2. Image obtained by fusion of preoperative magnetic resonance image and postoperative computed tomography. The image shows bilateral placement of electrodes in the posteroventral part of the globus pallidus internus.

second year following surgery. A reduction in slowness of movement and improvement in the muscle tone abnormality was observed in all patients. Axial dystonic postures and movements responded to DBS to a greater extent than oromandibular dystonia, fixed dystonic postures, or task-specific dystonias (such as writing dystonia). At the most recent follow-up, the clinical results were stable. One patient affected by symptomatic dystonia showed only transient improvement during the first month after surgery, and by the end of the follow-up period no benefit was observed. Cranial MRI confirmed the correct positioning of the electrodes. When stimulation was turned off, the patient subjectively experienced a worsening of symptoms, so it was decided to continue stimulation. DBS was effective in all patients who had suffered status dystonicus. Three patients showed complete disappearance of rapid hyperkinesias within the first week after surgery, so that discontinuation of sedation and ventilation was possible. In two patients, the improvement was slowly progressive. Discontinuation of sedation was possible within 3 months after surgery. After the disappearance of the status dystonicus, three of the five patients had improvements in their pre-existing clinical condition (before status dystonicus) ranging between 10 per cent and 38 per cent (mean 25 per cent) (Fig. 4).

In our series we observed two types of complication. The first was hardware-related, with migration of the electrode in three cases and pulse generator failure in six. The second was related to the surgical procedure, with infection in four cases (subcutaneous in three and sited around the electrode tip in one), and an intracranial haemorrhage around the electrode trajectory in one case. All the reported complications were successfully managed by replacement of the hardware or antibiotic treatment.

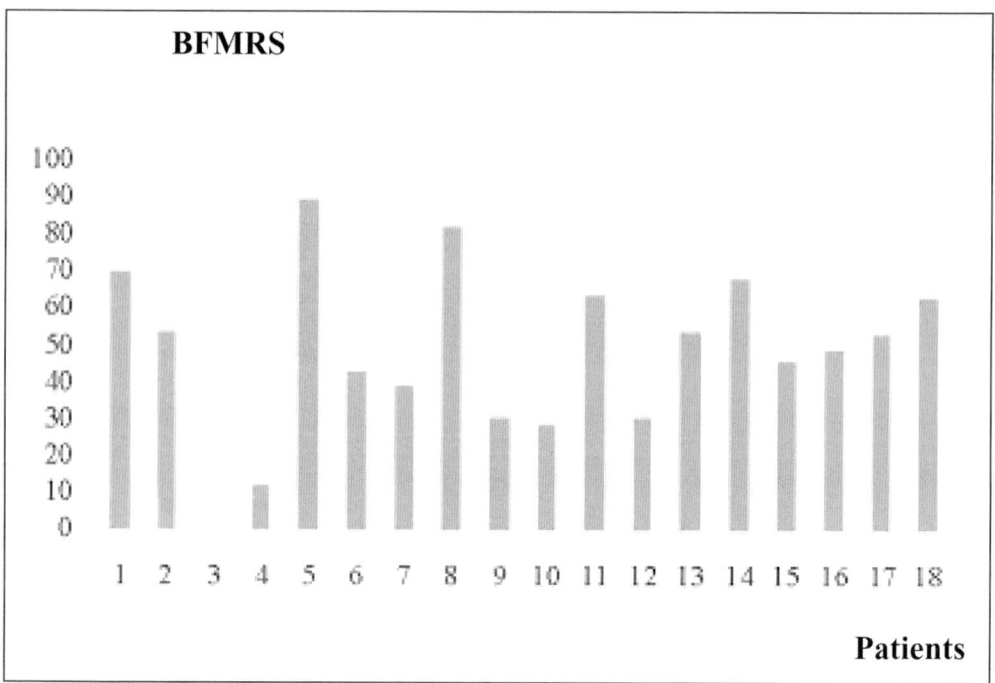

Fig. 3. Results of childhood-onset dystonia series after a mean follow-up of 2 years (patients with status dystonicus are not included).

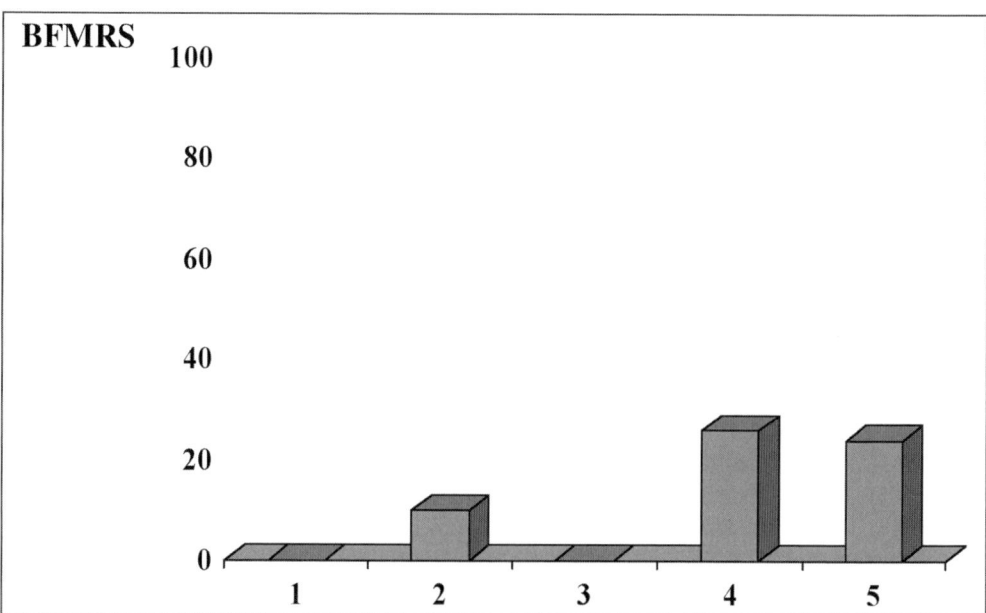

Fig. 4. Status dystonicus series treated by deep brain stimulation. After a mean follow up of 2 years from resolution of status dystonicus, an improvement in the pre-existing clinical condition (pre-status dystonicus) was observed in three patients. BFMRS, Burke-Fahn-Marsden dystonia rating scale.

Comment

In our series, DBS caused marked improvement of dystonia in all but one patient. This technique was particularly effective for axial and limb dystonic postures and movements, while oromandibular dystonia and fixed dystonic postures were modified to a lesser extent. The greatest benefit was observed in patients with primary dystonia, tardive dystonia, and status dystonicus; however, significant improvement was also observed in patients with symptomatic dystonia (Franzini et al., 2005; Zorzi et al., 2005) On the basis of our findings we also suggest that, besides aetiology, the type and distribution of dystonia may also influence the efficacy of DBS. While the reasons of DBS resistance remain to be clarified, it is important to report these cases for an accurate evaluation of the efficacy of DBS in dystonia. Furthermore, the patients of our series with smaller improvements had long disease durations with fixed dystonic postures and skeletal deformities, indicating that DBS must be considered at an early stage of the disease (Zorzi et al., 2005). Even without a statistically significant correlation between the duration of symptoms and outcome, we suggest that early surgery is necessary to avoid muscle contractures and skeletal deformities.

To our knowledge, apart from our reported series there has only been one report of DBS for the treatment of status dystonicus, which is a rare condition occurring in patients with various kinds of dystonia. The pathophysiology of this potentially life-threatening condition is unknown. Possible precipitating factors include intercurrent infections or discontinuation of therapy, but in most cases no cause is identifiable. Patients need intensive care unit management plus ventilation. They often develop metabolic complications such as rhabdomyolysis, and death is not infrequent. Hence DBS should be considered for the treatment of status dystonicus when conventional drugs are ineffective.

In conclusion, our data provide further evidence of the safety and efficacy of DBS in the treatment of childhood-onset dystonia of different aetiologies. Many issues remain to be clarified, such as the long-term effect of DBS, the selection criteria for patients in relation to the aetiology and the type of dystonia, and the timing of surgery. Further studies on larger series of patients are needed.

Video – Illustrative cases

Patient 1 (video 3, tracks 1 + 2) – A 7-year-old patient affected by DYT1 dystonia, two years from the onset. He has a generalized dystonia sparing the cranial muscles. Dystonic posturing of arms and dystonic movement of the right arm are evident. While standing, dystonia of the trunk and dystonic movement of the left limb are present. After 1 year from pallidal deep brain stimulation, he shows only slight dystonic posturing of arms and mild walking dystonia.

Patient 2 (video 3, tracks 3 + 4) – Patient affected by non-DYT1 primary dystonia. At the age of 6, one year from the onset of the disease, he shows a generalized dystonia mainly involving the axis and upper limbs. It is evident that a sensory trick is able to reduce the retrocollis.

The same patient after two years from pallidal deep brain stimulation: dystonia has markedly improved, and only slight dystonia of upper limbs and writing dystonia are left.

Patient 3 (video 3, tracks 5 + 6) – Patient affected by symptomatic dystonia associated with bilateral basal ganglia calcification. At the age of 12, he presented severe dystonia involving cranial muscles, trunk and upper limbs; dystonia is more evident on action and during walking.

At the age of 18, 4 years after pallidal deep brain stimulation, he shows a complete resolution of dystonia of the trunk and a great amelioration of arms dystonia.

Patient 4 (video 3, tracks 7 + 8) – An 8-year-old patient affected by non-DYT1 primary dystonia showing a status dystonicus. Continuous generalized dystonic movements, also involving cranial muscles, associated with more rapid, irregular hyperkinesias of variable amplitude are evident.

One week after pallidal deep brain stimulation, the dystonic movements and hyperkinesias have completely resolved.

References

Abosch, A. & Lozano, A. (2003): Stereotactic neurosurgery for movement disorders. *Can. J. Neurol. Sci.* **30** (Suppl. 1), S72–S82.

Benabid, A.L., Benazzous, A. & Pollak, P. (2002): Mechanisms of deep brain stimulation. *Mov. Disord.* **17** (Suppl. 3), S63–S68.

Coubes, P., Roubertie, A., Vayssiere, N., Hemm, S. & Echenne, B. (2000): Treatment of DYT1-generalised dystonia by stimulation of the internal globus pallidus. *Lancet* **355**, 2220–2221.

Fahn, S., Bressman, S. & Marsden, C.D. (1998): Classification of dystonia. *Adv. Neurol.* **78**, 1–10.

Ferroli, P., Franzini, A., Marras, C., Maccagnano, E., D'Incerti, L. & Broggi, G. (2004): A simple method to assess accuracy of deep brain stimulation electrode placement: pre-operative stereotactic CT + postoperative MR image fusion. *Stereotact. Funct. Neurosurg.* **82**, 14–19.

Franzini, A., Marras, C., Ferroli, P., Zorzi, G., Bugiani, O., Romito, L. & Broggi G. (2005): Long-term high-frequency bilateral pallidal stimulation for neuroleptic-induced tardive dystonia. Report of two cases. *J. Neurosurg.* **102**, 721–725.

Laitinen, L.V. (2004): Personal memories of the history of stereotactic neurosurgery. *Neurosurgery* **55**, 1420–1429.

Manji, H., Howard, R.S., Miller, D.H., Hirsch, N.P., Carr, L., Bhatia, K., Quinn, N. & Marsden, C.D. (1998): Status dystonicus: the syndrome and its management. *Brain* **121**, 243–252.

Rosenow, J., Das, K., Rovit, R.L. & Couldwell, W.T. (2002): Irving S. Cooper and his role in intracranial stimulation for movement disorders and epilepsy. *Stereotac. Funct. Neurosurg.* **78**, 95–112.

Vilensky, J.A., Sinish, P.R., Stone, J.L. & Gilman, S. (2005): The publications of Sir Victor Horsley: a listing and an assessment. *Neurosurgery* **57**, 581–584.

Zorzi, G., Marras, C., Nardocci, N., Franzini, A., Chiapparini, L., Maccagnano, E., Angelini, L., Caldiroli, D. & Broggi, G. (2005): Stimulation of the globus pallidus internus for childhood-onset dystonia. *Mov. Disord.* **20**, 1194–2000.

Chapter 10

Dopa-responsive dystonias/dyskinesias (DRDs): diagnosis and monitoring of the treatment

Vincenzo Leuzzi*, Teresa Giovanniello°, Carla Carducci°, Claudia Carducci° and Italo Antonozzi°

*Department of Psychiatric, Rehabilitative and Neurological Sciences of Developmental Age, University 'La Sapienza', via dei Sabelli 108, 00185 Rome, Italy;
°Department of Experimental Medicine and Pathology, University 'La Sapienza', viale Regina Elena 324, 00161 Rome, Italy
Vincenzo.Leuzzi@uniroma1.it

Summary

DOPA-responsive dystonias (DRD) form a heterogeneous group of syndromes characterized by biogenic amine synthesis deficiency. The phenotypic variability of these conditions, at a biochemical as well as a genetic level, makes the diagnosis difficult in many patients. The presence of hyperphenylalaninaemia is the principal diagnostic discriminator. Hyperphenylalaninaemia is present when an enzymatic disorder affects the liver enzyme phenylalanine hydroxylase, through involvement of cofactor BH4 biosynthesis/regeneration. Disorders that are not associated with hyperphenylalaninaemia are caused by deficiency of enzymes expressed mostly in the substantia nigra pars compacta (SNC) [tyrosine hydroxylase (TH), tryptophan hydroxylase (TPH)], or by the partial enzyme deficit involved in the synthesis of BH4, the consequences of which are limited to the SNC [GTP cyclohydrolase (GTP-CH)]. Responsiveness to L-DOPA treatment is suggestive but not diagnostic. Assay of biogenic amine metabolites and pterins in the liquor amnii remains the main diagnostic tool for the diagnosis of DRDs. A distinctive pattern of pterin and biogenic amine alterations suggests the presence of a specific disorder causing DRDs.

The disturbance of enzyme activity can be examined when the enzymes are expressed in the peripheral tissues, when their activity can be estimated [dihydropteridine reductase (DHPR), aromatic L-amino acid decarboxylase (AADC), 6-pyruvoyl-tetrahydropterin synthase (PTPS), GTP-CH, and sepiapterin reductase (SPR)]; however, some others cannot be studied (TH, TPH) because they are not expressed peripherally.

The metabolic pattern of CSF biogenic amines may also suggest the need for molecular genetic studies, though in a substantial proportion of subjects, mutations (GTP-CH deficit) cannot be found. Many patients suffering from DRD remain without an aetiological diagnosis in spite of extensive investigations. Nevertheless, several proteins involved in the synthesis and regulation of biogenic amines have still not been linked to any disease.

The aim of pharmacological treatment is to replete the biogenic amine deficit through oral supplementation with metabolic precursors (L-DOPA, 5-hydroxytryptophan), combined with the administration of drugs that limit the catabolism of the precursors and so increase their bioavailability.

Introduction

'Nine cases, including six familial cases, presented in this paper had dystonic posture and movements with onset in childhood. Although symptoms and evolutionary patterns were almost the same as those of DMD [*dystonia musculorum deformans*] there was a marked diurnal fluctuation of the symptoms. Even though the symptoms were progressive, they were alleviated completely by L-dopa...' (Segawa et al., 1976). This first description in the English literature of dopa-responsive dystonia (DRD) by Segawa and collaborators includes the main features of the disease: the hereditary pattern, precocious onset, progression of the disorder, diurnal fluctuation of the symptoms, and their complete responsiveness to L-dopa.

At about the same time but in a different field, other investigators (Bartholomé et al., 1975; Leeming & Smith, 1979) reported the first cases of 'malignant phenylketonuria (PKU)', referring to new forms of hyperphenylalaninaemia that were unresponsive to a phenylalanine-restricted diet and originated from a defect of synthesis or regeneration of tetrahydrobiopterine (BH4) – the cofactor of phenylalanine hydroxylase. Although these conditions presented a more severe phenotype than that reported by Segawa, were transmitted with a different hereditary pattern (autosomal recessive), and required a more complex therapeutic approach, they shared with the former the responsiveness to L-dopa. In 1994 such different clinical entities turned out to belong to a common family of disorders (Ichinose et al., 1994), when the genetic background of the syndrome of Segawa was ascribed to a disorder of the gene codifying for the enzyme guanosine triphosphate cyclohydrolase (GTP-CH) – the limiting enzyme in the synthesis of BH4. Starting from this seminal description, in the following few years a nosography of the genetic disorders of the dopaminergic system was proposed (Table 1). Not all the disorders included in Table 1 are responsive to L-dopa treatment, and only some of them manifest movement disorders (for a review, see De Vivo & Johnston, 2003). Moreover, further studies are necessary for a better understanding of the disorders associated with the defects of enzymes involved in the catabolism and transport of biogenic amines or with biogenic amine receptor defects.

Table 1. Disorders of monoamine neurotransmission

1. Disorders of BH4 synthesis and regeneration
2. Defects of the enzymes of monoamine biosynthesis
3. Defects of dopamine transport
4. Defects of dopamine catabolism
5. Defects of dopamine receptors

The L-dopa-responsive forms are classified as generalized or CNS-confined. If an enzyme disorder directly affects the liver enzyme phenylalanine hydroxylase, or affects it indirectly through involvement of biosynthesis/regeneration of cofactor BH4, this results in hyperphenylalaninaemia (Table 1). The presence of this biochemical marker is essential from a diagnostic point of view: patients with hyperphenylalaninaemia are detected by neonatal screening in a presymptomatic phase and undergo a specific diagnostic protocol aimed at detecting the disorders of cofactor metabolism. On the other hand, disorders that are not associated with hyperphenylalaninaemia are usually found in symptomatic subjects whose condition may evoke a number of different primary or secondary dystonias, thus requiring a more complex diagnostic work-up. The present review concerns the diagnosis of this last group of dopa-responsive disorders (Table 2).

Table 2. Genetic disorders of dopamine synthesis

Generalized disorders of BH4 metabolism (with HPA)	AR GTP-CH deficiency PTPS deficiency DHPR deficiency
CNS-confined disorders (without HPA)	AD and AR GTPCH deficiency PTPS deficiency SPR deficiency TH deficiency

AD, autosomal dominant; AR, autosomal recessive; CNS, central nervous system; DHPR, dihydropteridine reductase; GTP-CH, guanosine triphosphate cyclohydrolase; HPA, hyperphenylalaninaemia; PTPS, 6-pyruvoyl-tetrahydropterin synthase; SPR, sepiapterin reductase; TH, tyrosine hydroxylase.

Focusing on the disorders in Table 2, autosomal recessive GTP-CH deficiency is, as a general rule, associated with hyperphenylalaninaemia. However, phenylalanine has been reported to be normal in patients homozygous (Hwu et al., 1999; Nardocci et al., 2003) or compound heterozygous (Furukawa et al., 1998) for mutations on the *CGH1* gene. Also, autosomal recessive 6-pyruvoyl-tetrahydropterin synthase (PTPS) deficiency usually results in hyperphenylalaninaemia. Nevertheless the occurrence of an isolated central form of PTPS deficiency has been demonstrated (Blau et al., 2000), and because of a slight increase in phenylalanine, some patients may be misdiagnosed as having a mild defect of phenylalanine hydroxylase and discharged without an estimation of urinary pterins (Fiori et al., 2004).

Most of the disorders present with a heterogeneous clinical picture which includes the symptoms listed in Table 3, which vary according to the age of onset, the age of the patient, and the severity of the disease. One may conclude that disorders of neurotransmitter metabolism should be suspected in any child presenting with an encephalopathy and with normal neuroimaging where the illness cannot be ascribed to any alternative aetiology.

Table 3. Symptoms in dopa-responsive dystonias

- Prematurity
- Microcephaly
- Poor sucking
- ⇓ Spontaneous movements
- Floppiness (limb hypertonia, truncal hypotonia)
- Irritability, drowsiness, lethargy
- Temperature instability
- Pinpoint pupils, ptosis
- Infantile myoclonic epilepsy/epileptic encephalopathy
- Developmental delay
- Progressive mental retardation
- Neurological deterioration
- Hypokinesia
- Rigidity
- Distal chorea
- Hypersalivation
- ⇓ Somatic growth
- Swallowing difficulties
- Pyramidal tract dysfunction (spastic diplegia)
- Dystonia (± diurnal fluctuation)
- Myoclonus-dystonia syndrome
- MRI: normal/WM abnormalities/brain calcification (DHPR)/cerebral atrophy

DHPR, dihydropteridine reductase; MRI, magnetic resonance imaging; WM, white matter.

The pathways of biogenic amine synthesis and the enzymes which, if defective, result in L-dopa-responsive dystonia-dyskinesia syndromes are shown in Fig. 1. Table 4 gives the different diagnostic options for the diagnosis of these disorders, ordered by increasing complexity, specificity, and cost.

L-dopa trial

Responsiveness to L-dopa administration was a critical diagnostic marker in the first description of the Segawa syndrome. However, though attractive and inexpensive as a diagnostic test, the assessment of clinical improvement after this drug has several limitations. For example, the dose for the test has not been standardized; in a suspect case of classical Segawa syndrome in a young adult patient, a dose of ~ 10 mg/kg body weight (bw)/day of L-dopa combined with a peripheral inhibitor of aromatic amino-acid decarboxylase (benzerazide or carbidopa, 1.0 to 2.5 mg/kg bw/day) is suggested. In younger subjects, or in patients suffering from enzymatic disorders different from autosomal dominant GTP-CH deficit, the dosage should be lower. According to our experience, L-dopa is not well tolerated during the first years of life, often resulting in irritability, dosage peak myclonias and chorea, anorexia with loss of weight, regurgitation and diarrhoea, sleep disorders, and so on. The appearance of these symptoms can cause interruption of the pharmacological test before a definite clinical result can be observed. Moreover, in the case of a severely affected young patient, the pressure to make a definitive diagnosis is often not compatible with the time required for an L-dopa trial. Moreover, responsiveness to L-dopa is not a specific diagnostic test for disorders of biogenic amine metabolism, as other diseases such as juvenile parkinsonism may, at their onset, show a marked response to L-dopa treatment (Furukawa et al., 1996).

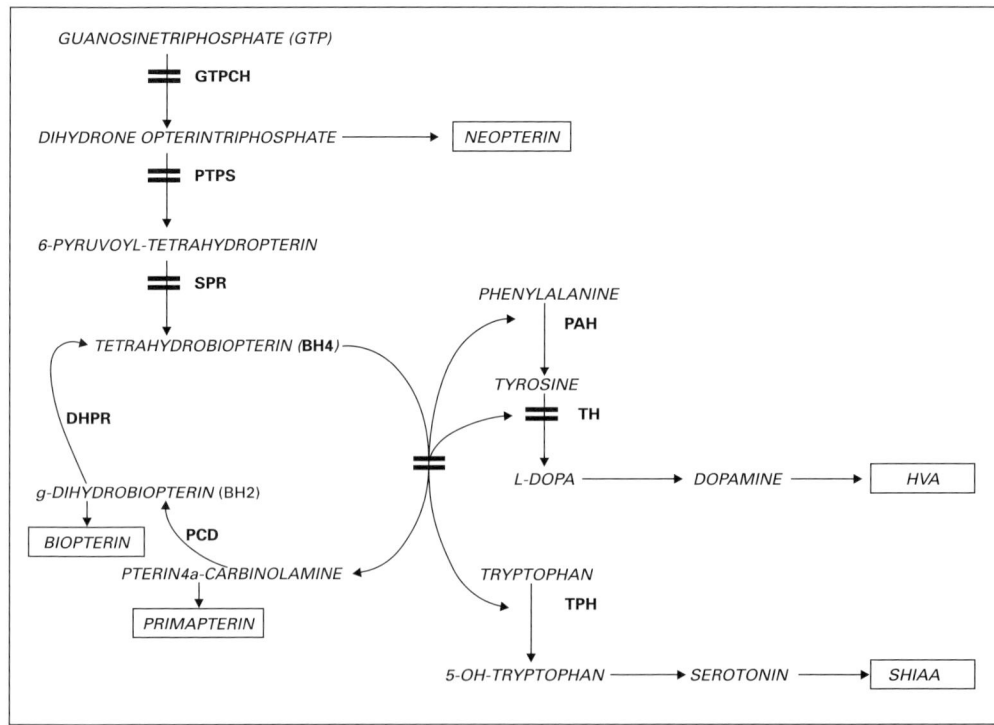

Fig. 1. Metabolic pathway. Biosynthesis of tetrahydrobiopterin and biogenic amines.

Table 4. Diagnostic options for dopa-responsive dystonias

- L-dopa test
- Blood prolactin assessment
- Pterin analysis in urine
- Phenylalanine loading test
- CSF analysis (pterins and biogenic amine metabolites)
- Genetic analysis
- Enzymatic assay

Prolactin assessment

Dopamine is the most important prolactin-inhibiting factor, and prolactin secretion is feedback-regulated through D2 receptors. Prolactin is released in a pulsatile manner, with 13 to 14 peaks a day and an interpulse interval of about 95 minutes. The main pulse amplitude represents a 58 per cent increase above the preceding nadir (Veldhuis & Johnson, 1998). Prolactin levels show a marked circadian variation with the maximum increase and decrease 4 hours after the onset of sleep (approximately 160 per cent of the 24-hour mean) and 6 hours after waking (40 per cent of the 24-hour mean), respectively (Frantz, 1978). The upper limit of the normal range is considered to be 500 mU/L (15 γ/L or 15 ng/mL) or, according to others, 800 mU/L (25 γg/L) (Bevan, 1991). Neuroendocrine dopaminergic neurons have a daily rhythm complementary to the prolactin rhythm (Freeman *et al.*, 2000). An increase in blood prolactin is reported in various neurotransmitter disorders affecting dopamine synthesis, such as PTPS, dihydropteridine reductase (DHPR) deficiency, and tyrosine hydroxylase (TH) deficiency (Birnbacher *et al.*, 1998; Blau *et al.*, 2001). In others [autosomal dominant (AD) and autosomal recessive GTP-CH and sepiapterin reductase (SPR) deficiencies], prolactin has not yet been systematically explored. In Parkinson's disease and other neurodegenerative disorders involving the dopaminergic system, prolactin remains normal.

In conclusion, prolactin assessment is an inexpensive, first-line test for brain dopamine defect. An increase in blood prolactin should alert one to a possible disorder of dopamine metabolism, but a normal prolactin does not rule out a DRD syndrome.

Phenylalanine loading test

The phenylalanine loading test was proposed by Hyland (Hyland *et al.*, 1997) as a possible non-invasive test for the diagnosis of dopa-responsive dystonia. The aim of the test is to detect a deficiency of BH4 synthesis by stressing hepatic (BH4-dependent) phenylalanine hydroxylase activity (Fig. 1) by oral loading with phenylalanine (100 mg/kg body weight). Blood is collected before phenylalanine administration and every hour for the 6 hours following the loading. Phenylalanine hydroxylase activity is assessed as the phenylalanine-to-tyrosine ratio (Phe/Tyr) at 4 hours after loading. Different values of the Phe/Tyr ratio have been reported as the critical threshold for diagnosis – for example: 4.5 (Saunders-Pullman *et al.*, 2000); 7.5 (Bandamann *et al.*, 2003); and 5.25 (Saunders-Pullman *et al.*, 2004). Figure 2 shows the trend of the Phe/Tyr ratio observed in normal controls and affected individuals. Our data suggest that the ratios obtained in the second and third hours may be most sensitive for detecting a defect in tyrosine synthesis and highlight the need for a more systematic study of diagnostic cut-off values. Moreover, although the sensitivity and specificity of the test is high, two false-negative cases (Saunders-Pullman *et al.*, 2004) and one false-positive case (Bandamann *et al.*, 2003) have been reported. To improve the reliability of the test, a peak blood phenylalanine value of

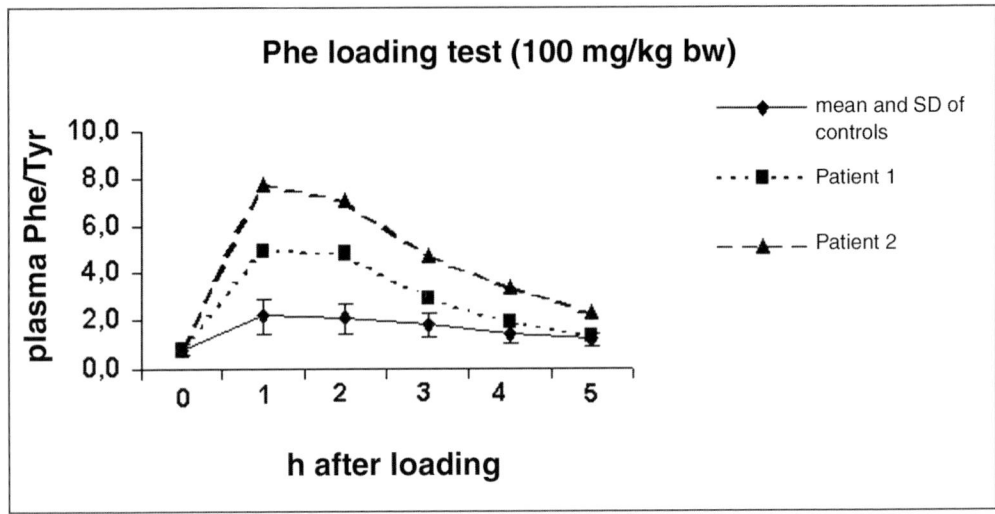

Fig. 2. The results of a phenylalanine loading test in two patients expressed as the phenylalanine to tyrosine ratio (Phe/Tyr), showing the effect of autosomal dominant GCH1 deficiency (genotype: patient 1, c.671A>G; patient 2, c.68C>T), and in a normal subject.

> 600 γmol/L coupled with evaluation of blood BH4 during the loading test (BH4 should rise as a result of the increase in blood phenylalanine) have been proposed (Saunders-Pullman et al., 2004). Finally, molecular analysis of the phenylalanine hydroxylase gene could improve the specificity of the test by excluding heterozygous carriers of phenylalanine hydroxylase mutations (about 1/100 in the general population). These additional examinations increase the cost of the test and reduce its practicality. Another obvious limiting factor is that the phenylalanine loading test is only capable of exploring defects in BH4 metabolism.

CSF examination

The assay of pterins and biogenic amine metabolites in the CSF is the gold standard for the diagnosis of DRDs. It allows the detection and full characterization of each disorder on the most appropriate metabolic grounds and thus makes it possible to carry out enzymatic and genetic studies in a specific direction. Moreover, it provides the metabolic coordinates for targeting the treatment and, with a clinical phenotype, is the basis for any genotype-phenotype correlations.

For the diagnosis of DRDs, the metabolites usually assessed in CSF are as follows:
- *neopterin*, the oxidation product of dihydroneopterine triphosphate, which reflects the activity of GTP-CH;
- *biopterin* (the oxidation product of q-dihydrobiopterin, 7,8-dihydrobiopterin, and BH4), which is a marker for BH4 synthesis and results from GTP-CH, PTPS, and SPR activities; it also denotes the regeneration activity (DHPR) of BH4, the intermediate products of which are q-dihydrobiopterin and 7,8-dihydrobiopterin (Fig. 1);
- *sepiapterin*, which is the disease marker of SPR deficiency (Zorzi et al., 2002);
- *homovanillic acid* (HVA), *3-methoxy-4-hydroxyphenylglycol* (MHPG), and *5-hydroxyindoleacetic acid* (5HIAA), which are catabolic products of dopamine, noradrenaline, and serotonin, respectively, and act as markers of these metabolites.

Table 5 summarizes the different patterns of pterin and biogenic amine alterations associated with each disorder causing DRDs. These patterns can be deduced from the knowledge of normal metabolic pathways, as schematised in Fig. 1.

GTP-CH is the initial and limiting step in the synthesis of BH4, and a defect in the enzyme results in a reduction in the concentrations of all pterins and dopamine and serotonin metabolites (HVA > 5HIAA). In the most severe form *(autosomal recessive GTP-CH deficiency)* neopterin and biopterin are both markedly reduced in the CSF (0.05 to 3 and 1.5 to 7.5 nmol/L, respectively; reference values, 9 to 35 and 10 to 70, respectively), as well as HVA and 5HIAA.

In *autosomal dominant GTP-CH1*, the pattern of metabolic alteration is the same though milder. Neopterin and biopterin are usually – but not invariably (Leuzzi *et al.*, 2002) – normal in the urine and reduced in the CSF (1.1 to 6.2 and 3.1 to 7.6 nmol/L, respectively). HVA and 5HIAA are mildly reduced in the CSF.

PTPS deficiency features high concentrations of neopterin, ranging from 5.0 to 51.2 mmol/mol creatine and only traces of biopterin (< 0.5 mmol/mol creatine) in urine and CSF (47 to 402 and 1.0 to 16.0 nmol/L, respectively), coupled with low levels of HVA and 5HIAA in the CSF (Hyland, 2003b).

In *SPR deficiency* (Bonafé *et al.*, 2001b), CSF neopterin is normal or high (14 to 51 nmol/L) while biopterin is definitely high (72 to 102 nmol/L), with a predominance of 7,8-dihydrobiopterin (BH2). Sepiapterin was assessed in two subjects and found to be high [5.6 and 11.4 nmol/L (normal < 0.5) (Zorzi *et al.*, 2002)]. Both HVA and 5HIAA are low in the CSF (Bonafé *et al.*, 2001b).

Finally in *TH deficiency*, pterins are normal in the urine and CSF, as is 5HIAA, while HVA and MHPG are selectively low (Hoffmann *et al.*, 2003).

Collection of CSF samples requires a meticulous technique to avoid possible blood contamination and the oxidation of neurotransmitter metabolites (immediate freezing of CSF in dry ice is necessary) (Hyland *et al.*, 1993). Moreover, as the concentration of biogenic amines have a rostro-caudal gradient, the first aliquot of CSF should be used for chemical analysis, while the last fractioned aliquot should be reserved for amine assessment (Hyland, 2003a).

Table 5. The patterns of pterin and biogenic amine metabolites in different dopa-responsive dystonias

Defect	CSF metabolite concentrations						
	Biopterin	BH2	Neopterin	Sepiapterin	HVA	5HIAA	HVA/5HIAA
AD GTP-CH	↓	N	↓	N	±↓	±↓	±↓
AR GTP-CH	↓↓	N	↓↓	N	↓	↓	↓↓↓
PTPS	↓	N	↑↑	N	↓	↓	↓↓
SPR	↑	↑	N↑	↓	↓	↓↓	
TH	N	N	N	N	↓↓	N	↓↓↓↓

AD, autosomal dominant; AR, autosomal recessive; BH2, dihydrobiopterin; GTP-CH, guanosine triphosphate cyclohydrolase; HVA, homovanillic acid; N, normal; PTPS, 6-pyruvoyl-tetrahydropterin synthase; SPR, sepiapterin reductase; TH, tyrosine hydroxylase; 5HIAA, 5-hydroxyindoleacetic acid.

Limitations of CSF analysis

CSF sampling is an invasive procedure and not easily repeatable in children. Conflicting results can arise from concurrent viral infections (the CSF neopterin concentration increases during viral infections) or as a result of drug administration. Moreover, the interpretation of borderline values – sometimes found in the mildest forms of enzyme defects – can be difficult and may require the examination of a second sample.

Finally, shipping frozen CSF to the few reference laboratories capable of undertaking this examination implies further risk as far as the reliability of the results is concerned.

Molecular analysis

The *GCH1*, *PTPS*, *SPR*, and *TH* genes have been characterized, cloned, and sequenced. There is a great alleleic heterogeneity and a high rate of spontaneous mutation, especially in the *GCH1* gene (Ichinose *et al.*, 1999). Although genetic analysis remains the best confirmatory diagnostic test when the clinical presentation of a disease is associated with a specific biochemical alteration, the diagnostic approach to DRDs cannot be based on the results of genetic analyses for several reasons. First, in a substantial number of DRD patients, genetic analysis fails to detect alterations in the candidate gene (*GCH1* gene alterations cannot be found in as many as 40 per cent of individuals affected by autosomal dominant DRD). Second, only some of the patients have been studied at the RNA or protein level (Hirano *et al.*, 1996); where a mutation is not found in either the coding region or the exon-intron boundaries, it may lie in the untranslated or regulatory regions of the gene (Segawa *et al.*, 2003). Finally, a large genomic deletion of one or more exons of the gene can occur. With respect to the other disorders, seven of 20 cases of autosomal recessive GTP-CH deficiency, 44 of 298 cases of PTPS deficiency, and seven of 14 cases of SPR deficiency have so far been characterized at the genetic level (Figs. 3-7).

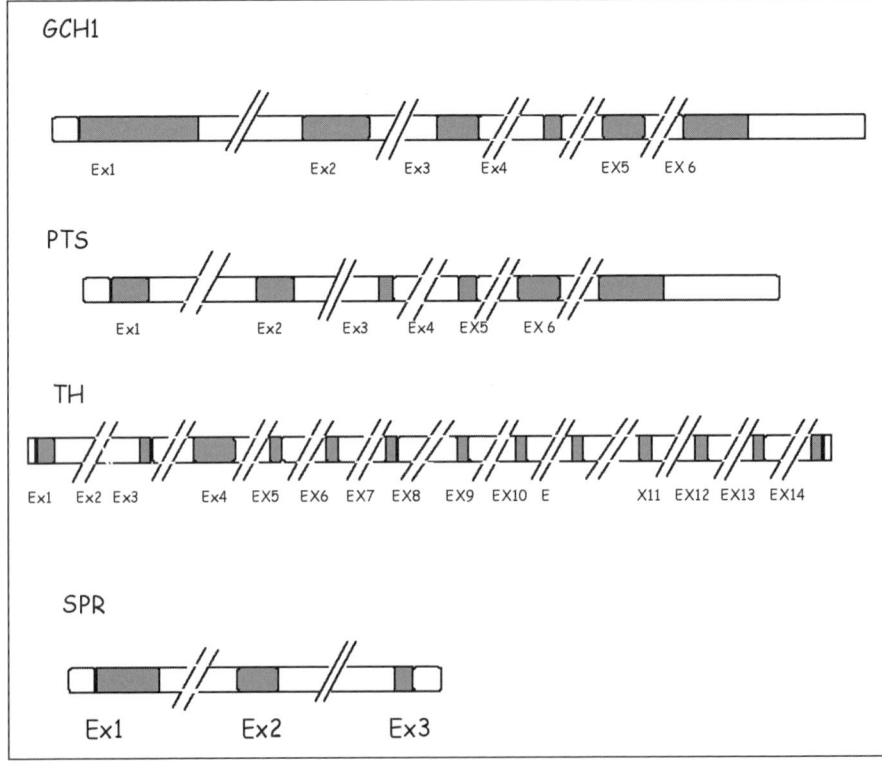

Fig. 3. Genomic structure of GCH1, PTS, TH and SPR genes.

Chapter 10   Dopa-responsive dystonias/dyskinesias (DRDs): diagnosis and monitoring of the treatment

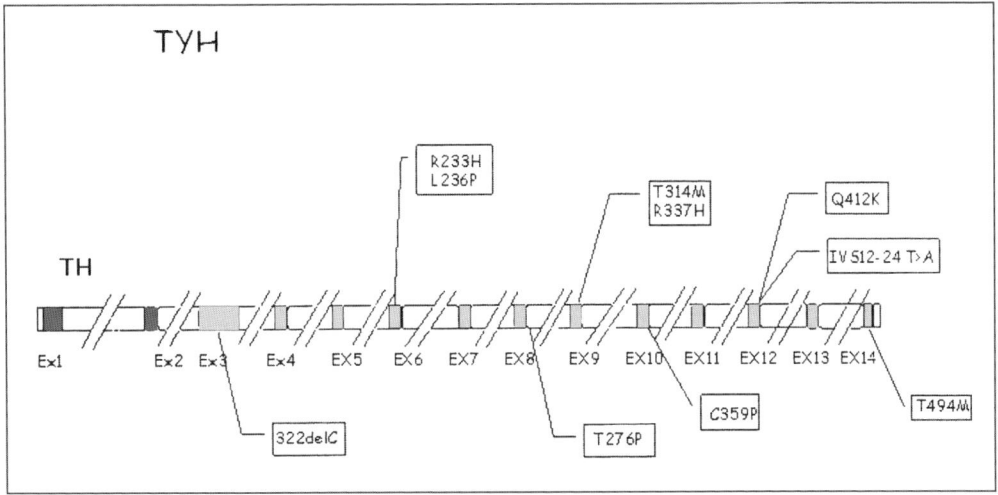

Fig. 4. Genomic structure and mutation detected in human TH gene. Mutations are listed in HGMD (http://www.hgmd.cf.ac.uk).

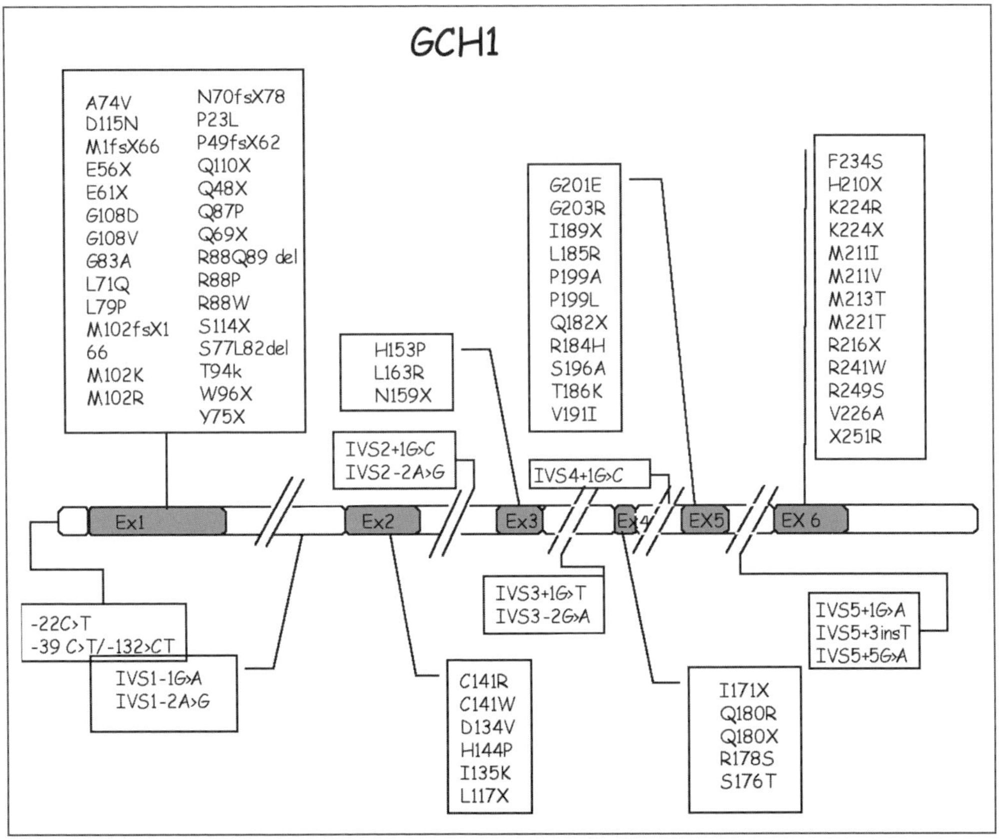

Fig. 5. Genomic structure and mutation detected in human GCH1 gene. Mutations are listed in HGMD (http://www.hgmd.cf.ac.uk).

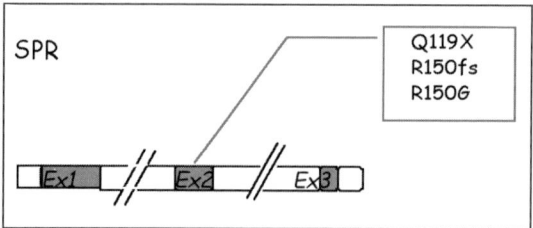

Fig. 6. Genomic structure and mutation detected in human SPR gene. Mutations are listed in HGMD (http://www.hgmd.cf.ac.uk).

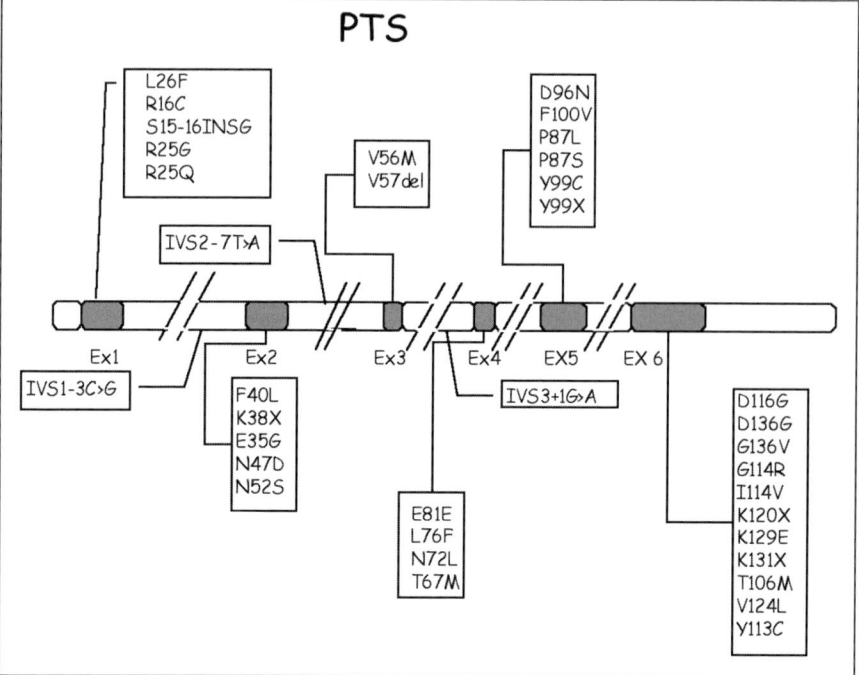

Fig. 7. Genomic structure and mutation detected in human PTS gene. Mutations are listed in HGMD (http://www.hgmd.cf.ac.uk).

All 21 TH-deficient patients reported so far have had their mutations on the TH gene, encompassing a mutation in the promoter region of the gene. Nevertheless, we have observed several patients with clinical and CSF patterns suggestive of TH deficiency in whom no mutations on the TH gene were found.

Enzymatic activity

The activity of GTPCH1, PTPS, and SPR can be assessed in cytokine-stimulated (GTP-CH) and unstimulated (PTPS, SPR) fibroblasts (Bonafé et al., 2001a). As a TH assay in accessible material is not available at present, CSF analysis and the identification of DNA mutations remains the only way to confirm the diagnosis of TH deficiency. For the other diseases, the assay of enzymatic activity is an important tool for exploring the link between genotype and the biochemical phenotype. However, from a diagnostic point of view, this should be reserved for the small number of cases in whom no mutation has been found on the candidate gene or where the pathogenic value of a previously unreported genetic alteration needs to be substantiated. A further limiting factor is that very few laboratories around the world are at present capable of undertaking this analysis. Figure 7 shows the result of GTP-CH activity assessed in a patient with Segawa disease, compared with a normal control.

As for other neurological conditions caused by inherited metabolic alterations, DRDs show an intrinsic fluctuation of symptoms which can sometimes complicate the assessment of pharmacological treatment. The pharmacokinetics of dopaminergic drugs also contribute to this clinical fluctuation, making evaluation of treatment difficult. Clinical observation before and during treatment remains crucial in evaluating the efficacy of treatment in most patients with DRDs. In subjects with classical autosomal dominant Segawa disease the response to treatment is usually striking and clinical improvement reliably reflects the effect of the treatment. This is also true for milder late-onset forms of autosomal recessive Segawa disease (TH and SPR defects). On the other hand, the clinical evaluation of treatment may not be straightforward in patients with the early-onset severe forms of TH and PTPS deficiency. In these individuals the need to restore the biogenic amines quickly is sometimes not compatible with the time required to detect an unequivocal clinical improvement. Moreover, young patients do not tolerate the precursors of biogenic amines well, and suffer from on/off phenomena, peak-dose dyskinesias, marked irritability, sleep disorders, vomiting and diarrhoea with resulting loss of weight, and so on – all of which can hamper the attainment of an adequate therapeutic dose of the drugs. In these situations other biological markers must be monitored to check for the restoration of biogenic amines in the CNS. Prolactin levels decrease as the central dopaminergic status improves and so can reflect the efficacy of the pharmacological treatment (Spada et al., 1996). Prolactin concentrations are decreased by D2-receptor agonists such as bromocriptine and pramipexole but without necessarily resulting in clinical improvement. Nevertheless, assessment of serum prolactin combined with careful clinical observation may be a useful marker of the restoration of biogenic amines in the CNS. Serial CSF assessment of biogenic amine metabolites is certainly the most direct approach to evaluating the effect of pharmacological treatment. Being an invasive procedure, it should be reserved for patients whose clinical condition cannot be adequately monitored by clinical observation or prolactin concentration – for example, in children under 1 year of age, when biogenic amine depletion needs to be quickly corrected, physiological hyperprolactinaemia is present. In any case, the CSF results should be always assessed in parallel with the clinical status – the aim of treatment is to improve the clinical symptoms, not necessarily to normalize the CSF biogenic amine concentrations; in our experience, in patients with early and severe forms of TH or PTPS defects, these two aims may not always coincide. Finally, when monoamine oxidase inhibitors or (central) catechol-*O*-methyltransferase (COMT) is given, HVA, 5HIAA, and MHPG are not reliable indicators of biogenic amine repletion and so CSF monitoring should be avoided.

References

Bandmann, O., Goertz, M., Zschocke, J., Deuschl, G., Jost, W., Hefter, H., Muller, U., Zofel, P., Hoffmann, G. & Oertel, W. (2003): The phenylalanine loading test in the differential diagnosis of dystonia. *Neurology* **60**, 700–702.

Bartholomé, K., Lutz, P. & Bickel, H. (1975): Determination of phenylalanine hydroxylase activity in patients with phenylketonuria and hyperphenylalaninemia. *Pediatr. Res.* **9**, 899–903.

Bevan, J.S. (1991): Interpreting prolactin levels: implications for the management of large pituitary lesions. *Br. J. Neurosurg.* **5**, 3–6.

Birnbacher, R., Scheibenreiter, S., Blau, N., Bieglmayer, C., Frisch, H. & Waldhauser, F. (1998): Hyperprolactinemia, a tool in treatment control of tetrahydrobiopterin deficiency: endocrine studies in an affected girl. *Pediatr. Res.* **43**, 472–477.

Blau, N., Scherer-Oppliger, T., Baumer, A., Riegel, M., Matasovic, A., Schinzel, A., Jaeken, J. & Thöny, B. (2000): Isolated central form of tetrahydrobiopterin deficiency associated with hemizygosity on chromosome 11q and a mutant allele of PTPS. *Hum. Mutat.* **16**, 54–60.

Blau, N., Thöny, B., Cotton, R. & Hyland, K. (2001): Disorders of tetrahydrobiopterin and related biogenic amines. In: *The metabolic and molecular basis of inherited disease*, 8th ed., eds. C.R. Scriver, W.R. Sly, B. Childs, *et al.*, pp. 1725–1776. New York: McGraw-Hill.

Bonafé, L., Thöny, B., Leimbacher, W., Kierat, L. & Blau, N. (2001a): Diagnosis of dopa-responsive dystonia and other tetrahydrobiopterin disorders by the study of biopterin metabolism in fibroblasts. *Clin. Chem.* **47**, 477–485.

Bonafé, L., Thöny, B., Penzien, J.M., Czarnecki, B. & Blau, N. (2001b): Mutations in the sepiapterine reductase gene cause a novel tetrahydrobiopterin-dependent monoamine-neurotransmitter deficiency without hyperphenylalaninemia. *Am. J. Hum. Genet.* **69**, 269–277.

De Vivo, D.C. & Johnston, M.V. (2003): Pediatric neurotransmitter diseases. *Ann. Neurol.* **54** (Suppl. 6).

Fiori, L., Blau, N., Zenga, A., Riva, E. & Giovannini, M. (2004): Diagnosis of severe PTPS deficiency in a 28-year-old lawyer with normal IQ. *J. Inherit. Metab. Dis.* **27** (Suppl. 1).

Frantz, A.G. (1978): Prolactin. *N. Engl. J. Med.* **298**, 201–207.

Freeman, M.E., Kanyicska, B., Lerant, A. & Nagy, G. (2000): Prolactin: structure, function, and regulation of secretion. *Physiol. Rev.* **80**, 1523–1631.

Furukawa, Y., Mizuno, Y. & Narabayas, H. (1996): Early-onset parkinsonism with dystonia. Clinical and biochemical differences from hereditary progressive dystonia or DOPA-responsive dystonia. *Adv. Neurol.* **69**, 327–337.

Furukawa, Y., Kish, S.J., Bebin, E.M., Jacobson, R.D., Fryburg, J.S., Wilson, W.G., Shimadzu, M., Hyland, K. & Trugman, J.M. (1998): Dystonia with motor delay in compound heterozygotes for GTP-cyclohydrolase I gene mutations. *Ann. Neurol.* **44**, 10–16.

Hirano, M., Tamaru, Y., Ito, H., Matsumoto, S., Imai, T. & Ueno, S. (1996): Mutant GTP cyclohydrolase I mRNA levels contribute to dopa-responsive dystonia onset. *Ann. Neurol.* **40**, 796–798.

Hoffmann, G.F., Assmann, B., Bräutigam, C., Dionisi-Vici, C., Häussler, M., de Klerk, G.B.C., Naumann, M., Steenbergen-Spanjers, G.C.H., Strassburg, H.-M. & Wevers, R.A. (2003): Tyrosine hydroxylase deficiency causes progressive encephalopathy and dopa-responsive dystonia. *Ann. Neurol.* **54** (Suppl. 6), S56–S65.

Hwu, W.L., Wang, P.J., Hsiao, K.J., Wang, T.R., Chiou, Y.W. & Lee, Y.M. (1999): Dopa-responsive dystonia induced by a recessive GTP cyclohydrolase I mutation. *Hum. Genet.* **105**, 226–230.

Hyland, K. (2003a): The lumbar puncture for diagnosis of pediatric neurotransmitter diseases. *Ann. Neurol.* **54** (Suppl. 6), S13–S17.

Hyland, K. (2003b): Disorders of neurotransmitter metabolism. In: *Physician's guide to the laboratory diagnosis of metabolic diseases*, eds. N. Blau, M. Duran, M.E. Blaskovics & K.M. Gibson, pp. 107–122. Berlin: Springer-Verlag.

Hyland, K., Surtees, R.A., Heales, S.J., Bowron, A., Howells, D.W. & Smith, I. (1993): Cerebrospinal fluid concentrations of pterins and metabolites of serotonin and dopamine in a paediatric reference population. *Pediatr. Res.* **34**, 10–14.

Hyland, K., Fryburg, J.S., Wilson, W.G., Bebin, E.M., Arnold, L.A., Gunasekera, R.S., Jacobson, R.D., Rost-Ruffner, E. & Trugman, J.M. (1997): Oral phenylalanine loading in dopa-responsive dystonia: a possible diagnostic test. *Neurology* **48**, 1290–1297.

Ichinose, H., Ohye, T., Takahashi, E., Seki, N., Hori, T., Segawa, M., Nomura, Y., Endo, K., Tanaka, H. & Tsuji, S. (1994): Hereditary progressive dystonia with marked diurnal fluctuation caused by mutations in the GTP cyclohydrolase I gene. *Nat. Genet.* **8**, 236–242.

Ichinose, H., Suzuki, T., Inagaki, H., Ohye, T. & Nagatsu, T. (1999): Molecular genetics of dopa-responsive dystonia. *Biol. Chem.* **380**, 1355–1364.

Leeming, R.J. & Smith, I. (1979): Atypical PKU with normal phenylalanine hydroxylase and dihydropteridine reductase activity in vitro. *Arch. Dis. Child.* **54**, 166–167.

Leuzzi, V., Carducci, C., Carducci, C., Cardona, F., Artiola, C. & Antonozzi, I. (2002): Autosomal dominant GTP-CH deficiency presenting as a dopa-responsive myoclonus-dystonia syndrome. *Neurology* **59**, 1241–1243.

Nardocci, N., Zorzi, G., Blau, N., Fernandez Alvarez, E., Sesta, M., Angelini, L., Pannacci, M., Invernizzi, F. & Garavaglia, B. (2003): Neonatal dopa-responsive extrapyramidal syndrome in twins with recessive GTPCH deficiency. *Neurology* **60**, 335–337.

Saunders-Pullman, R., Hyland, K. & Blau, N. (2000): Phenylalanine loading in the diagnosis of DRD: the necessity for measuring biopterins. *Ann. Neurol.* **48**, 466.

Saunders-Pullman, R., Blau, N., Hyland, K., Zschocke, J., Nygaard, T., Raymond, D., Shanker, V., Mohrmann, K., Arnold, L., Tabbal, S., De Leon, D., Ford, B., Brin, M., Chouinard, S., Ozelius, L., Klein, C. & Bressman, S. (2004): Phenylalanine loading as a diagnostic test for DRD: interpreting the utility of the test. *Mol. Genet. Metab.* **83,** 207–210.

Segawa, M., Hosaka, A., Miyagawa, F., Nomura, Y. & Imai, H. (1976): Hereditary progressive dystonia with marked diurnal fluctuation. *Adv. Neurol.* **14,** 215–233.

Segawa, M., Nomura, Y. & Nsishyama, N. (2003): Autosomal dominant guanosine triphosphate cyclohydrolase I deficiency (Segawa disease). *Ann. Neurol.* **54** (Suppl. 6), S32–S45.

Spada, M., Ferraris, S., Ferrero, G.B., Sartore, M., Lanza, C., Perfetto, F., de Sanctis, L., Dompe, C., Blau, N. & Ponzone, A. (1996): Monitoring treatment in tetrahydrobiopterin deficiency by serum prolactin. *J. Inherit. Metab. Dis.* **19,** 231–233.

Veldhuis, J.D. & Johnson, M.L. (1988): Operating characteristics of the hypothalamo-pituitary-gonadal axis in men: circadian, ultradian, and pulsatile release of prolactin and its temporal coupling with luteinizing hormone. *J. Clin. Endocrinol. Metab.* **67,** 116–123.

Zorzi, G., Redweik, U., Trippe, H., Penzien, J.M., Thony, B. & Blau, N. (2002): Detection of sepiapterin in CSF of patients with sepiapterin reductase deficiency. *Mol. Genet. Metab.* **75,** 174–177.

Chapter 11

Clinical and aetiological spectrum of dopa-responsive syndromes

Giovanna Zorzi, Federica Zibordi, Daniele Ghezzi[*], Chiara Barzaghi[*], Barbara Garavaglia[*] and Nardo Nardocci

Unit of Child Neuropsychiatry, Fondazione IRCCS Istituto Neurologico 'C. Besta', via Celoria 11, 20133 Milan, Italy;
[*] *Unit of Molecular Neurogenetics, Fondazione IRCCS Istituto Neurologico 'C. Besta', via Celoria 11, 20133 Milan, Italy*
nnardocci@istituto-besta.it
Video 4

Summary

Dopa-responsive syndromes comprise a heterogeneous group of genetic conditions characterized by L-dopa responsiveness. These disorders arise as a result of defects in one of the enzymes involved in the synthesis of dopamine and serotonin, and are referred to as neurotransmitter disorders. They are currently classified according to the presence or absence ('central forms') of hyperphenylalaninaemia. The neurotransmitter disorders with hyperphenylalaninaemia are caused by defects in BH4, the cofactor for functioning of the rate-limiting enzymes in the synthesis of dopamine and serotonin. The clinical picture is that of a severe encephalopathy with psychomotor retardation, swallowing difficulties, abnormal movements, and seizures. Neurotransmitter disorders without hyperphenylalaninaemia involve defects both in BH4 metabolism and in the enzymes involved in the synthesis of biogenic amines, and include dominant guanosine triphosphate cyclohydrolase I (GTP-CH) deficiency and tyrosine hydroxylase (TH) deficiency. The clinical picture is characterized by dystonia and parkinsonism, but atypical presentations, signs of more diffuse central nervous system involvement, or extraneurological symptoms may be observed. In most patients, treatment leads to a complete resolution of symptoms, so early diagnosis is mandatory. We describe the clinical features – from both personal experience and a review of published reports – and the diagnosis.

Introduction

Dopa-responsive syndromes constitute a broad spectrum of neurological conditions with different types of movement disorders (dystonia, parkinsonism, myoclonus, and so on), sometimes combined with signs and symptoms of a more diffuse central nervous system involvement.

Biochemically, these disorders are characterized by low levels of serotonin or dopamine, or both, in the cerebral spinal fluid, and they are currently included among the neurotransmitter disorders (Swoboda & Hyland, 2002). The clinical features depend on the severity and the pattern of neurotransmitter deficiency. Supplementation therapy with neurotransmitter precursors may lead to the complete resolution of symptoms in some patients.

Synthesis of serotonin and dopamine

Dopamine and serotonin are formed from tryptophan and tyrosine by the two enzymes tryptophan hydroxylase (TPH: EC 1.14.16.4) and tyrosine hydroxylase (TH, EC 1.1.16.2), both rate-limiting for the synthesis of these neurotransmitters; L-dopa and 5-hydroxytryptophan are then decarboxylated by the pyridoxine-dependent aromatic amino-acid decarboxylase (AADC, EC 4.1.1.28) into the active neurotransmitters. Dopamine is further hydroxylated by the enzyme dopamine ß-hydroxylase (DBH, EC 1.14.17.1) to form norepinephrine. The main routes of catabolism of serotonin lead to the formation of acidic metabolites by aldehyde dehydrogenase (EC 1.2.1.3) and monoamine oxidase (MAO, EC 1.4.3.4). The major CNS metabolite of dopamine is homovanillic acid (HVA) and of serotonin, 5-hydroxyindoleacetic acid (5-HIAA); their concentrations are thought to reflect the turnover of dopamine and serotonin.

Tetrahydrobiopterin (BH4) is the essential cofactor for the enzymes TH, TPH, and phenylalanine-3-hydroxylase (PAH). BH4 is synthesized from guanosine triphosphate (GTP) in a multistep pathway catalysed by the rate limiting enzyme GTP-cyclohydrolase I (GTP-CH, EC 3.5.4.16), 6-pyruvoyltetrahydropterin synthase (PTPS, EC 4.6.1.10), and sepiapterin reductase (SR, EC: 1.1.1.153). Two additional enzymes are involved in the regeneration of BH4: pterin-4a-carbinolamine dehydratase (PCD, EC 4.2.1.96) and dihydropteridine reductase (DHPR, EC 1.6.99.7).

Classification of neurotransmitter disorders

Neurotransmitter disorders can be placed in two main categories (Table 1), depending on whether or not there is hyperphenylalaninaemia (Swoboda & Hyland, 2002).

Table 1. Classification of neurotransmitter disorders

With hyperphenylalaninaemia Autosomal recessive GTP-CH deficiency, 14q22.1-22.2 PTPS deficiency, 11q22.3-23.3 DHPR deficiency, 4p15.31
Without hyperphenylalaninaemia Autosomal dominant GTP-CH deficiency, 14q22.1-22.2 TH deficiency, 11p15.5 AADC deficiency, 7p11 SR deficiency, 2p14-p12

AADC, aromatic amino-acid decarboxylase; DHPR, dihydropteridine reductase; GTP-CH, guanosine triphosphate cyclohydrolase I; PTPS, 6-pyruvoyltetrahydropterin synthase; SR, sepiapterin reductase; TH, tyrosine hydroxylase.

Neurotransmitter disorders with hyperphenylalaninaemia

These arise as a result of a defect in BH4 metabolism and all are recessively inherited. Patients are usually identified at newborn screening for raised levels of phenylalanine. The clinical picture is one of a severe encephalopathy with psychomotor retardation, swallowing difficulties, abnormal movements, and seizures (Blau *et al.*, 2001a). Patients with initially normal levels of phenylalanine or a milder clinical picture are also described (Blau *et al.*, 2001a; Nardocci *et al.*, 2003). The diagnosis can be confirmed by enzymatic or genetic assays (Bonafè *et al.*, 2001). Treatment with neurotransmitter precursors (L-dopa, 5-HIAA) and BH4 can improve the neurological symptoms but does not usually prevent encephalopathy from developing.

Neurotransmitter disorders without hyperphenylalaninaemia

These include both defects in BH4 metabolism and defects in the enzymes involved in the synthesis of biogenic amines. The clinical features and diagnostic aspects of the two main central forms, autosomal dominant GTP-CH deficiency and TH deficiency, will be described in detail.

Autosomal dominant GTP-CH deficiency

In 1971 Segawa and his co-workers described a unique type of progressive dystonia with onset in childhood. They called this new entity hereditary progressive dystonia. It showed marked diurnal fluctuation and there was a dramatic response to L-dopa. The distinct features were dominant inheritance with a female predominance, onset in childhood with gait dystonia, a progressive course with the later appearance of parkinsonian features, worsening of symptoms towards evening, and a dramatic and persistent response to low doses of L-dopa. The authors postulated that the pathogenesis of the disease was a hypofunction of the dopaminergic system (Segawa *et al.*, 1971).

In 1993 the gene locus was mapped to chromosome 14 by linkage analysis, and one year later Ichinose and co-workers found mutations in the CGH-1 gene (Ichinose *et al.*, 1994). Our knowledge of the biochemical disturbances and the genetic defect has led to a better understanding of the disorder, now named autosomal dominant GTP-CH deficiency.

For an illustration of this condition, see video 4, track 1 *(details at the end of this chapter).*

Clinical features

The classical clinical presentation of autosomal dominant GTP-CH deficiency is gait dystonia of childhood onset, subsequently spreading to the arms, trunk, and sometimes the craniocervical region. Asymmetrical involvement is often observed. Brisk tendon reflexes and ankle clonus are common, while parkinsonian features (rigidity, postural tremor) may appear later during the course of the disease. Symptoms typically are worse in the evening and treatment with low doses of L-dopa causes their complete and persistent remission without side effects. There are no mental or psychological abnormalities, and no autonomic nervous system dysfunction. The disease has an autosomal dominant inheritance with a female predominance (Segawa *et al.*, 1971).

After the discovery of the causative gene, many patients with atypical clinical presentations have been described; the diagnosis of autosomal dominant GTP-CH in clinical practice continues to be a challenge and misdiagnosis of this treatable disorder is not infrequent (Bandmann & Wood, 2002).

Because of the low penetrance of the gene, a family history can be unrevealing or suggest a recessive mode of inheritance. In our series of nine patients from five families, dominant inheritance was evident only in one family, and three patients were apparently sporadic (Garavaglia *et al.*, 2004).

Age at onset is variable, from as early as 1 year to over 50 years (Segawa *et al.*, 2003). Patients with very early-onset can present with motor delay and may be misdiagnosed as having cerebral palsy (Nygaard *et al.*, 1994; Furukawa *et al.*, 1998). In some children, delayed development of language and deceleration of linear growth have also been noted (Segawa *et al.*, 2003).

Patients with onset after the second decade tend to have dystonia and postural tremor in the upper limbs initially, and those with adult onset present mainly with parkinsonian features, indicating that the clinical presentation is age-dependent (Segawa *et al.*, 2003). Atypical presentations with focal dystonia, paroxysmal dystonia, or myoclonic dystonia have also been reported in some cases (Bandmann et al., 1998; Leuzzi et al., 2002; Segawa et al., 2003; Garavaglia et al., 2004).

Diurnal fluctuations are absent in at least 25 per cent of patients with autosomal dominant GTP-CH, and it is known that worsening of symptoms with fatigue and sleep relief may also be experienced by patients with other types of dystonia (Bandmann & Wood, 2002).

An excellent response to L-dopa is the rule and before the possibility of genetic testing the diagnosis of autosomal dominant GTP-CH deficiency was based upon this pharmacological test (Nygaard et al., 1991). Patients may not respond completely or immediately to treatment, or may require higher doses (Bandmann & Wood, 2002). Rarely, a worsening of symptoms has been reported (Grimes et al., 2002). We have observed one patient with GTP-CH deficiency in whom treatment with L-dopa caused severe side effects; in this patient anticholinergic agents were of great benefit, as reported in several other patients (Jarman et al., 1997; Garavaglia et al., 2004). Treatment with L-dopa needs to be given at sufficiently high dosage for an appropriate length of time – we suggest that children start with 1 mg/kg/d, increasing to 10 mg/kg/d and continuing for at least 3 months.

Genetic and biochemical aspects

The disease is caused by mutations in the *CGH-1* gene. Up to now, more than 90 independent mutations – mainly point mutations – have been discovered throughout all the exons and in the splicing regions (Blau et al., 2001b). Most patients carry one heterozygous mutation, but there are also cases of compound heterozygosity. There is no evidence of a correlation between a given mutation and a clinical phenotype.

The diagnosis can also be based on biochemical investigations. CSF analysis reveals low levels of HVA and pterins (biopterin and neopterin), while 5-HIAA may be normal or only slightly reduced (Blau et al., 2001c). GTP-CH activity measured in mononuclear blood cells or fibroblasts is reduced by more than 50 per cent because of the dominant negative effect of the mutation (Bonafè et al., 2001). Additional diagnostic tests such as a phenylalanine loading test may be helpful, but false-negative and false-positive cases are not infrequent (Saunders-Pullman et al., 2004).

Approximately 60 to 80 per cent of patients with a dopa-responsive dystonia syndrome have mutations of the *CGH-1* gene, in line with our experience. Mutations in other causative genes responsible for dopa-responsive dystonia have been discovered, such as the parkin, tyrosine hydroxylase, and more recently the sepiapterin reductase genes, indicating that dopa-responsive dystonia is a syndrome with wide genetic heterogeneity that is not yet fully defined (Segawa et al., 2003; Steinberg et al., 2004).

In clinical practice, *CGH-1* negative patients should undergo measurement of neurotransmitters and pterins in the CSF. The CSF profile is an essential indicator of which gene has to be screened. Despite biochemical alterations indicating GTP-CH deficiency, a few patients have been reported without any detectable mutations in the *CGH-1* gene. One possible explanation for this is the presence of mutations in non-coding regions of the gene or large genomic deletions which are undetectable by the currently employed laboratory techniques. Mutations in unknown regulatory genes capable to modify the CGH-1 function can also be postulated (Segawa et al., 2003).

Tyrosine hydroxylase deficiency

Tyrosine hydroxylase (TH) deficiency was first described in 1995 as the second genetic cause of a dopa-responsive dystonia syndrome (Ludecke *et al.*, 1995). The disease was subsequently described in isolated patients under different names, such as 'autosomal recessive L-dopa responsive dystonia', 'L-dopa responsive infantile parkinsonism', or 'L-dopa responsive spastic paraplegia' (Hoffmann *et al.*, 2003).

For an illustration of this condition, see video 4, track 2 *(details at the end of this chapter).*

Clinical features

The disease has different phenotypes, ranging from exercise-induced dystonia to progressive dystonia with tremor, and spastic paraplegia responding to L-dopa. Recently, new patients with a more severe phenotype unresponsive to treatment have been reported, adding a progressive neurometabolic encephalopathy to the concept of TH as a form of dopa-responsive dystonia (Hoffmann *et al.*, 2003). A recent review of published reports has shown that most patients with TH deficiency present with severe encephalopathy with little or no response to L-dopa. Our experience in the neuropaediatric department of the Besta Institute, spanning the previous 5 years, confirms these data – we have followed up four patients affected by TH deficiency who exemplify the severe clinical presentation of the disease.

The clinical features of our four cases are summarized in Table 2. The family history was unrevealing except in one case (patient 1), who had an older sister who died at the age of 3 years from undiagnosed progressive encephalopathy. Age of onset of the disease was very early, within the first months of life in all cases. Psychomotor retardation, failure to thrive, hypotonia, and hypokinesia were the presenting symptoms. Two patients experienced birth anoxia (patients 1 and 2) and were initially diagnosed as having cerebral palsy. After the age of 6 months, additional neurological signs and symptoms suggestive of catecholamine deficiency appeared in all four children. Episodes of abnormal posturing and movements lasting for several hours, occurring towards the evenings and relieved by sleep, episodes of unexplained fever, and oculogyric crises were noted. The neurological picture in these children was not characterized by dystonia as the predominant feature but was dominated by parkinsonian signs (hypomimia, hypotonia, hypokinesia, and absence of postural control). The disease was progressive in all cases. Neurotransmitter metabolites in the CSF were measured and a marked reduction of HVA was detected, consistent with TH deficiency (Brautigam *et al.*, 1999). Treatment with L-dopa was started in all patients. Three of the four children responded to this, but the degree of clinical amelioration was variable, from moderate to excellent. Unlike patients with GTP-CH deficiency, all children with TH in our series experienced side effects from L-dopa treatment, such as hyperkinesia and irritability, so the drug had to be given at very low dosage initially (0.2 to 0.5 mg/kg/d). These side effects limited the possibility of achieving dosages above 2-3 mg/kg/d in two patients (patients 2 and 4), and in one patient (patient 3) they were so severe that the drug had to be withdrawn.

Genetic and biochemical aspects

The disease is caused by homozygous mutations in the *TH* gene, and some patients are compound heterozygotes. Most of the mutations described are isolated, but a common one (the 'R233H' mutation) has been found in the Dutch population. Expression studies have shown that the residual activity of the mutated enzyme is variable and correlates with the severity of the clinical phenotype (Hoffmann *et al.*, 2003).

Table 2. Clinical features of the four patients with TH deficiency

Symptoms	PATIENT 1	PATIENT 2	PATIENT 3	PATIENT 4
Family history	–	+	–	–
Fetal distress	+	+	–	–
Onset of neurological symptoms	4 months	3 months	3 months	2 months
Failure to thrive	++	+	++	++
Mental retardation	+	+	++	+
Motor retardation	++	++	++	++
Loss of postural reflexes	++	++	++	++
Rigidity	–	–	++	–
Hypotonia	++	++	++	++
Hypokinesia	++	++	+	+
Hypomimia	++	++	+	+
Dystonia	+	+	++	++
Feeding problems	++	–	++	++
Bilateral ptosis	–	–	++	–
Oculogyric crises	++	++	–	+
Paroxysmal dyskinesias	++	++	++	++
Disturbances of body temperature	++	++	++	–
Diurnal fluctuations	+	+	+	–
Progressive course	++	++	++	+
Response to L-dopa	+	++	–	+

Analysis of the CSF reveals severe impairment of dopamine synthesis in TH patients. HVA is markedly reduced, while 5-HIAA and pterins are normal. Methoxy-4-hydroxy-phenylglycol (MHPG), the major end product of norepinephrine and epinephrine, is also reduced in the CSF. All the other metabolic investigations in blood and urine – such as tyrosine, phenylalanine, and pterins – are normal. Plasma prolactin is usually raised in TH patients (Brautigam et al., 1999; Hoffmann et al., 2003).

Conclusions

Dopa-responsive syndromes comprise a heterogeneous group of diseases characterized clinically by responsiveness to L-dopa treatment and biochemically by low levels of serotonin and dopamine metabolites in the CSF. Early diagnosis is mandatory as supplementation treatment may lead to a complete remission of symptoms. The clinical features are variable, including abnormal movements and a wide range of non-motor symptoms related to neurotransmitter dysfunction which have not yet been systematically investigated. Diagnosis may require complex biochemical and genetic investigations, but in a small proportion of patients no definite genetic alteration is uncovered. Further studies on larger series of patients are needed for better delineation of the clinical phenotype, and to define the genetic aetiology.

Video – Illustrative cases

Autosomal dominant GTPCH deficiency (<u>video 4, track 1</u>) – Patient with autosomal dominant GTP-deficiency, with onset of the disease at the age of 3. Generalized dystonia becomes associated with rigidity, evident during walking, and a writing dystonia at 7 years of age.

After 1 week with L-dopa treatment, the neurological examination reveals a clear reduction of dystonia. In the last part, the 14-year-old patient, still under L-dopa treatment (5 mg/kg/ per day), presents only a slight writing dystonia.

TH deficiency (<u>video 4, track 2</u>) – A 6-year-old patient with TH deficiency, showing hypokinesia, hypomimia, and brief episodes of forced upward eye deviation, consisting in oculogyric crises. During voluntary actions, dystonic posturing of arms is evident.

In the second part of the video, a paroxysmal event is shown, starting with an oculogyric crisis, soon followed by oromandibular dykinesias and hyperkinesias of arms.

References

Bandmann, O., Marsden, C.D. & Wood, N.W. (1998): Atypical presentation of Dopa-responsive dystonia. *Adv. Neurol.* **78**, 283–290.

Bandmann, O. & Wood, N.W. (2002): Dopa-responsive dystonia: the story so far. *Neuropediatrics* **33**, 1–5.

Blau, N., Thony, B., Cotton, R.G.H. & Hyland, K. (2001a): Disorders of tetrahydrobiopterin and related biogenic amines. In: *The metabolic and molecular bases of inherited disease*, 8th ed., eds. B. Childs, K.W. Kinzler & B. Vogelstein, pp. 1725–1776. New York: McGraw-Hill.

Blau, N., Thony, B. & Dianzani, I. (2001b): Database of mutations causing tetrahydrobiopterin deficiency: http://www.bh4.org/biomdb1.html/

Blau, N., Bonafè, L. & Thony, B. (2001c): Tetrahydrobiopterin deficiencies without hyperphenylalaninemia: diagnosis and genetics of dopa-responsive dystonia and sepiapterin reductase deficiency. *Mol. Genet. Metab.* **74**, 172–185.

Bonafè, L., Thony, B., Leimbacher, W., Kierat, L. & Blau, N. (2001): Diagnosis of dopa-responsive dystonia and other tetrahydrobiopterin disorders by the study of biopterin metabolism in fibroblasts. *Clin. Chem.* **47**, 477–485.

Brautigam, C., Steenbergen-Spanjers, G.C.H., Hoffmann, G.F., Dionisi-Vici, C., van den Heuvel, L.P.W.J., Smeitink, J.A.M. & Wevers, R.A. (1999): Biochemical and molecular genetic characteristics of the severe form of tyrosine hydroxylase deficiency. *Clin. Chem.* **12**, 2073–2078.

Furukawa, Y., Kish, S.J., Bebin, E.M, Jacobson, R.D., Fryburg, J.S., Wilson, W.G., Shimadzu, M., Hyland, K. & Trugman, J.M. (1998): Dystonia with motor delay in compound heterozygotes for GTP-cyclohydrolase I gene mutation. *Ann. Neurol.* **4**, 10–16.

Garavaglia, B., Invernizzi, F., Agostoni Carbone, M.L., Viscardi, V., Saracini, F., Ghezzi, D., Zeviani, M., Zorzi, G. & Nardocci, N. (2004): GTP-cyclohydrolase I gene mutations in patients with autosomal dominant and recessive GTP-CH1 deficiency: identification and functional characterization of four novel mutations. *J. Inher. Metab. Dis.* **27**, 455–463.

Grimes, D.A., Barclay, C.L., Duff, J., Furukawa, Y. & Lang, A. (2002): Phenocopies in a large GCH1 mutation positive family with dopa-responsive dystonia: confusing the picture? *J. Neurol. Neurosurg. Psychiatry* **72**, 801–804.

Hoffmann, G.F., Assmann, B., Brautigam, C., Dionisi-Vici, C., Haussler, M., de Klerk, J.B.C., Naumann, M., Steenbergen-Spanjers, G.C.H., Strassburg, H.M. & Wevers, R.A. (2003): Tyrosine hydroxylase deficiency causes progressive encephalopathy and dopa-nonresponsive dystonia. *Ann. Neurol.* **54** (Suppl. 6), S56–S65.

Ichinose, H., Ohye, T., Takahashi, E., Seki, N., Hori, T., Segawa, M., Nomura, Y., Endo, K., Tanaka, H., Tsuji, S., Fujita, K. & Nagatsu, T. (1994): Hereditary progressive dystonia with marked diurnal fluctuation caused by mutations in the GTP cyclohydrolase I gene. *Nat. Genet.* **8**, 236–242.

Jarman, P.R., Bandmann, O., Marsden, C.D. & Wood, N.W. (1997): GTP cyclohydrolase I mutations in patients with dystonia responsive to anticholinergic drugs. *J. Neurol. Neurosurg. Psychiatry* **63**, 304–308.

Leuzzi, V., Carducci, C., Carducci C., Cardona, F., Artiola, C. & Antonozzi, I. (2002): Autosomal dominant GTP-CH deficiency presenting as a dopa-responsive myoclonus dystonia syndrome. *Neurology* **59**, 1241–1243.

Ludecke, B., Dworniczak, B. & Bartholomè, K. (1995): A point mutation in the tyrosine hydroxylase gene associated with Segawa syndrome. *Hum. Genet.* **95**, 123–125

Nardocci, N., Zorzi, G., Blau, N., Fernandez-Alvarez, E., Sesta, M., Angelici, L., Pannacci, M., Invernizzi, F. & Garavaglia, B. (2003): Neonatal dopa-responsive extrapyramidal syndrome in twins with recessive GTPCH deficiency. *Neurology* **60**, 335–337.

Nygaard, T.G., Marsden, C.D. & Fahn, S. (1991): Dopa-responsive dystonia: long-term treatment and prognosis. *Neurology* **41**, 174–181.

Nygaard, T., Waran, S., Levine, R., Naini, A. & Chutorian, A. (1994): Dopa-responsive dystonia simulating cerebral palsy. *Pediatr. Neurol.* **11**, 236–240.

Saunders-Pullman, R., Blau, N., Hyland, K., Zschocke, J., Nygaard, T., Raymond, D., Shanker, V., Mohrmann, K., Arnold, L., Tabbai, S., deLeon, D., Ford, B., Brin, M., Chouinard, S., Ozelius, L., Klein, C. & Bressman, S.B. (2004): Phenylalanine loading as a diagnostic test for DRD: interpreting the utility of the test. *Mol. Genet. Metab.* **83**, 207–212

Segawa, M., Nomura, Y. & Nishiyama, N. (2003): Autosomal dominant guanosine triphosphate cyclohydrolase I deficiency (Segawa disease). *Ann. Neurol.* **54** (Suppl. 6), S32-S45.

Segawa, M., Ohmi, K., Itoh, S., Aoyama, M. & Hayakama, H. (1971): Childhood basal ganglia disease with remarkable response to L-dopa: hereditary basal ganglia disease with diurnal fluctuation [in Japanese]. *Shinryo* (Tokio) **24**, 667–672.

Steinberg, D., Blau, N., Goriunov, D., Bitsch, J., Zuker, M., Hummel, S. & Muller, U. (2004): Heterozygous mutation in 5'-untranslated region of sepiapterin reductase gene (SPR) in a patient with dopa-responsive dystonia. *Neurogenetics* **5**, 187–190.

Swoboda, K.J. & Hyland, K. (2002): Diagnosis and treatment of neurotransmitter-related disorders. *Neurol. Clin. North Am.* **20**, 1143–1161.

Chapter 12

Sydenham's chorea

Francisco Cardoso

Movement Disorders Clinic, Neurology Service, Department of Internal Medicine, The Federal University of Minas Gerais, Av. Pasteur 89/1107, 30150-290 Belo Horizonte, MG, Brazil
cardosofe@terra.com.br
Video 5

Summary

The incidence of Sydenham's chorea (SC) has steadily decreased in the past few decades. Nevertheless, it remains the most common cause of acute chorea in children worldwide and is still a major public health problem in underdeveloped areas. Recent data show that the clinical picture of SC involves motor (chorea, decreased muscle tone, bradykinesia, tics) and non-motor features (especially obsessive-compulsive behaviour, and reports of attention-deficit and hyperactivity disorder). SC is thought to be caused by an autoimmune reaction induced by group-A β-haemolytic streptococci (GABHS). The weight of evidence favours the hypothesis that antibodies induced by GABHS cross-react with specific basal ganglia epitopes; however, details of the pathogenesis remain to be determined. It has been proposed that a similar mechanism accounts for the development of tics, obsessions, and other clinical features in a certain group of patients without SC. As there is no specific biological marker of SC, its diagnosis is clinical. Its treatment involves the use of antichoreic drugs (valproic acid is regarded as the first line treatment, with neuroleptics being used when the former fails) and prophylaxis of GABHS infections with penicillin or sulphonamides. There is growing evidence that immunosuppression with corticosteroids benefits selected patients. Recent studies with prospective follow up of patients with SC have shown that a significant proportion either have recurrence of chorea or never go into remission.

Introduction

'Chorea' (derived from the Latin *choreus* meaning 'dance') describes abnormal involuntary movements that are brief, random, usually distal, and without purpose. First described in the Middle Ages, the most common illness was perhaps a psychogenic movement disorder, but some cases were probably the postinfectious chorea known now as Sydenham's chorea (SC). My aim in the present chapter is to provide an overview of SC, the most common movement disorder associated with bacterial infection. The chapter contains a summary of my clinical and research experiences with SC. Details of the methods used in the studies can be found in articles published by our group which are cited in the text. I also provide a review of the literature on the subject.

Epidemiology

The incidence of rheumatic fever and SC in the USA and Western Europe has declined since World War II as result of improved health care, increased antibiotic usage, and lower virulence of streptococcal strains (Quinn, 1989). This fall is demonstrated by the finding that the annual age-adjusted incidence rate of initial attacks of rheumatic fever per 100,000 children declined from 3.0 in 1970 to 0.5 in 1980 in Fairfax County (Virginia, USA) (Schwartz et al., 1983). Furthermore, Nausieda and colleagues (1980) showed that SC accounted for 0.9 per cent of children's admissions to hospitals in Chicago before 1940, while between 1950 and 1980 the number fell to 0.2 per cent. Despite the fall in incidence, SC remains the most common cause of acute chorea in children worldwide, and there have been recent outbreaks of rheumatic fever with chorea in the USA and Australia (Ayoub, 1992; Ryan et al., 2000). Rheumatic fever remains a significant public health problem in developing areas, particularly within the low-income population. For instance, at the Movement Disorders Clinic of the Federal University of Minas Gerais (FUMG) SC accounts for 64 per cent of all patients with chorea, far exceeding conditions such as Huntington's disease and others. At the northern tip of the Northern Territory of Australia, an area predominantly inhabited by Aboriginal people, the point prevalence of rheumatic fever was 9.6 per 1000 people aged 5 to 14 years in 1995 (Carapetis et al., 1996). SC occurs in about 26 per cent of patients with rheumatic fever (Cardoso et al., 1997). The clinical manifestations may vary among people of differing ethnic backgrounds (Carapetis & Currie, 1999).

Clinical findings

The usual age at onset of SC is 8 to 9 years, but there are reports of patients developing chorea during the third decade of life. In most series there is a female preponderance (Cardoso et al., 1997). Typically, patients develop the disease 4 to 8 weeks after an episode of group-A β-haemolytic streptococcal (GABHS) pharyngitis. It is worth mentioning that SC has not been reported after streptococcal infection of the skin. The chorea, characterized by a random and continuous flow of contractions, spreads rapidly and becomes generalized, though in 20 per cent of cases it remains lateralized as hemichorea (Nausieda et al., 1980; Cardoso et al., 1997). The movement disorder is characterized by a random and continuous flow of contractions, which can be seen in the videoclip on the accompanying DVD (track 1). This shows a girl with recent onset of involuntary movements of the left side of the body. On neurological examination, in addition to left hemichorea she had decreased muscle tone, bradykinesia, and decreased verbal fluency.

Motor impersistence is common and is particularly noticeable during tongue protrusion and ocular fixation. The muscle tone is usually decreased; in severe and rare cases (1.5 per cent of all patients seen at the FUMG Movement Disorders Clinic) this is so pronounced that the patient may become bedridden *(chorea paralytica)*. Patients often show other neurological and non-neurological symptoms and signs. There are reports of the common occurrence of tics in SC. I find it virtually impossible to distinguish simple tics from fragments of chorea. Even vocal tics – reported to be present in 70 per cent or more of patients with SC in one study (Mercadante et al., 1997) – are not simple to diagnose in patients with hyperkinesias. Those physicians experienced with movement disorders are well aware that involuntary vocalizations may result from dystonia or chorea of the pharynx and larynx. This has been described, for instance, in subjects with oromandibular dystonia or Huntington's disease (Jankovic, 2001).

Under these circumstances the vocalization lacks the subjective feeling (premonitory urge or sensory tic) so characteristic of idiopathic tic disorders such as Tourette's syndrome. In a cohort of 120 SC patients followed up at our unit, we have identified complex tics in fewer than 4 per cent of cases. There is evidence that many patients with active chorea have hypometric saccades, and a few also develop oculogyric crises. Dysarthria is common, and Gowers had already recognized during the 19th century that SC patients have a 'disinclination to speak.' In fact, a recent case-control study of patients at the FUMG Movement Disorders Clinic described a pattern of decreased verbal fluency that reflected reduced phonetic but not semantic output (Cunningham et al., 2006). This result suggests dysfunction of the dorsolateral prefrontal-basal ganglia circuit. Studying adults with SC, we have extended this finding, showing that many functions dependent of the prefrontal area are impaired in these patients. Our conclusion was that SC should be included among the causes of dysexecutive syndrome (Cardoso et al., 2005a). In a recent survey of 100 patients with rheumatic fever, half of whom had chorea, we found that migraine was more frequent in SC (21.8 per cent) than in normal controls (8.1 per cent) ($p = 0.02$) (Teixeira et al., 2005a). This is similar to what has been described in Tourette's syndrome (Kwack et al., 2003). In the older literature, there are also references to papilloedema, central retinal artery occlusion, and seizures in a few patients with SC.

Recently, attention has been drawn to behavioural abnormalities. Swedo and colleagues (Swedo et al., 1998) found obsessive-compulsive behaviour in five of 13 SC patients, three of whom met criteria for obsessive-compulsive disorder, whereas no patient in the rheumatic fever group presented with obsessive-compulsive behaviour. In another study of 30 patients with SC, Asbahr and colleagues (Asbahr et al., 1998) showed that 70 per cent of their subjects presented with obsessions and compulsions, while 16.7 per cent met criteria for obsessive-compulsive disorder. None of 20 patients with rheumatic fever without chorea had obsessions or compulsions (Asbahr et al., 1998). Similar findings were reported in a more recent study showing that patients with rheumatic fever but without chorea had more obsessions and compulsions than healthy controls (Mercadante et al., 2000). In that study, however, the actual percentage of SC patients who had obsessive-compulsive disorder was not made clear. As the authors stated that the frequency of obsessive-compulsive disorder was similar in patients with and without rheumatic fever, one can presume that about 12 per cent of the 22 SC patients met criteria for this condition. Mercadante and colleagues (2000) also tackled the issue of hyperactivity and attention deficit disorder in SC and found that 45 per cent of their 22 patients met criteria for this condition. Recently, Maia et al. from our unit investigated behavioural abnormalities in 50 healthy subjects, 50 patients with rheumatic fever without chorea, and 56 patients with SC (Maia et al., 2005). These investigators found that obsessive-compulsive behaviour, obsessive-compulsive disorder, and attention-deficit and hyperactivity disorder were more common in the SC group (19 per cent, 23.2 per cent, and 30.4 per cent, respectively) than in healthy controls (11 per cent, 4 per cent, and 8 per cent) or in patients with rheumatic fever but without chorea (14 per cent, 6 per cent, and 8 per cent). They also showed that obsessive-compulsive behaviour resulted in very little interference with activities of daily living.

There is one note of caution over the interpretation of data on hyperactivity in SC. Comparing patients with acute and persistent SC, attention-deficit hyperactivity disorder was significantly more common in the latter (50 vs. 16 per cent). There was also a trend towards more obsessive-compulsive behaviour and obsessive-compulsive disorder among subjects with more prolonged forms of SC, but the difference did not reach statistical significance. As there is no biological marker used in the current diagnostic criteria (DSM-IV), it is not always easy to differentiate restlessness associated with chorea from the true hyperactivity of attention-deficit hyperactivity disorder. A recent investigation showed that the peripheral nervous system is not targeted in SC (Cardoso et al., 2005b). Finally, it must be borne in mind that SC is a major manifestation of rheumatic fever: 60 to 80 per cent of patients with SC have cardiac involvement, particularly mitral valve dysfunction, whereas the association with arthritis is less common, being present in only 30 per cent of cases. In approximately 20 per cent of the patients, chorea is the sole finding (Cardoso et al., 1997).

The finding that behavioural problems are common in patients with rheumatic fever and chorea contributed to the view that Sydenham's chorea is a model for childhood autoimmune neuropsychiatric disorders (Swedo, 1994). PANDAS (Paediatric Autoimmune Neuropsychiatric Disorders associated with Streptococcal infection) is a controversial concept, according to which infection with group-A β-haemolytic streptococci may induce tics, obsessive-compulsive behaviour, and other neuropsychiatric disturbances. The following working diagnostic criteria for this condition have been proposed:

- the presence of obsessive-compulsive disorder or a tic disorder;
- prepubertal symptom onset;
- episodic course of symptom severity;
- association with group-A β-haemolytic streptococcal infections;
- association with neurological abnormalities.

According to a description of 50 patients who met these criteria, the onset of tics and obsessive-compulsive disorder was at a mean age 6.3 years and 7.4 years, respectively. The same study also noted 'significant psychiatric comorbidity': emotional lability, separation anxiety, night-time fears, and bedtime rituals, cognitive deficits, and oppositional behaviours (Swedo et al., 1988). There is a growing list of neurological symptoms and signs related to streptococcal infections: dementia, dystonia, encephalitis lethargica-like syndrome, motor stereotypies, myoclonus, opsoclonus, parkinsonism, paroxysmal dyskinesia, restless leg syndrome, and tremor (Cardoso, 2005). At present, however, there is no conclusive evidence that anti-basal-ganglia antibodies induced by streptococci play a significant role in the pathogenesis of tic disorders.

Aetiology and pathogenesis

Group-A β-haemolytic streptococci are the causative agents of SC and related disorders. Taranta and Stollerman established the casual relationship between infection with GABHS and the occurrence of SC (Taranta & Stollerman, 1956). Based on the assumption of molecular mimicry between streptococcal and central nervous system antigens, it has been proposed that the bacterial infection in genetically predisposed subjects leads to the formation of cross-reactive antibodies that disrupt basal ganglia function. Such circulating antibodies have been shown to be present in 50 to 90 per cent of patients with SC (Husby et al., 1976; Cardoso, 2002a). A specific epitope of streptococcal M proteins that cross-reacts with basal ganglia has been identified (Bronze & Dale, 1993). In a recent study of patients seen at the FUMG Movement Disorders Clinic, we showed that all patients with active SC have titres of circulating serum anti-basal-ganglia antibodies – demonstrated by enzyme linked immunosorbent assay and western blotting – that are higher than in controls. In subjects with persistent SC (duration of disease more than 2 years despite the best medical treatment), the difference was less striking (Church et al., 2002). It must be emphasized that the biological value of the anti-basal-ganglia antibodies remains to be determined. However, a recent study suggested that they may interfere with neuronal function: Kirvan et al. (2003) showed that IgM from a patient with SC induced the expression of calcium-dependent calmodulin in a culture of neuroblastoma cells. Although an interesting finding, this study has limitations. First, it was an *in vitro* investigation, employing an artificial paradigm that does not necessarily reflect the situation observed in human patients; second, the antibody was obtained from a single patient; and third, the investigators studied IgM, whereas all other investigations of anti-basal-ganglia antibodies in SC have detected IgG. Our finding that there is a linear correlation between the increase in intracellular calcium levels in PC12 cells and anti-basal-ganglia antibody titre in the serum from SC patients suggests that these antibodies have a pathogenic role (Teixeira *et al.*, 2005d).

Although some investigations suggest that susceptibility to rheumatic chorea is linked to human leucocyte-antigen-linked antigen expression (Ayoub *et al.*, 1986), a more recent study failed to identify any relation between SC and human leucocyte antigen class I and class II alleles (Donadi *et al.*, 2000). The genetic marker for rheumatic fever and related conditions would be the B-cell alloantigen D8/17 (Feldman *et al.*, 1993). Despite repeated reports by the group that developed the assay claiming its high specificity and sensitivity (Eisen *et al.*, 2001; Harel *et al.*, 2002), findings of other investigators suggest that the D8/17 marker lacks specificity and sensitivity. For instance, Kaur *et al.* (1998) showed that the discriminating power of monoclonal antibody against D8/17 was relatively low among patients with rheumatic fever of northern Indian ethnic origin. Studying Caucasians in the USA, Murphy and colleagues (Murphy *et al.*, 2001) showed that 65.6 per cent of their patients with obsessive-compulsive disorder or chronic tic disorder and 8.3 per cent of controls tested positive for D8/17. In the Netherlands, Jansen *et al.* (2002) found that only a minority of their patients with post-GABHS arthritis had an increase in D8/17-positive lymphocytes.

Because of difficulties with the molecular mimicry hypothesis in accounting for the pathogenesis of SC, there have been recent studies addressing the role of immune cellular mechanisms in this condition. When investigating sera and CSF samples from SC patients from the FUMG Movement Disorders Clinic, Church *et al.* (2003) found an increase in cytokines that take part in the Th2 (antibody-mediated) response – interleukins 4 (IL-4) and 10 (IL-10) – in sera from patients with acute SC relative to those with persistent SC. They also described raised IL-4 and IL-10 in 31 per cent of the CSF samples from acute SC patients, whereas just IL-4 was raised in the CSF of persistent SC. The investigators concluded that SC is characterized by a Th2 response. However, as they also found a rise in IL-12 in acute SC, and as, more recently, we have described increased concentrations of the chemokines CXCL9 and CXCL10 in sera from patients with acute SC (Teixeira *et al.*, 2004), we conclude that Th1 (cell-mediated) mechanisms may also be involved in the pathogenesis of this disorder.

Some investigators have suggested that streptococcal infection induces vasculitis in medium-sized vessels, leading to neuronal dysfunction. Such vascular lesions could be produced by anti-phospholipid antibodies. There is also a suggestion that cellular immune mechanisms participate in the pathogenesis of streptococcus-related movement disorders. However, most of these findings have not been replicated to date. Currently, the weight of evidence suggests that the pathogenesis of SC is related to circulating cross-reactive antibodies. More recently, it has been shown that streptococcus-induced antibodies can be associated with a form of acute disseminated encephalomyelitis characterized by a high frequency of dystonia and other movement disorders, as well as by basal ganglia lesions on neuroimaging (Dale *et al.*, 2001). Antineural and antinuclear antibodies have also been found in patients with Tourette's syndrome but their relation to previous streptococcal infection remains equivocal (Morshed *et al.*, 2001).

Diagnosis

The current diagnostic criteria of SC are a modification of the Jones criteria: chorea with acute or subacute onset and lack of clinical and laboratory evidence of an alternative cause are mandatory findings. The diagnosis is further supported by the presence of additional major or minor manifestations of rheumatic fever (Committee of Rheumatic Fever, Endocarditis, and Kawasaki Disease, 1992; Cardoso et al., 1997; Cardoso et al., 1999). Recently, the first validated scale to rate SC has been published. The UFMG Sydenham's Chorea Rating Scale was designed to provide a detailed quantitative description of the performance of activities of daily living, behavioural abnormalities, and motor function of patients with SC. It comprises 27 items, each being scored from 0 (no symptom or sign) to 4 (severe disability or finding) (Teixeira et al., 2005c).

Several conditions may present with clinical manifestations similar to SC (Table 1) (Cardoso, 2004). The most important differential diagnosis is systemic lupus erythematosus (SLE), in which up to 2 per cent of patients may develop chorea. From a clinical point of view, the majority of patients with this condition will have other non-neurological manifestations such as arthritis, pericarditis, other forms of serositis, and skin abnormalities. Moreover, the neurological picture of SLE tends to be more complex and may include psychosis, seizures, other movement disorders, and even changes in mental state and conscious level. Only in rare instances will chorea, with a tendency to spontaneous remissions and recurrences, be an isolated manifestation of SLE. The difficulty in distinguishing these two conditions is increased by the finding that at least 20 per cent of patients with SC show recurrence of the movement disorder. Eventually, patients with SLE will develop other features, meeting the diagnostic criteria for that condition (Bakdash et al., 1999). Primary antiphospholipid antibody syndrome is differentiated from SC by the absence of other clinical and laboratory features of rheumatic fever as well as by the usual association with repeated abortions, venous thrombosis, other vascular events, and the presence of typical laboratory abnormalities. Encephalitides, either caused by direct viral invasion or by an immune-mediated postinfectious process, can also cause chorea. This usually happens in younger children. The clinical picture is more diversified and includes seizures, pyramidal signs, and impairment of psychomotor development. There are laboratory abnormalities suggestive of the underlying condition. Drug-induced choreas are readily distinguished by a careful history demonstrating a temporal relation between onset of the movement disorder and exposure to the agent.

Children and young adults with chorea should undergo a complete neurological examination and laboratory investigations to assess the various causes of chorea, as there is no specific biological marker of SC. The aim of the diagnostic workup in patients suspected of having rheumatic chorea is threefold: first, to find evidence of a recent streptococcal infection or acute phase reaction; second, to search for cardiac injury associated with rheumatic fever; and third, to rule out alternative causes. Tests for acute phase reactants (erythrocyte sedimentation rate, C-reactive protein, leucocytosis), other blood tests (rheumatoid factor, mucoproteins, protein electrophoresis), and supportive evidence of a preceding streptococcal infection (increased antistreptolysin-O, antiDNAse-B, or other antistreptococcal antibodies; positive throat culture for group A streptococcus; recent scarlet fever) are much less helpful in SC than in other forms of rheumatic fever owing to the long latent period between the infection and the onset of the movement disorder. A raised antistreptolysin O titre may be found in populations with a high prevalence of streptococcal infection. Furthermore, the antistreptolysin O titre declines if the interval between infection and rheumatic fever is more than 2 months. Anti-DNase-B titres,

Table 1. Differential diagnosis of Sydenham's chorea – causes of acquired chorea

Category	Cause
Immunological	Systemic lupus erythematosus Antiphospholipid antibody syndrome Henoch-Schönlein purpura
Infectious	Neurosyphilis Tuberculosis HIV Measles Influenza Cytomegalovirus Epstein-Barr virus (mononucleosis) *Borrelia burgdorferi* (Lyme disease) Varicella Prion
Drugs	Sympathomimetics Neuroleptics (tardive dyskinesia) Cocaine Antiepileptic drugs
Miscellaneous	Anoxic encephalopathy Endocrine dysfunction (*e.g.*, hyperthyroidism) Metabolic disturbance (*e.g.*, hyperglycaemia) Post-pump chorea Moyamoya disease

however, may remain elevated for up to 1 year after streptococcal pharyngitis. Heart evaluation (Doppler echocardiography) is mandatory because carditis is found in up to 80 per cent of cases of SC. Cardiac lesions are the main source of serious morbidity in SC. Serological studies for SLE and primary antiphospholipid antibody syndrome must be done to rule out these conditions. Electroencephalography has little importance in the work-up of these patients, showing only non-specific generalized slowing both acutely and after clinical recovery. Spinal fluid analysis is usually normal, but there may be a slight increase in the lymphocyte count. In general, neuroimaging will help to rule out structural causes such as Moyamoya disease. Computed tomography of the brain invariably fails to show abnormalities. Similarly, cranial magnetic resonance imaging is often normal, although there are case reports of reversible hyperintensity in the basal ganglia area. In one study, Giedd and colleagues (1995) found increased signal in only two of 24 patients, although morphometric techniques showed that mean values for the dimensions of the striatum and the pallidum exceeded those of controls. Unfortunately, these findings are of little help on an individual basis because there was an extensive overlap between controls and patients. Positron emission tomography and SPECT imaging may prove useful in the evaluation, showing transient increases in striatal metabolism during the acute phase of the illness (Goldman *et al.*, 1993; Weindl *et al.*, 1993; Lee *et al.*, 1999). Recently, Barsottini and colleagues (2002) showed that six of 10 patients with SC had hyperperfusion of the basal ganglia. This contrasts with other choreic disorders (such as Huntington's disease), which are associated with hypometabolism. However, a recent investigation of seven patients with SC showed hyperperfusion in two, while the remaining five had hypometabolism (Citak *et al.*, 2004). It is possible that the inconsistencies in these studies reflect heterogeneity of the patient population. In our own unit, we have found hypermetabolism of the basal ganglia on SPECT during acute SC, whereas patients with persistent chorea often display hypometabolism in this area. Increasing interest is now directed towards autoimmune markers that may be useful for diagnosis, though a test for antineuronal antibodies is not yet commercially available, being currently used only for research purposes. Preliminary evidence suggests that these antibodies are not specific for SC. Similarly, the low sensitivity and specificity of the alloantigen D8/17 renders it unsuitable for the diagnosis of this condition.

Prognosis and complications

Older reports describe SC as a rather benign self-limited condition that goes into remission after a few months (Nausieda et al., 1980). Careful prospective follow-up of patients in the past few years has shown, however, that in up to half the cases chorea remains active 2 years after onset. Moreover, despite the regular use of secondary prophylaxis, recurrences of the movement disorders are observed in up to 50 per cent of subjects (Cardoso et al., 1999; Korn-Lubetzki et al., 2004). Interestingly, in many of the recurrences there is a lack of association either with streptococcal infection or even with anti-basal-ganglia antibodies (Harrison et al., 2004; Korn-Lubetzki et al., 2004). The most serious problem in patients with SC is the occurrence of valvulopathy and other cardiac problems. The importance of this complication is illustrated by the finding that in areas where rheumatic fever is endemic, 70 per cent of cardiac operations performed are to treat these complications (Cardoso, 2002a).

Management

There are no controlled studies of the symptomatic treatment of SC, and the reader must be aware that all the recommendations made here are for off-label use of the cited drugs. My first choice is valproic acid at an initial dose of 250 mg once a day. This is increased during a two week period to 250 mg three times a day. If the response is not satisfactory, the dose can be increased gradually to 1500 mg a day. As this drug has a rather slow onset of action, I usually wait two weeks before concluding that a regimen is ineffective. A recent study showed that carbamazepine (15 mg/kg per day) is as effective as valproic acid (20 to 25 mg/kg per day) in inducing remission of chorea (Genel et al., 2002).

If the patient fails to respond to valproic acid, the next option is a neuroleptic agent. Pimozide – a potent dopamine D2 receptor blocker – is usually effective at controlling the hyperkinesias. Although pimozide-induced atrioventricular block has been described, this complication has not been seen in the more than 100 patients with SC followed at the FUMG Movement Disorders Clinic and Paediatric Cardiology Service. The usual initial regimen is 1 mg twice a day. If chorea is still troublesome after two weeks, the dose is increased to 2 mg twice a day. Neuroleptics are the first choice of treatment in the rare patients who present with *chorea paralytica*. Dopamine D2 receptor blockers must be used with great caution in patients with SC. After observing the development of parkinsonism, dystonia, or both in patients treated with neuroleptics, we undertook a case-control study comparing the response to these drugs in patients with SC and Tourette's syndrome. We showed that 5 out of 100 patients with chorea developed extrapyramidal complications, whereas these were not observed among patients with tics matched for age and dose of neuroleptics (Teixeira et al., 2003).

There are no published guidelines on the discontinuation of antichoreic agents. My personal policy is to attempt a gradual decrease in the dose (25 per cent reduction every two weeks) after the patient has been free of chorea for at least a month. Finally, the most important measure in the treatment of patients with SC is secondary prophylaxis with penicillin or, if there is allergy, a sulphonamide up to the age of 21 years. If the onset occurs after this age, the recommendation is to maintain prophylaxis indefinitely (Cardoso, 2002b).

There is some controversy over the role of immunosuppression in the management of SC. Despite reports of the effectiveness of prednisone in suppressing chorea, this drug is only used when there is associated severe carditis. There are a few reports describing the value of plasma exchange or intravenous immunoglobulins in SC. The potential complications and high cost of these latter forms of treatment preclude their recommendation, particularly in view of the efficacy of the other drugs described above. In my practice, intravenous methylprednisolone is reserved for patients with persistent disabling chorea refractory to antichoreic agents. We recently reported that I.V. methylprednisolone in a dose of 25 mg/kg per day for children and 1 g/day for adults given for 5 days, followed by 1 mg/kg per day of prednisone orally is an effective and well tolerated form of treatment for patients with SC refractory to conventional treatment with antichoreic drugs and penicillin (Cardoso *et al.*, 2003; Teixeira *et al.*, 2005b). At least one other group has replicated our findings of a good response to steroids in selected patients with SC (Barash *et al.*, 2005).

Prevention

Prompt treatment of streptococcal pharyngitis with appropriate antibiotics has lowered the incidence of SC. Once the diagnosis of rheumatic chorea is established, the patient must receive secondary prophylaxis with penicillin, or in patients with allergy, a sulphonamide. This has been shown to decrease the risk of neurological or cardiac problems with subsequent streptococcal infections (Mason *et al.*, 1991). The recommendation of the World Health Organisation is to maintain the secondary prophylaxis up to the age of 21 years. In instances where the diagnosis of SC is made after this age, the policy is less clear. Because of the potential seriousness of cardiac lesions, our own recommendation is to maintain prophylaxis indefinitely. Patients with a history of SC should be informed of the possible re-emergence of chorea during pregnancy or with use of oral contraceptives.

Conclusions

Despite the decline in its incidence, SC remains as the most common cause of acute chorea in children worldwide. It has been firmly established that it is a complex neuropsychiatric condition, involving motor, sensory, and behavioural abnormalities. Although SC is an immune-mediated complication of streptococcal infection, details of its pathogenesis remain uncertain. Treatment with valproic acid, neuroleptics, or in selected instances corticosteroids is effective in the majority of cases. In a substantial proportion of patients, however, the illness may run a prolonged course.

Acknowledgments: I would like to express my gratitude to my collaborators in the studies cited in this article. Special thanks to Antonio Lúcio Teixeira Jr, MD, PhD, Débora Palma Maia, MD, MSc, Mauro César Quintão Cunningham, MD, MSc, Rogério Beato, MD, Andrew Lees, MD, FRCP, and Mr Antonio Carlos Bittencourt.

References

Asbahr, F.R., Negrao, A.B., Gentil, V., Zanetta, D.M., da Paz, J.A., Marques-Dias, M.J. & Kiss, M.H. (1998): Obsessive-compulsive and related symptoms in children and adolescents with rheumatic fever with and without chorea: a prospective 6-month study. *Am. J. Psychiatry* **155**, 1122–1124.

Ayoub, E.M. (1992): Resurgence of rheumatic fever in the United States. The changing picture of a preventable illness. *Postgrad. Med.* **92**, 133–142.

Ayoub, E.M., Barrett, D.J., Maclaren, N.K. & Krischer, J.P. (1986): Association of class II human histocompatibility leukocyte antigens with rheumatic fever. *J. Clin. Invest.* **77**, 2019–2026.

Bakdash, T., Goetz, C.G., Singer, H.S. & Cardoso, F. (1999): A child with recurrent episodes of involuntary movements. *Mov. Disord.* **14**, 146–154.

Barash, J., Margalith, D. & Matitiau, A. (2005): Corticosteroid treatment in patients with Sydenham's chorea. *Pediatr. Neurol.* **32**, 205–207.

Barsottini, O.G., Ferraz, H.B., Seviliano, M.M. & Barbieri, A. (2002): Brain SPECT imaging in Sydenham's chorea. *Braz. J. Med. Biol. Res.* **35**, 431–436.

Bronze, M.S. & Dale, J.B. (1993): Epitopes of streptococcal M proteins that evoke antibodies that cross-react with human brain. *J. Immunol.* **151**, 2820–2828.

Carapetis, J.R. & Currie, B.J. (1999): Rheumatic chorea in northern Australia: a clinical and epidemiological study. *Arch. Dis. Child.* **80**, 353–358.

Carapetis, J.R., Wolff, D.R. & Currie, B.J. (1996): Acute rheumatic fever and rheumatic heart disease in the top end of Australia's Northern Territory. *Med. J. Aust.* **164**, 146–149.

Cardoso, F. (2002a): Chorea gravidarum. *Arch. Neurol.* **59**, 868–870.

Cardoso, F. (2002b): Infectious and transmissible movement disorders. In: *Parkinson's disease and movement disorders*, 4th ed., eds. J. Jankovic & E. Tolosa, pp. 930-940. Baltimore: Williams and Wilkins.

Cardoso, F. (2004): Chorea: non-genetic causes. *Curr. Opin. Neurol.* **17**, 433–436.

Cardoso, F. (2005): Tourette syndrome: autoimmune mechanism. In: *Pediatric movement disorders. Progress in understanding*, eds. E. Fernández-Alvarez, A. Arzimanoglou & E. Tolosa, pp. 23-46. Paris: John Libbey Eurotext.

Cardoso, F., Silva, C.E. & Mota, C.C. (1997): Sydenham's chorea in 50 consecutive patients with rheumatic fever. *Mov. Disord.* **12**, 701–703.

Cardoso, F., Vargas, A.P., Oliveira, L.D., Guerra, A.A. & Amaral, S.V. (1999): Persistent Sydenham's chorea. *Mov. Disord.* **14**, 805–807.

Cardoso, F., Maia, D.P., Cunningham, M.C. & Valença, G. (2003): Treatment of Sydenham's chorea with corticosteroids. *Mov. Disord.* **18**, 1374–1377.

Cardoso, F., Beato, R., Siqueira, C.F. & Lima, C.F. (2005a): Neuropsychological performance and brain SPECT imaging in adult patients with Sydenham's chorea. *Neurology* **64** (Suppl. 1), A76.

Cardoso, F., Dornas, L., Cunningham, M. & Oliveira, J.T. (2005b): Nerve conduction study in Sydenham's chorea. *Mov. Disord.* **20**, 360–363.

Church, A.J., Cardoso, F., Dale, R.C., Lees, A.J., Thompson, E.J. & Giovannoni, G. (2002): Anti-basal ganglia antibodies in acute and persistent Sydenham's chorea. *Neurology* **59**, 227–231.

Church, A.J., Dale, R.C., Cardoso, F., Candler, P.M., Chapman, M.D., Allen, M.L., Klein, N.J., Lees, A.J. & Giovannoni, G. (2003): CSF and serum immune parameters in Sydenham's chorea: evidence of an autoimmune syndrome? *J. Neuroimmunol.* **136**, 149–153.

Citak, E.C., Gucuyener, K., Karabacak, N.I., Serdaroglu, A., Okuyaz, C. & Aydin, K. (2004): Functional brain imaging in Sydenham's chorea and streptococcal tic disorders. *J. Child Neurol.* **19**, 387–390.

Committee of Rheumatic Fever, Endocarditis, and Kawasaki Disease. Guidelines for diagnosis of rheumatic fever, Jones criteria, 1992 update. Special Writing Group of the Committee of Rheumatic Fever, Endocarditis, and Kawasaki Disease of the Council on Cardio-Vascular Disease of the Young of the American Heart Association. (1992): Guidelines for the diagnosis of rheumatic fever. *JAMA* **268**, 2069–2073.

Cunningham, M.C.Q., Maia, D.P., Teixeira, A.L. & Cardoso, F. (2006): Sydenham's chorea is associated with decreased verbal fluency. *Parkinsonism Relat. Disord.* **13**, 165–167.

Dale, R.C., Church, AJ., Cardoso, F., Goddard, E., Cox, T.C., Chong, W.K., Williams, A., Klein, N.J., Neville, B.G., Thompson, E.J. & Giovannoni, G. (2001): Poststreptococcal acute disseminated encephalomyelitis with basal ganglia involvement and auto-reactive antibasal ganglia antibodies. *Ann. Neurol.* **50**, 588–595.

Donadi, E.A., Smith, AG., Louzada-Junior, P., Voltarelli, J.C. & Nepom, G.T. (2000): HLA class I and class II profiles of patients presenting with Sydenham's chorea. *J. Neurol.* **247**, 122–128.

Eisen, J.L., Leonard, H.L., Swedo, S.E., Price, L.H., Zabriskie, J.B., Chiang, S.Y., Karitani, M. & Rasmussen, S.A. (2001): The use of antibody D8/17 to identify B cells in adults with obsessive-compulsive disorder. *Psychiatry Res.* **104**, 221–225.

Feldman, B.M., Zabriskie, J.B., Silverman, E.D. & Laxer, R.M. (1993): Diagnostic use of B-cell alloantigen D8/17 in rheumatic chorea. *J. Pediatr.* **123**, 84–86.

Genel, F., Arslanoglu, S., Uran, N. & Saylan, B. (2002): Sydenham's chorea: clinical findings and comparison of the efficacies of sodium valproate and carbamazepine regimens. *Brain. Dev.* **24**, 73–76.

Giedd, J.N., Rapoport, J.L., Kruesi, M.J., Parker, C., Schapiro, M.B., Allen, A.J., Leonard, H.L., Kaysen, D., Dickstein, D.P., Marsh, W.L. et al. (1995): Sydenham's chorea: magnetic resonance imaging of the basal ganglia. *Neurology* **45**, 2199–2202.

Goldman, S., Amrom, D., Szliwowski, H.B., Detemmerman, D., Goldman, S., Bidaut, L.M., Stanus, E. & Luxen, A. (1993): Reversible striatal hypermetabolism in a case of Sydenham's chorea. *Mov. Disord.* **8**, 355–358.

Harel, L., Zeharia, A., Kodman, Y., Straussberg, R., Zabriskie, J.B. & Amir, J. (2002): Presence of the d8/17 B-cell marker in children with rheumatic fever in Israel. *Clin. Genet.* **61**, 293–298.

Harrison, N.A., Church, A., Nisbet, A., Rudge, P. & Giovannoni, G. (2004): Late recurrences of Sydenham's chorea are not associated with anti-basal ganglia antibodies. *J. Neurol. Neurosurg. Psychiatry* **75**, 1478–1479.

Husby, G., Van De Rijn, U., Zabriskie, J.B., Abdin, Z.H. & Williams, R.C. (1976): Antibodies reacting with cytoplasm of subthalamic and caudate nuclei neurons in chorea and acute rheumatic fever. *J. Exp. Med.* **144**, 1094–1110.

Jankovic, J. (2001): Differential diagnosis and etiology of tics. *Adv. Neurol.* **85**, 15–29.

Jansen, T.L., Hoekstra, P.J., Bijzet, J., Limburg, P.C. & Griep, E.N. (2002): Elevation of D8/17-positive B lymphocytes in only a minority of Dutch patients with post-streptococcal reactive arthritis (PSRA): a pilot study. *Rheumatology* **41**, 1202–1203.

Kaur, S., Kumar, D., Grover, A., Khanduja, K.L., Kaplan, E.L., Gray, E.D. & Ganguly, N.K. (1998): Ethnic differences in expression of susceptibility marker(s) in rheumatic fever/rheumatic heart disease patients. *Int. J. Cardiol.* **64**, 9–14.

Kirvan, C.A., Swedo, S.E., Heuser, J.S. & Cunningham, M.W. (2003): Mimicry and autoantibody-mediated neuronal cell signaling in Sydenham chorea. *Nat. Med.* **9**, 914–920.

Korn-Lubetzki, I., Brand, A. & Steiner, I. (2004): Recurrence of Sydenham chorea: implications for pathogenesis. *Arch. Neurol.* **61**, 1261–1264.

Kwack. C., Vuong, K.D. & Jankovic, J. (2003): Migraine headache in patients with Tourette syndrome. *Arch. Neurol.* **60**, 1595–1598.

Lee, P.H., Nam, H.S., Lee, K.Y., Lee, B.I. & Lee, J.D. (1999): Serial brain SPECT images in a case of Sydenham's chorea. *Arch. Neurol.* **56**, 237–240.

Maia, D.P., Teixeira, A.L., Cunningham, M.C.Q. & Cardoso, F. (2005): Obsessive compulsive behavior, hyperactivity and attention-deficit disorder in Sydenham's chorea. *Neurology* **64**, 1799–1801.

Mason, T., Fisher, M. & Kujala, G. (1991): Acute rheumatic fever in West Virginia: not just a disease of children. *Arch. Intern. Med.* **151**, 133–136.

Mercadante, M.T., Campos, M.C., Marques-Dias, M.J., Miguel, E.C. & Leckman, J. (1997): Vocal tics in Sydenham's chorea. *J. Am. Acad. Child Adolesc. Psychiatry* **36**, 305–306.

Mercadante, M.T., Busatto, G.F., Lombroso, P.J., Prado, L., Rosario-Campos, M.C., do Valle, R., Marques-Dias, M.J., Kiss, M.H., Leckman, J.F. & Miguel, E.C. (2000): The psychiatric symptoms of rheumatic fever. *Am. J. Psychiatry* **157**, 2036–2038.

Morshed, S.A., Parveen, S., Leckman, J.F., Mercadante, M.T., Bittencourt Kiss, M.H., Miguel, E.C., Arman, A., Yazgan, Y., Fujii, T., Paul, S., Peterson, B.S., Zhang, H., King, R.A., Scahill, L. & Lombroso, P.J. (2001) : Antibodies against neural, nuclear, cytoskeletal, and streptococcal epitopes in children and adults with Tourette's syndrome, Sydenham's chorea, and autoimmune disorders. *Biol Psychiatry* **50**, 566–577.

Murphy, T.K., Benson, N., Zaytoun, A., Yang, M., Braylan, R., Ayoub, E. & Goodman, W.K. (2001): Progress toward analysis of D8/17 binding to B cells in children with obsessive compulsive disorder and/or chronic tic disorder. *J. Neuroimmunol.* **120**, 146–151.

Nausieda, P.A., Grossman, B.J., Koller, W.C., Weiner, W.J. & Klawans, H.L. (1980): Sydenham's chorea: an update. *Neurology* **30**, 331–334.

Quinn, R.W. (1989): Comprehensive review of morbidity and mortality trends for rheumatic fever, streptococcal disease, and scarlet fever: the decline of rheumatic fever. *Rev. Infect. Dis.* **11**, 928–953.

Ryan, M., Antony, J.H. & Grattan-Smith, P.J. (2000): Sydenham's chorea: a resurgence of the 1990s? *J. Pediatr. Child Health* **36**, 95–96.

Schwartz, R.H., Hepner, S.I. & Ziai, M. (1983): Incidence of acute rheumatic fever. A suburban community hospital experience during the 1970s. *Clin. Pediatr.* **22,** 798–801.

Swedo, S.E. (1994): Sydenham's chorea. A model for childhood autoimmune neuropsychiatric disorders. *JAMA* **272,** 1788–1791.

Swedo, S.E., Leonard, H.L., Garvey, M., Mittleman, B., Allen, A.J., Perlmutter, S., Lougee, L., Dow, S., Zamkoff, J. & Dubbert, B.K. (1998): Paediatric autoimmune neuropsychiatric disorders associated with streptococcal infections: clinical description of the first 50 cases. *Am. J. Psychiatry* **155,** 264–271.

Taranta, A. & Stollerman, G.H. (1956): The relationship of Sydenham's chorea to infection with group A streptococci. *Am. J. Med.* **20,** 1970–1978.

Teixeira, A.L., Cardoso, F., Maia, D.P. & Cunningham, M.C. (2003): Sydenham's chorea may be a risk factor for drug induced parkinsonism. *J. Neurol. Neurosurg. Psychiatry* **74,** 1350–1351.

Teixeira, A.L., Cardoso, F., Souza, A.L. & Teixeira, M.M. (2004): Increased serum concentrations of monokine induced by interferon-gamma/CXCL9 and interferon-gamma-inducible protein 10/CXCL-10 in Sydenham's chorea patients. *J. Neuroimmunol.* **150,** 157–162.

Teixeira, A.L., Meira, F.C., Maia, D.P., Cunningham, M.C. & Cardoso, F. (2005a): Migraine headache in patients with Sydenham's chorea. *Cephalalgia* **25,** 542–544.

Teixeira, A.L., Maia, D.P. & Cardoso, F. (2005b): Treatment of acute Sydenham's chorea with methyl-prednisolone pulse-therapy. *Parkinsonism Relat. Disord.* **11,** 327–330.

Teixeira, A.L., Maia, D.P. & Cardoso, F. (2005c): UFMG Sydenham's chorea rating scale (USCRS): reliability and consistency. *Mov. Disord.* **20,** 585–591.

Teixeira, A.L., Guimarães, M.M., Romano-Silva, M.A. & Cardoso, F. (2005d): Serum from Sydenham's chorea patients modifies intracellular calcium levels in PC12 cells by a complement-independent mechanism. *Mov. Disord.* **20,** 843–845.

Weindl, A., Kuwert, T., Leenders, K.L., Poremba, M., Grafin von Einsiedel, H., Antonini, A., Herzog, H., Scholz, D., Feinendegen, L.E. & Conrad, B. (1993): Increased striatal glucose consumption in Sydenham's chorea. *Mov. Disord.* **8,** 437–444.

Chapter 13

Opsoclonus-myoclonus syndrome

Michael R. Pranzatelli

National Paediatric Myoclonus Center, Division of Child and Adolescent Neurology, Departments of Neurology and Paediatrics, Southern Illinois University School of Medicine, P.O. Box 19643, Springfield, Illinois 62794-9643, USA
mpranzatelli@siumed.edu

Summary

Opsoclonus-myoclonus syndrome (OMS) is a rare, often multiphasic, autoimmune disorder, known to be associated with neuroblastoma. The tumour's high incidence of spontaneous regression and viral-like prodrome even in bona fide neuroblastoma cases makes it likely that all cases are paraneoplastic. The typically low tumour grade and excellent tumour survival should not falsely reassure those managing the paraneoplastic syndrome, which causes serious neurodevelopmental morbidity. Late recognition and inadequate treatment of OMS are largely responsible for poor outcome, predisposing to relapse during drug tapering or infections. Tumour resection is not a sufficient treatment for OMS and should not delay immunotherapy. The recent finding that B-cells (CD19+, CD5+) and T-cells (HLA-DR+, CD8+, and γδ+) are expanded in the cerebrospinal fluid in OMS indicates lymphocyte recruitment into the central nervous system. These cellular abnormalities correlate with neurological severity, serving as new biomarkers of disease activity that will allow evidence-based and selective treatments. Various autoantibodies to post-synaptic densities or unidentified brain antigens have been found, but there is no single antibody marker for OMS. Immunological treatments include corticotropin, corticosteroids, intravenous immunoglobulins, immunosuppressants, chemotherapy, monoclonal antibody therapy (rituximab), plasma exchange, and immunoadsorption. Combination immunotherapy has decided advantages over monotherapy. Other treatments aimed at alleviating the co-morbid features of OMS – such as rage and sleep problems, obsessive-compulsive and attention-deficit disorders – should be used adjunctively with immunotherapy. Recognition that children with OMS often require comprehensive treatment for years helps families, schools, and medical providers work toward the best possible long term outcome.

Background

Opsoclonus-myoclonus syndrome (OMS) is a rare but important movement disorder (Kinsbourne, 1962). In the typical case, a toddler develops acutely a constellation of neurological abnormalities that rapidly progress over days to a few weeks (Tate *et al.*, 2005). The diagnosis is straightforward once opsoclonus, or conjugately darting eyes, appears. However, this may be one of the later features of the syndrome. This results in a misdiagnosis of acute cerebellar ataxia in a majority of cases (Tate *et al.*, 2005). The child's extreme irritability and characteristic age vulnerability should prompt a search for occult neuroblastoma (Solomon

& Chutorian, 1968). Besides opsoclonus, myoclonus, and ataxia, affected children show rage, impaired sleep, expressive language impairment (dysarthria to anarthria), and hyperacusis (Pranzatelli *et al.*, 2005a). Later sequelae can include obsessive-compulsive disorder, attention-deficit hyperactivity disorder, cognitive impairment, and oppositional defiant disorder (Tate *et al.*, 2005). In contrast to the neurological disaster, the prognosis for surviving the tumour is excellent in OMS compared with neuroblastoma without OMS (Altmann & Baehner, 1976).

The National Pediatric Myoclonus Center is now a world centre for the evaluation and treatment of children with OMS. Our database now includes 180 cases. The purpose of founding this organization was to advocate for children with OMS and to recruit enough subjects for basic research and clinical trials. Otherwise, this disorder is too rare for fruitful investigation to develop a cure. Over the more than 20 years the centre has been in operation, we have observed patterns that challenge old concepts about this disorder.

The belief that OMS can be caused either by a tumour or by a virus is based on series in which a diagnosis of neuroblastoma was made in only about 50 per cent of OMS cases (Bolthauser *et al.*, 1979; Talon & Stoll, 1985), despite the use of modern imaging techniques (Shalaby-Rana *et al.*, 1997; Boubaker *et al.*, 2003). However, recent evidence challenges the view that there are two different aetiologies. On the grounds of logic it appears improbable that an identical syndrome should be produced by two disparate aetiologies. Even an experienced examiner would not be able to tell whether a given child did or did not have a tumour on neurological grounds. It is true that some viral illnesses have been documented in children with OMS (Kuban *et al.*, 1983; McMinn *et al.*, 2001). These include infections with both DNA and RNA viruses. However, are these the primary aetiological factors or secondary triggers? Neuroblastoma is notorious for spontaneous involution; no other tumour has such a propensity (Everson & Cole, 1966; Nishihara *et al.*, 2002). The possibility exists, therefore, that children may have already had a neuroblastoma by the time their clinical symptoms prompt a search for the tumour, but the tumour has been eradicated by the immune system. The argument for this is based on the high degree of lymphocytic infiltration in neuroblastomas (Martin & Beckwith, 1968), especially those that are associated with OMS (Cooper *et al.*, 2001). Also, the distribution of onset age does not differ between groups (Fig. 1). Whether or not a tumour is found may not affect outcome (Hammer *et al.*, 1995).

We also have gathered data that OMS is not a uniform disease (Pranzatelli, 2005). There appear to be subgroups on both clinical and immunological grounds. Clinically, there are children who have a monophasic course and with conventional treatment undergo complete remission. Some may be misdiagnosed as acute cerebellar ataxia and are not treated. The more common scenario is the child who has one or more relapses, prompted either by infection or attempts to taper steroids or corticotropin. Whether these children have a multiphasic *versus* a monophasic illness that was never successfully eradicated is unclear. A third group of children has relapsing-progressive disease. Mental retardation and significant motor and behavioural/cognitive disability is characteristic of this group (Papero *et al.*, 1995; Mitchell *et al.*, 2002).

Constructing a working hypothesis

In building a hypothesis of aetiopathophysiology, one must begin with the tumour – neuroblastoma is the only commonly occurring tumour in OMS – and work toward the neural structures presumed to be involved (Pranzatelli, 2000a). The assumption, which is backed by some data, is that an onconeuroantigen found both on the tumour and the neuroembryologically-related nerve cells provokes an autoimmune disorder, which is a case of 'friendly fire' on the

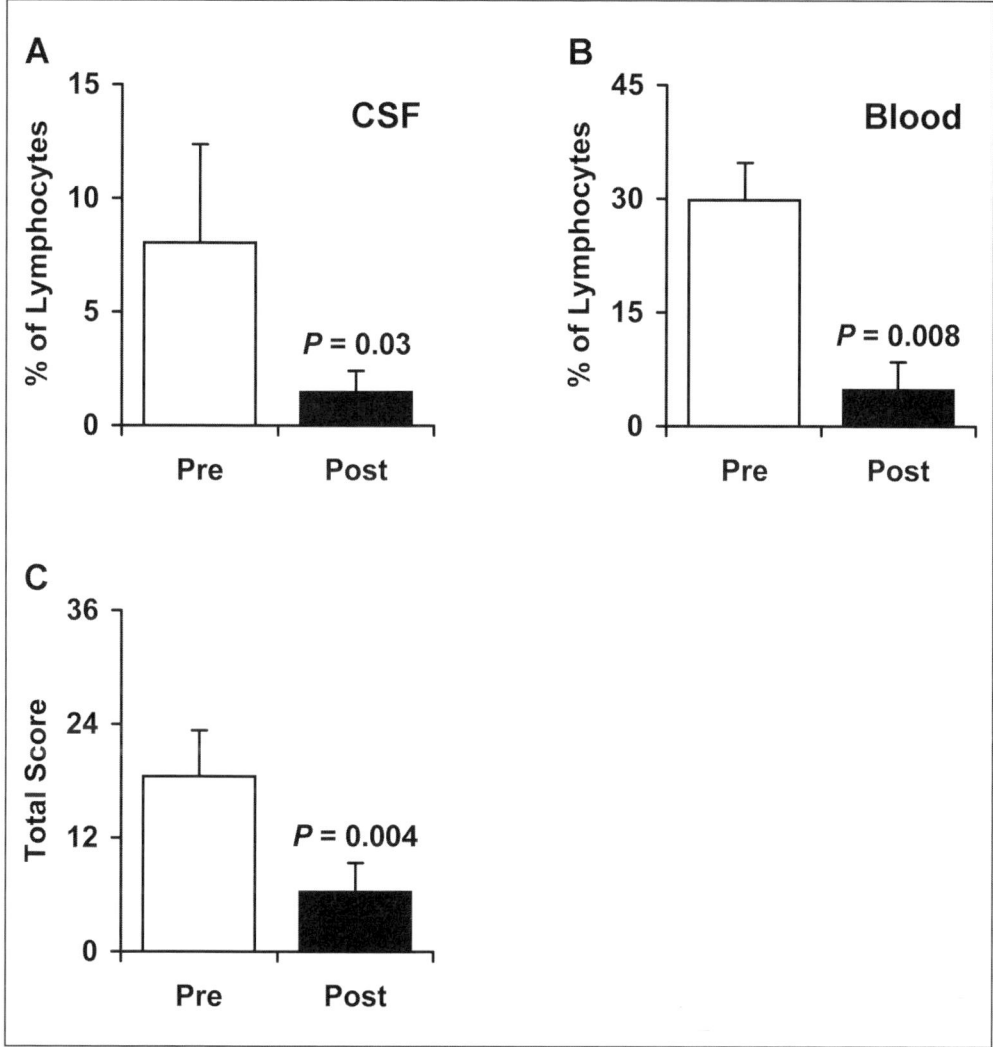

Fig. 1. Frequency plot of age at opsoclonus-myoclonus syndrome (OMS) onset in all OMS cases (upper) and according to presumed aetiology (lower). Note: The no-tumour and tumour groups were not significantly different.

brain (Pranzatelli, 2000b). The cerebellum is surely a primary target in the disease, but whether it explains all the features is less clear (Pranzatelli, 1992). The cerebellum plays a role in language development (Lieberman, 2002) and motor learning (Marr, 1969; Lalonde & Botez, 1990). Some behavioural or affective symptoms may be cerebellar in origin (Hamilton et al., 1983; Botez et al., 1989; Riva & Giorgi, 2000). As with myoclonus (Chase & Morales, 1990), the mechanisms of saccadic eye movements are said to be located in the brain stem (Fuchs et al., 1985), but the contrary view is that the origin is cerebellar (Wertenbaker et al., 1981). Cognitive impairment and attention-deficit disorder imply more frontal cerebral involvement, either as a result of frontal cerebellar connections or because of direct effects of the immune system on these more remote sites. In an adult with infant-onset OMS, we found cerebellar vermis atrophy 41 years after the disease onset (Pranzatelli *et al.*, 2002a). The patient had clinical gait ataxia as well as truncal and appendicular ataxia. Cerebellar atrophy has also been reported in some children with OMS (Hayward *et al.*, 2001), but is not typical. Using conventional proton magnetic resonance spectroscopy, however, no abnormal cerebellar spectra have been identified (Kuhn *et al.*, 2002). In summary, it would seem that a neuroblastoma can result in at least a cerebellar injury, especially involving the vermis.

We further hypothesized that there were two immunological defects. First, the tumour escapes immune surveillance, in that it is allowed to grow. In some children it grows so large that it is inoperable. In others, however, the tumour may be only a few mm in size. There may be some genetic vulnerability to this, but there is no simple Mendelian inheritance. Family members with OMS, including twins, have been reported; however, there are complex immunoregulatory genes that would be difficult to track down. The second defect is that once the immune system does find the neuroblastoma, then there seems to be an overreaction on some level. Fortunately, this is uncommon, occurring in only three to four per cent of all neuroblastomas. However, in those individuals, immune system dysregulation occurs, or else a state of autoimmunity. Secondary factors may further promote the development of an autoimmune disorder. CNS lymphocyte recruitment appears to be associated with the neuropsychological abnormalities. There may or may not be initial cerebrospinal fluid (CSF) pleocytosis. There is no evidence of any major cerebellar oedema or mass lesion. In most cases, head magnetic resonance imaging (MRI) is normal.

The currently favoured immunological hypothesis of OMS is that it is humorally-mediated. This is due in part to various putative autoantibodies that have been described, and also to a lack of studies on T-cells and other lymphocytes. Anti-Hu antibody was found in children with neuroblastoma without OMS, and in paraneoplastic OMS (Manley *et al.*, 1995). More recently, it has become apparent that anti-Hu has more to do with neuroblastoma than it does with OMS (Antunes *et al.*, 2000; Rudnick *et al.*, 2001). Both IgM and IgG autoantibodies to high-molecular-weight neurofilament and other smaller antigens have also been reported (Connolly *et al.*, 1997). Commercial screening for 'paraneoplastic' autoantibodies in children with OMS is not productive (Pranzatelli *et al.*, 2002b). All these studies employed Western blots. More recently, a different technique was used and various other autoantigens were detected, but no particular autoantigen was found in every case of OMS studied (Bataller *et al.*, 2003). In no study has a relation between autoantibody titres and neurological severity been found. Although paraneoplastic autoantibodies have been injected into experimental animals, no signs of OMS developed – hence there is no animal model of OMS. Also, because most children with OMS do not die from their condition, there have been limited post-mortem studies. In some cases, there is evidence of brain inflammation (Tuchman *et al.*, 1989; Clerico *et al.*, 1993), but no abnormalities were found in others (Kinsbourne, 1962; Ziter *et al.*, 1979). As a result, the autoantibody hypothesis of OMS is in question.

CSF and blood lymphocyte subset abnormalities in OMS

About a decade ago, we proposed that both B- and T-cells entered the brain once activated by the peripheral disease induction, to compromise brain function by producing autoantibodies or inflammatory cytokines, or by direct cell-to-cell toxicity (Pranzatelli, 1996). Thereby, normal immune cell trafficking (Hickey, 1999) can progress to lymphocyte recruitment (Hafler *et al.*, 1985; Sun, 1993). We were able to validate this hypothesis by undertaking immunophenotyping of CSF lymphocytes through flow cytometry (FACS) (Pranzatelli *et al.*, 2004a). Our initial focus was on the same cell types that are known to infiltrate neuroblastomas and to be involved in the body's defence against tumours, such as natural killer cells and γδ T-cells, conventional T-cells, and B-cells. Four different monoclonal antibody probes were used per assay tube.

This was a cross-sectional study, so individuals at any stage in their disease were included. Our population base involved a mixture of ages, ranging from infants to school-aged children. Half had chronic disease, about 20 per cent were acute, and the others were subacute. About half the children had moderate disease, about 20 per cent were severe, and the rest were moderate-to-severe. There was a slight excess of children in whom no tumour had been found. The INNS tumour stages ranged from stage 1 – the vast majority – to stage 3 (only a small percentage). Most of the tumours were located in the abdomen or thorax; a few were in the pelvis. Almost half the patients had previously received cyclophosphamide. Some had received multi-agent chemotherapy; others had received no chemotherapy. The tumour type was mostly neuroblastoma, with about 25 per cent of the cases being ganglioneuroblastoma. Each of the patients was videotaped, and the videotape was scored by a trained, blinded observer using the OMS Evaluation Scale (Pranzatelli et al., 2001). This is a 12-item scale rated from 0 to 3, with a maximum abnormality score of 36 (Table 1). This scale is meant to be used widely to provide objective documentation of the motor abnormalities of OMS.

Table 1. Evaluation scale of motor performance in opsoclonus-myoclonus syndrome

Item No.	Description
1	Walking: side-to-side imbalance
2	Walking: front-to-back imbalance
3	Walking: wide base
4	Instability while standing (feet apart)
5	Difficulty achieving standing position
6	Truncal instability while sitting
7	Targeting difficulty
8	Difficulty grasping with one hand
9	Difficulty with pincer grasp
10	Abnormal eye movements while tracking (fixation)
11	Abnormal eye movements while resting
12	Speech abnormality (dysarthria)

Videotapes were made to include a segment of each item needed for scoring. Each item is scored from 0 to 3 as follows: 0, normal; 1, mild; 2, moderate; 3, severe.

We found many abnormalities in the CSF. The frequency of CD4+ helper/inducer cells was decreased. The percentage of CD8+ cytotoxic/suppressor T-cells was increased. This resulted in a reduction in the CD4/CD8 ratio. In some individuals this was profound, resulting in a ratio of < 1:1 instead of the normal 3:1. There were no abnormalities in the frequency of killer-like T-cells and natural killer cells. The frequency of CD19+ B-cells was increased significantly. There also was an increase in percentage of γδ T-cells (unconventional T-cells). Using the OMS evaluation scale to assess mild, moderate, and severe levels of abnormality, comparisons were made between the three OMS groups. CD4+ T-cells decreased significantly with severity while the frequency of CSF B-cells (Fig. 2) and γδ T-cells increased with severity. There was substantial variability in the degree of cellular abnormality. Exploring the B-cell hypothesis further, we found that B-cell expansion was more prevalent in the acute cases (Fig. 3) and tended to decrease over time (Pranzatelli et al., 2004b). In chronic symptomatic cases, however, the percentage did not return to normal. We also examined T-cell activation in maturation markers. The only abnormality was an increase in HLA-DR+ or activated T-cells. No other cell abnormalities correlated with severity.

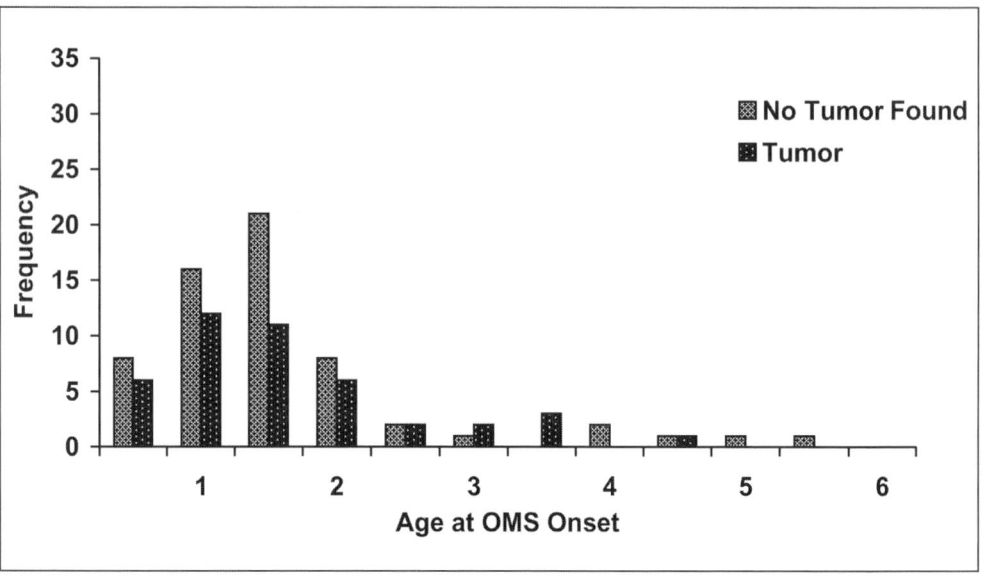

Fig. 2. Relation of neurological severity to percentage of B-cells in CSF. As an aid to clinical interpretation, neurological severity was defined as mild if the videotape total score was =12, moderate if 13–24, and severe if 25–36. Controls are shown for comparison. Asterisk signifies significant difference compared with controls. Cross indicates significant difference among severity categories, p < 0.05 by Duncan test. From left to right, n = 18, 16, 14, and 6.

Analysis of different treatment groups yielded novel observations. Conventional immunotherapy, such as steroids or intravenous immunoglobulin, did not result in a significant difference between groups. Children who had previously been treated with cyclophosphamide or multi-agent chemotherapy for their tumours did not have a different CSF immunophenotype from those who had not been so treated. These data indicated that, while conventional treatments and standard cancer chemotherapy may work by different mechanisms, they had not prevented the persistence of neurological problems that resulted in patients coming to our centre.

We then did a study to determine whether the distribution of peripheral blood mononuclear cells was altered in paraneoplastic OMS (Pranzatelli et al., 2004c). All groups were age- and sex-matched. Seventeen children with OMS but without a demonstrated tumour were compared with 17 with OMS in whom a tumour had been found, and there were 17 neurological controls. The blood mirrored some but not all of the immunological abnormalities found in the CSF. For instance, the CD4+ T-cell subset was smaller both in relative and absolute size compared with the controls. As a result, the CD4/CD8 ratio was also reduced. The absolute but not the relative size of the γδ T-cell subset was significantly reduced. There were no abnormalities of NK cells or NK-like T-cells, or of either naive or memory T-cells. Unfortunately, there were

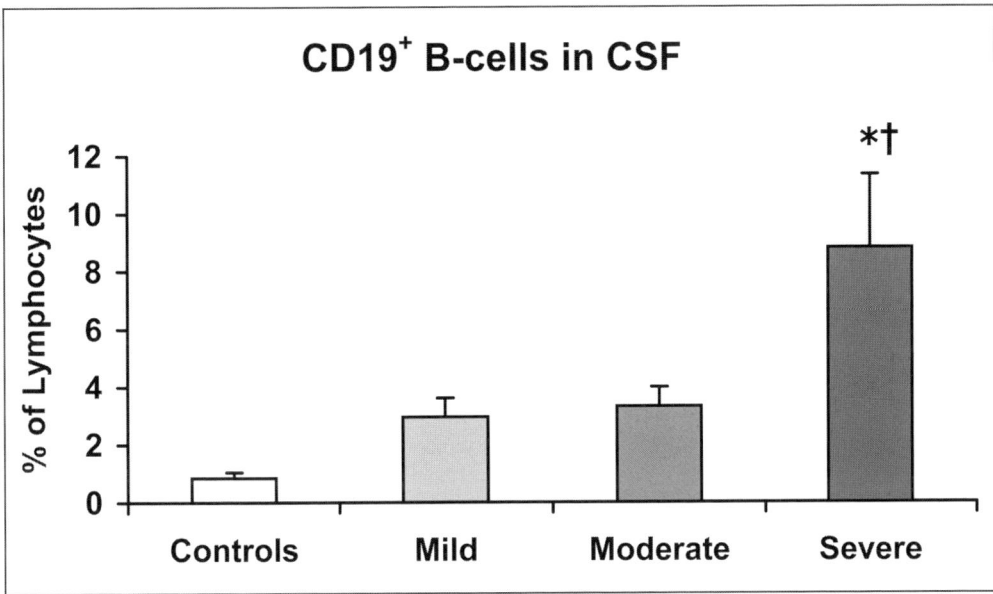

Fig. 3. Relation of syndrome duration to the percentage of CSF B-cells. The syndrome duration category was defined as acute if ≤ 3 months, subacute if 3–12 months, and chronic if >1 year. Controls are shown for comparison. Asterisk signifies significant difference compared with controls. Cross indicates significant difference among duration categories, $p < 0.05$ by Duncan test. From left to right, n = 18, 8, 10, and 18. As a point of comparison, neurological severity (total score) also varied with the duration of the illness ($F_{2,51} = 4.6; p = 0.014$, ANOVA). Scores in the chronic phase (11.8 ± 8.8) were about half those in the acute and subacute phases ($p < 0.05$, Duncan's test).

no significant abnormalities of CD19+ B-cells or activated T-cells, which had been very abnormal in the CSF. Previous chemotherapy for neuroblastoma did not alter the frequency of CD4+ T-cells. When the groups of OMS cases with or without a tumour were combined, we were able to show that chemotherapy decreased both the relative and the absolute size of the CD19+ B-cell subset and had only a small effect on the T-cell subsets. We concluded that blood lymphocyte subset analysis reflected the changes in conventional CD4 and CD8+ T-cells, but not B-cells. It remains to be demonstrated by longitudinal studies whether these T-cell abnormalities could play a role as treatment markers. Such longitudinal studies are ongoing at our centre.

Departing from FACS, we took another approach in the search for evidence of cellular immune activation in OMS (Pranzatelli *et al.*, 2004d). Neopterin is a known indicator of cellular immune activation in a variety of disorders. Its concentration in the CSF has been shown to be a more reliable marker of inflammation involving the central nervous system than serum levels. Neopterin was measured by reverse-phase high-performance liquid chromatography. CSF concentrations of neopterin were raised compared with controls. The increase in neopterin was most marked in acute and untreated patients, and the magnitude of the increase was similar to that reported for central nervous system viral infections. No differences were found between the children who did and did not have a demonstrable tumour. Previous studies on CSF neopterin showed that it increases after allogenic T-cell activation, but monocytes and macrophages can also be induced to produce neopterin by cytokines. Neopterin was not a sensitive biomarker of disease activity in OMS because some children with OMS, despite having neurological abnormalities, did not have a raised neopterin concentration. This may have been a result of previous immunotherapy, as this was a cross-sectional study. Although neopterin is not sensitive enough to serve as a clinical biomarker of disease activity, it does support the autoimmune hypothesis of OMS.

Therapeutic innovations

Given data on various putative autoantibodies in OMS, we focused on the B-cell autoaggression as our primary hypothesis. The next step was to determine whether any immunotherapies were available that eradicated CSF B-cells, and what the effect of such treatment would be on the clinical course. In the USA, rituximab was approved by the FDA in 1997 for the treatment of B-cell lymphoma. Its safety profile seemed acceptable and it had previously been used in children for various haematological autoimmune disorders, such as idiopathic thrombocytopenic purpura. Our centre was the first to report the use of rituximab in paediatric OMS (Pranzatelli *et al.*, 2003; Pranzatelli *et al.*, 2005b). We found that this agent was very efficient at eradicating B-cells in the blood, as had been known previously. However, we also found that it significantly reduced the numbers of B-cells in the CSF (Fig. 4) (Pranzatelli *et al.*, 2005b). Many patients had undetectable B-cells after treatment. Since then, we have seen a few children who did not respond, and a few who needed re-treatment a year later. But for most, rituximab exerted a lasting beneficial effect on the frequency of CSF B-cells. The relation between clinical and immunological effects was a reduction in total score on the OMS Evaluation Scale (Table 1) (Pranzatelli *et al.*, 2001). Before treatment, the average total score was in the moderate severity range, whereas after therapy, it was in the mild severity category.

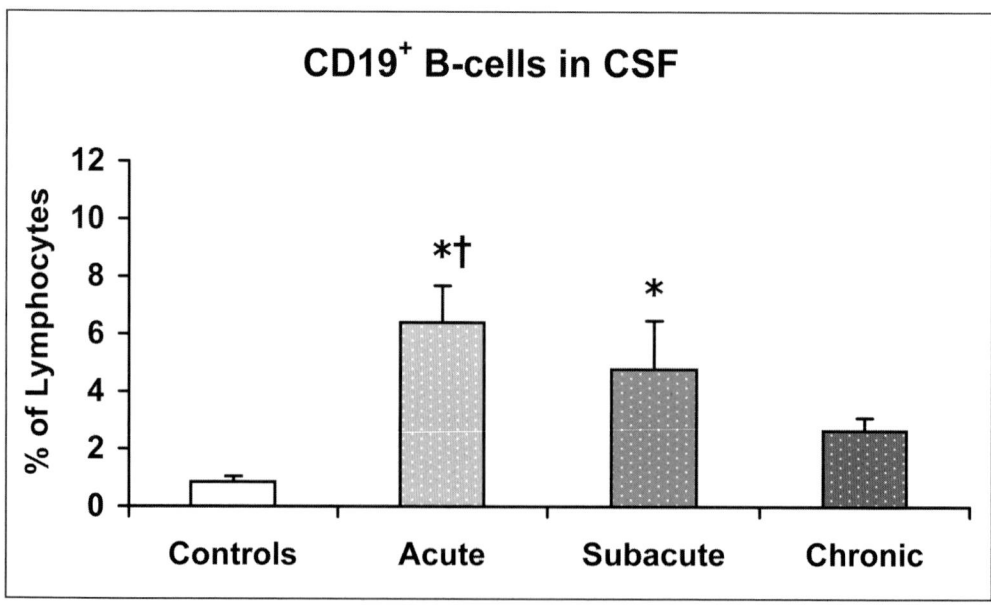

Fig. 4. *Effects of rituximab on CSF B-cells and severity of opsoclonus-myoclonus syndrome. Six months after completion of rituximab infusions, CSF (A) and blood B cells (B) were depleted. The total score (C) decreased from the upper limit of moderate to the upper limit of mild categories. Clinical severity was classified as mild if the total score was = 12, moderate if 13–24, and severe if 25–36.*

The choice of immunological agents and the overall strategy of using these as a treatment remains one of the greatest controversies in OMS (Table 2). Corticotropin (ACTH), intravenous immunoglobulins (IVIg), and corticosteroids are the typical conventional agents (Sugie *et al.*, 1992; Petruzzi & DeAlarcon, 1995; Pranzatelli, 1996; Veneselli *et al.*, 1998; Blaes, 2002). Plasma exchange and immunoadsorption are still under investigation (Batchelor *et al.*, 1998; Yiu *et al.*, 2001). In our experience, high-dose ACTH (Pranzatelli *et al.*, 1998) is superior to corticosteroids (Emir *et al.*, 2003), but there are no controlled trials. Having seen the pitfalls of using single or even dual conventional therapies in children with moderately severe to severe disease, we no longer accept them as adequate treatment. Others have had similar negative experiences (Koh *et al.*, 1994; Pohl *et al.*, 1996). This is not to say that corticosteroids, IVIg, or ACTH cannot be used alone in the mildest of cases. We believe that the moderately severe and severe cases should have chemotherapy as the third agent. To determine what type of chemotherapy should be used, we rely heavily on the results of CSF lymphocyte immunophenotyping. We devised this approach because FACS is available at most major medical centres, so the procedure could be adopted globally. Each flow cytometry centre can develop its own control data. If flow cytometry is not available, the clinical rule of thumb is that when a child does not return completely to normal on ACTH therapy, there is always significant underlying autoimmune disease. Because no conventional agent affects the frequency of pathological lymphocytes in the CSF, and presumably in the brain, the child is at risk of ongoing brain injury and relapse when the conventional agents are tapered or removed.

Table 2. Immunotherapies for opsoclonus-myoclonus syndrome

Category	Agents
Biological agents	Corticotropin (ACTH) Intravenous immunoglobulins (IVIg) Rituximab
Drugs	Oral corticosteroids Intravenous dexamethasone (pulse dosing) Cyclophosphamide 6-Mercaptopurine Methotrexate Azathioprine Mycophenolate mofetil*
Pheresis	Plasmapheresis Immunoadsorption

Treatment categories and types of agents may be combined.
*Not for use in patients with CSF B-cell expansion.

Some clinicians use a wait-and-watch approach. Sometimes no treatment is begun until months after tumour resection, based on the belief that resection alone will stop OMS. In fact, two thirds of such cases will not improve or will deteriorate after surgery (Tate *et al.*, 2005). At this point a single agent is initiated. If the child does not improve, a second conventional agent may be added. Some will consider the use of chemotherapy, but many will not. Children who do not have a tumour are at greatest risk of not being offered chemotherapy for their neurological syndrome. This is unfortunate. We believe there is a window of opportunity for successfully eradicating the underlying autoimmune disease without allowing permanent brain injury to occur. Once mental retardation develops, there is no going back. No one knows exactly how long the window of opportunity is open, so we are proponents of front-end therapy. At our centre, the combination that we most commonly use is ACTH, IVIg, and rituximab. In the most difficult cases, secondary agents or approaches may be necessary as well, depending on the initial response.

Others are evaluating a protocol that combines oral corticosteroids with IVIg and cyclophosphamide. In a pilot study (Pranzatelli *et al.*, 2005c), we found that cyclophosphamide did have anti-B-cell properties in the CSF. However, it usually did not reduce B-cells to normal levels at the doses used in this protocol. We recommended that dose-response studies be carried out before the cyclophosphamide protocol is used internationally. Finally, we have encountered some children with severe disease who require the use of multiple types of chemotherapy over a few to several years to put their disease into remission. Mycophenolate mofetil, which has replaced azathioprine in inflammatory diseases, does not reduce the frequency of CSF B-cells in OMS (Pranzatelli *et al.*, 2005d).

Conclusions

Several conclusions can be drawn from these data. OMS is characterized by multiple immunological abnormalities. These abnormalities involve B- and T-cells, sometimes persisting for years, and showed significant individual variability. We were able to demonstrate that CSF B- and T-cell recruitment is directly linked to neurological dysfunction. We speculated that this may account for relapses and disease progression in OMS, and that B- and T-cells are useful biomarkers of disease activity in this disorder. The observation that the tumour and no-tumour-found groups were not immunologically different on the basis of CSF cellular abnormalities cannot be ignored. These data imply that OMS is paraneoplastic until proven otherwise, and that the neurological syndrome should not be treated differently depending on whether one does or does not find an underlying tumour. The data also clearly indicate that tumour therapy, including both tumour resection and conventional cancer chemotherapy, is insufficient as treatment for the paraneoplastic disorder, at least in those individuals who have persistent symptoms. As a result, there is a need for more selective and potent agents. Our centre is currently very active in developing innovative treatment strategies.

References

Altmann, A.J. & Baehner, R.L. (1976): Favorable prognosis for survival in children with coincident opso-myoclonus and neuroblastoma. *Cancer* **37**, 846–852.

Antunes, N.L., Khakoo, Y., Matthay, K.K., Seeger, R.C., Stram, D.O., Gerstner, E., Abrey, L.E. & Dalmau, J. (2000): Antineuronal antibodies in patients with neuroblastoma and paraneoplastic opsoclonus-myoclonus. *J. Pediatr. Hematol. Oncol.* **22**, 315–320.

Bataller, L., Rosenfeld, M.R., Graus, F., Vilchez, J.J., Cheung, N.K. & Dalmau, J. (2003): Autoantigen diversity in the opsoclonus-myoclonus syndrome. *Ann. Neurol.* **53**, 347–353.

Batchelor, T.T., Platten, M. & Hochberg, F.H. (1998): Immunoadsorption therapy for paraneoplastic syndromes. *J. Neurooncol.* **40**, 131–136.

Blaes, F. (2002): Immunotherapeutic approaches to paraneoplastic neurological disorders. *Expert Opin. Biol. Ther.* **2**, 419–430.

Bolthauser, E., Deonna, T. & Hirt, H.R. (1979): Myoclonic encephalopathy of infants or 'dancing eyes syndrome.' *Helv. Paediatr. Acta* **34**, 119–133.

Botez, M.I., Botez, T., Elie, R. & Attig, E. (1989): Role of the cerebellum in complex human behavior. *Ital. J. Neurol. Sci.* **10**, 291–300.

Boubaker, A. & Bischof Delaloye, A. (2003): Nuclear medicine procedures and neuroblastoma in childhood. Their value in the diagnosis, staging and assessment of response to therapy. *Q. J. Nucl. Med.* **47**, 31–40.

Chase, M.H. & Morales, F.R. (1990): The atonia and myoclonia of active (REM) sleep. *Annu. Rev. Psychol.* **41**, 557–584.

Clerico, A., Tenore, A., Bartolozzi, S., Remotti, D., Ruco, L., Dominici, C., Properzi, E. & Castello, M.A. (1993): Adrenocorticotropic hormone-secreting ganglioneuroblastoma associated with opsomyoclonic encephalopathy: a case report with immunohistochemical study. *Med. Pediatr. Oncol.* **21**, 690–694.

Connolly, A.M., Pestronk, A., Mehta, S., Pranzatelli, M.R. & Noetzel, M.J. (1997): Serum autoantibodies in childhood opsoclonus-myoclonus syndrome: an analysis of antigenic targets in neural tissues. *J. Pediatr.* **130**, 878–884.

Cooper, R., Khakoo, Y., Matthay, K.K., Lukens, J.N., Seeger, R.C., Stram, D.O., Gerbing, R.B., Nakagawa, A. & Shimada, H. (2001): Opsoclonus-myoclonus-ataxia syndrome in neuroblastoma: histopathologic features – a report from the children's cancer group. *Med. Pediatr. Oncol.* **36**, 623–629.

Emir, S., Akyuz, C. & Buyukpamukcu, M. (2003): Treatment of the neuroblastoma-associated opsoclonus-myoclonus-ataxia (OMA) syndrome with high-dose methylprednisolone [letter]. *Med. Pediatr. Oncol.* **40,** 139.

Everson, T.C. & Cole, W.H. (1966): Spontaneous regression of neuroblastoma. In: *Spontaneous regression of cancer*, eds. T.C. Everson & W.H. Cole, p. 88. Philadelphia: WB Saunders.

Fuchs, A.F., Kaneko, C.R.S. & Seudder, C.A. (1985): Brainstem control of saccadic eye movements. *Annu. Rev. Neurosci.* **8**, 307–337.

Hafler, D.A., Fox, D.A., Manning, M.E., Schlossman, S.F., Reinherz, E.L. & Weiner, H.L. (1985): In vivo activated T lymphocytes in the peripheral blood and cerebrospinal fluid of patients with multiple sclerosis. *N. Eng. J. Med.* **312**, 1405–1411.

Hamilton, N.G., Frick, R.B., Takahasi, T. & Hopping, M.W. (1983): Psychiatric symptoms and cerebellar pathology. *Am. J. Psychiatry* **140**, 1322–1326.

Hammer, M.S., Larsen, M.B. & Stack, C.V. (1995): Outcome of children with opsoclonus-myoclonus regardless of etiology. *Pediatr. Neurol.* **13**, 21–24.

Hayward, K., Jeremy, R.J., Jenkins, S., Barkovich, A.J., Gultekin, S.H., Kramer, J., Crittenden, M. & Matthay, K.K. (2001): Long-term neurobehavioral outcomes in children with neuroblastoma and opsoclonus-myoclonus-ataxia syndrome: relationship to MRI findings and anti-neuronal antibodies. *J. Pediatr.* **139**, 552–559.

Hickey, W.F. (1999): Leukocyte traffic in the central nervous system: the participants and their roles. *Semin. Immunol.* **11**, 125–137.

Kinsbourne, M. (1962): Myoclonic encephalopathy of infants. *J. Neurol. Neurosurg. Psychiatry* **25**, 221–276.

Koh, P.S., Raffensperger, J.G., Berry, S., Larsen, M.B., Johnstone, H.S., Chou, P., Luck, S.R., Hammer, M. & Cohn, S.L. (1994): Long-term outcome in children with opsoclonus-myoclonus and ataxia and coincident neuroblastoma. *J. Pediatr.* **125**, 712–716.

Kuban, K.C., Ephros, M.A., Freeman, R.L., Laffell, L.B. & Bresnan, M.J. (1983): Syndrome of opsoclonus-myoclonus caused by Coxsackie B3 infection. *Ann. Neurol.* **13**, 69–71.

Kuhn, M.J., Pranzatelli, M.R. & Langheim, J.M. (2002): MR Spectroscopy in children with opsoclonus-myoclonus syndrome. *Proceedings of the 40th Annual Meeting of the American Society of Neuroradiology*, p. 233.

Lalonde, R. & Botez, M.I. (1990): The cerebellum and learning processes in animals. *Brain. Res. Rev.* **15**, 325–332.

Lieberman, P. (2002): On the nature and evolution of the neural bases of human language. *Am. J. Phys. Anthropol.* **35** (Suppl.), 36–62.

Manley, G.T., Smitt, P.S., Dalmau, J. & Posner, J.B. (1995): Hu antigens: reactivity with Hu antibodies, tumor expression, and major immunogenic sites. *Ann. Neurol.* **38**, 102–110.

Marr, D. (1969): A theory of cerebellar cortex. *J. Physiol. (Lond.)* **202**, 437–470.

Martin, E.F. & Beckwith, J.B. (1968): Lymphoid infiltrates in neuroblastoma: their occurrence and prognostic significance. *J. Pediatr. Surg.* **3**, 161–164.

McMinn, P., Stratov, I., Nagarajan, L. & Davis, S. (2001): Neurological manifestations of enterovirus 71 infection in children during an outbreak of hand, foot, and mouth disease in Western Australia. *Clin. Infect. Dis.* **32**, 236–242.

Mitchell, W.G., Davalos-Gonzalez, Y., Brumm, V.L., Aller, S.K., Burger, E., Turkel, S.B., Borchert, M.S., Hollar, S. & Padilla S. (2002): Opsoclonus-ataxia caused by childhood neuroblastoma: developmental and neurologic sequelae. *Pediatrics* **109**, 86–98.

Nishihira, H., Toyoda, Y., Tanaka, Y., Ijiri, R., Aida, N., Takeuchi, M., Ohnuma, K., Kigasawa, H., Kato, K. & Nishi, T. (2002): Natural course of neuroblastoma detected by mass screening: a 5-year prospective study at a single institution. *J. Clin. Oncol.* **18**, 3012–3017.

Papero, P.H., Pranzatelli, M.R., Margolis, C.J., Tate, E., Wilson, L.A. & Glass, P. (1995): Neurobehavioral and psychosocial functioning of children with opsoclonus-myoclonus syndrome. *Dev. Med. Child. Neurol.* **37**, 915–932.

Petruzzi, J.M. & DeAlarcon, P.A. (1995): Neuroblastoma-associated opsoclonus-myoclonus treated with intravenously administered immune globulin G. *J. Pediatr.* **127**, 328–329.

Pohl, K.R.E., Pritchard, J. & Wilson, J. (1996): Neurological sequelae of the dancing eye syndrome. *Eur. J. Pediatr.* **155**, 237–244.

Pranzatelli, M.R. (1992): The neurobiology of opsoclonus-myoclonus. *Clin. Neuropharmacol.* **15**, 186–228.

Pranzatelli, M.R. (1996): The immunopharmacology of the opsoclonus-myoclonus syndrome. *Clin. Neuropharmacol.* **19**, 1–47.

Pranzatelli, M.R. (2000a): Paraneoplastic syndromes: an unsolved murder. *Semin. Pediatr. Neurol.* **7**, 118–130.

Pranzatelli, M.R. (2000b): Friendly fire. *Discover* April, 35–36.

Pranzatelli, M.R. (2005): Opsoclonus-myoclonus-ataxia. In: *Pediatric movement disorders*, eds. E. Fernandez-Alvarez, A. Arzimanoglou & E. Tolosa, pp. 120–136. Paris: John Libbey Eurotext.

Pranzatelli, M.R., Huang, Y., Tate, E., Goldstein, D.S., Holmes, C.S., Goldstein, E.M., Ketner, K., Kinast, M., Lange, B.M., Sanz, A., Shevell, M.I., Stanford, R.E. & Taff, I.P. (1998): Monoaminergic effects of high-dose corticotropin in corticotropin-responsive pediatric opsoclonus-myoclonus. *Mov. Disord.* **13**, 522–528.

Pranzatelli, M.R., Tate, E.D., Galvan, I. & Wheeler, A. (2001): Controlled pilot study of piracetam for pediatric opsoclonus-myoclonus. *Clin. Neuropharmacol.* **24**, 352–357.

Pranzatelli, M.R., Tate, E.D., Kinsbourne, M., Caviness, V.S. & Mishra, B. (2002a): Forty-one year follow-up of childhood-onset opsoclonus-myoclonus: cerebellar atrophy, multiphasic relapses, response to IVIG. *Mov. Disord.* **17**, 1387–1390.

Pranzatelli, M.R., Tate, E.D., Wheeler, A., Bass, N., Gold, A.P., Griebel, M.L., Gumbinas, M., Heydemann, P.T., Holt, P.J., Jacob, P., Kotagal, S., Minarcik, C.J. & Schub, H.S. (2002b): Screening for autoantibodies in children with opsoclonus-myoclonus-ataxia. *Pediatr. Neurol.* **27**, 384–387.

Pranzatelli, M.R., Tate, E.D., Travelstead, A.L. & Verhulst, S.J. (2003): CSF B-cell expansion in opsoclonus-myoclonus: effect of rituximab, an anti-B-cell monoclonal antibody. *Neurology* **60** (Suppl. 1), A395.

Pranzatelli, M.R., Travelstead, A., Tate, E.D., Allison, T.J., Moticka, E.J., Franz, D.N., Nigro, M.A., Parke, J.T., Stumpf, D.A. & Verhulst, S.J. (2004a): B- and T-cell markers in pediatric opsoclonus-myoclonus syndrome: immunophenotyping of CSF lymphocytes. *Neurology* **62**, 1526–1532.

Pranzatelli, M.R., Travelstead, A.L., Tate, E.D., Allison, T.J. & Verhulst, S.J. (2004b): CSF B-cell expansion in opsoclonus-myoclonus syndrome: a biomarker of disease activity. *Move. Disord.* **19**, 770–777.

Pranzatelli, M.R., Travelstead, A., Tate, E.D., Allison, T.J., Lee, N.D., Fisher, J. & Jasty, R. (2004c): Immunophenotype of blood lymphocytes in neuroblastoma-associated opsoclonus-myoclonus. *J. Pediatr. Hematol. Oncol.* **26**, 718–723.

Pranzatelli, M.R., Hyland, K., Tate, E.D., Arnold, L.A., Allison, T.J. & Soori, G.S. (2004d): Evidence of cellular immune activation in children with opsoclonus-myoclonus: cerebrospinal fluid neopterin. *J. Child. Neurol.* **19**, 919–924.

Pranzatelli, M.R., Tate, E.D., Dukart, W.S., Flint, M.J., Hoffman, M.T. & Oksa, A.E. (2005a): Sleep disturbance and rage attacks in opsoclonus-myoclonus syndrome: response to trazodone. *J. Pediatr.* **147**, 372–378.

Pranzatelli, M.R., Tate, E.D., Travelstead, A.L. & Longee, D. (2005b): Immunologic and clinical response to rituximab in a child with opsoclonus-myoclonus syndrome. *Pediatrics* **115**, e115–e119.

Pranzatelli, M.R., Tate, E.D., Travelstead, A.L., Allison, T.J., Grana, N., Parkhurst, J. & Russell, C. (2005c): Cyclophosphamide therapy in pediatric opsoclonus-myoclonus. *Ann. Neurol.* **58** (Suppl. 9), S90.

Pranzatelli, M.R., Tate, E.D., Travelstead, A.L., Bennett, H.J., Halthore, S.N., Kerstan, P., Sharpe, S. & Taub, J.W. (2005d): Mycophenolate reduces CSF T-cell activation and is a steroid sparer in opsoclonus-myoclonus syndrome. *Ann. Neurol.* **58** (Suppl. 9), S111.

Riva, D. & Giorgi, C. (2000): The cerebellum contributes to higher functions during development. *Brain* **123**, 1051–1061.

Rudnick, E., Khakoo, Y., Antunes, N.L., Seeger, R.C., Brodeur, G.M., Shimada, H., Gerbing, R.B., Stram, D.O. & Matthay, K.K. (2001): Opsoclonus-myoclonus-ataxia syndrome in neuroblastoma: clinical outcome and antineuronal antibodies – a report from the Children's Cancer Group Study. *Med. Pediatr. Oncol.* **36**, 612–622.

Shalaby-Rana, E., Majd, M., Andrich, M.P. & Movassaghi, N. (1997): In-11 pentetreotide scintigraphy in patients with neuroblastoma. Comparison with I-131 MIBG, N-Myc oncogene amplification, and patient outcome. *Clin. Nucl. Med.* **22**, 315–319.

Solomon, G.E. & Chutorian, A.M. (1968): Opsoclonus and occult neuroblastoma. *N. Engl. J. Med.* **279**, 475–477.

Sugie, H., Sugie, Y., Akimoto, H., Endo, K., Shirai, M. & Ito, M. (1992): High-dose IV human immunoglobulin in a case with infantile opsoclonus polymyoclonia syndrome. *Acta. Paediatr.* **18**, 371–372.

Sun, J.B. (1993): Autoreactive T and B cells in nervous system diseases. *N. Engl. J. Med.* **345**, 340–350.

Talon, P. & Stoll, C. (1985): Opso-myoclonus syndrome of infancy. New observations. Review of literature (110 cases). *Pédiatrie* **40**, 441–449.

Tate, E.D., Allison, T., Pranzatelli, M.R. & Verhulst, S.J. (2005): Neuroepidemiologic trends in 105 US cases of pediatric opsoclonus-myoclonus syndrome. *J. Pediatr. Oncol. Nurs.* **22**, 8–19.

Tuchman, R.F., Alvarez, L.A., Kantrowitz, A.B., Moser, F.G., Llena, J. & Moshe, S.L. (1989): Opsoclonus-myoclonus syndrome: correlation of radiographic and pathologic observations. *Neuroradiology* **31**, 250–252.

Veneselli, E., Conte, M., Biancheri, R., Acquaviva, A. & De Bernardi, B. (1998): Effect of steroid and high-dose immunoglobulin therapy on opsoclonus-myoclonus syndrome occurring in neuroblastoma. *Med. Pediatr. Oncol.* **30**, 15–17.

Wertenbaker, C., Behrens, M.M., Hunter, S.B. & Plank, C.R. (1981): Opsoclonus – a cerebellar disorder? *Neuroophthalmology* **2**, 73–84.

Yiu, V.W., Kovithavongs, T., McGonigle, L.F. & Ferreira, P. (2001): Plasmapheresis as an effective treatment for opsoclonus-myoclonus syndrome. *Pediatr. Neurol.* **24**, 72–74.

Ziter, F.A., Bray, P.F. & Cancilla, P.A. (1979): Neuropathological findings in a patient with neuroblastoma and myoclonic encephalopathy. *Arch. Neurol.* **36**, 51.

Chapter 14

Pantothenate kinase-associated neurodegeneration

Susan J. Hayflick

*Departments of Molecular and Medical Genetics, Pediatrics and Neurology,
Oregon Health & Science University, L103, 3181 SW Sam Jackson Park Rd, Portland,
Oregon 97239-3098, USA*
hayflick@ohsu.edu
Video 6

Summary

Neurodegeneration with brain iron accumulation (NBIA) comprises a heterogeneous group of progressive disorders that share the feature of high basal ganglia iron.
Pantothenate kinase-associated neurodegeneration (PKAN) is an autosomal recessive form of NBIA. PKAN is caused by mutations in the pantothenate kinase 2 gene *(PANK2)*, which lead to a range of phenotypes that vary by age of onset and predominant symptoms. Clinical features of PKAN include dystonia, pigmentary retinopathy, behavioural and psychiatric disturbances, parkinsonism, speech difficulties, and acanthocytosis. Though molecular testing can confirm a diagnosis of PKAN, this disorder is strongly suspected by the finding of characteristic changes on magnetic resonance imaging showing excess iron in the globus pallidus. Though the precise cellular effect of deficient pantothenate kinase 2 remains unclear, studies suggest that this mitochondrial form of the key regulatory enzyme in coenzyme A biosynthesis is critical for the maintenance of cell membrane integrity and defences against reactive oxygen species.
The link between pantothenate kinase 2 deficiency and the accumulation of iron in the basal ganglia is not yet understood. Despite this, the discovery of the genetic basis of PKAN has led to ideas for rational treatments that await clinical testing once a sensitive outcome measure of disease progression can be validated.

Introduction

Normally iron is regionally distributed throughout the mammalian brain. Regions of high iron content include the globus pallidus, the red nucleus, and the substantia nigra. Brain iron accumulates with age and as a secondary feature of disease pathogenesis in common neurological disorders including Parkinson's disease and Alzheimer's disease. The primary function of physiological iron in the CNS and the basis for its regional distribution remain important unanswered questions.

Single-gene disorders are useful for identifying genes which, when defective, perturb critical physiological processes. Brain iron homeostasis is altered in a several common diseases as well as in a few rare Mendelian disorders. As single-gene disorders can be dissected down to their molecular basis, these latter conditions can reveal both disease pathophysiology and the normal cellular processes that underlie the disease.

The Mendelian disorders in which iron accumulates in the brain include aceruloplasminaemia, neuroferritinopathy, infantile neuroaxonal dystrophy, and pantothenate kinase-associated neurodegeneration (PKAN). This review will focus on PKAN and what has been learned about its features since the discovery of the gene.

Genetics

PKAN is an autosomal recessive disorder associated with mutations in the *PANK2* gene (Zhou et al., 2001). The disease was mapped to chromosome 20p13 in 1996 and the culprit gene identified in 2001. *PANK2* comprises seven exons with disease-causing mutations found in every case. There is a loose correlation between genotype and phenotype, with mutations that are predicted to generate no functional protein leading to the more severe classical form of the disease. Several polymorphisms within the *PANK2* gene have also been characterized. Consortium data on *PANK2* sequence variants are valuable for interpreting clinical test results and are available from the author.

Biochemical basis of disease

With the gene discovery came new insights into the metabolic basis of PKAN.

PANK2 is one of four human genes predicted to encode a pantothenate kinase. It is distinguished from *PANK1*, *PANK3*, and *PANK4* by encoding a mitochondrial targeting signal. Pantothenate kinase is the key regulatory enzyme in the synthesis of coenzyme A, and PANK2 is the mitochondrial form of this enzyme (Zhou et al., 2001; Johnson et al., 2004). The hypothesized effect of deficient mitochondrial pantothenate kinase is defective lipid metabolism, which is predicted to result in impaired membrane homeostasis and repair (Zhou et al., 2001; Johnson et al., 2004).

The mechanism whereby PANK2 deficiency leads to basal ganglia iron accumulation remains unclear. Based on predictions of the metabolic impact of defective PANK2 and on the observation of raised brain concentrations of cysteine in patients with probable PKAN (Perry et al., 1985), we proposed a hypothesis for iron accumulation (Zhou et al., 2001). In normal brain, non-haem iron accumulates regionally and is at highest concentration in the medial globus pallidus and the substantia nigra pars reticulata, the two regions most severely affected in PKAN. Phosphopantothenate, the product of pantothenate kinase, normally condenses with cysteine in the next step in CoA synthesis. In PKAN, phosphopantothenate is deficient, theoretically leading to cysteine accumulation. N-Pantothenoyl-cysteine and panteheine – also substrates for phosphorylation by pantothenate kinase and both containing cysteine – are also predicted to accumulate. Cysteine binds iron effectively. Therefore we predict that the iron present in PKAN is in association with the accumulation of these cysteine-containing substrates. Though iron accumulation is not primary in PKAN, iron dyshomeostasis is very likely to contribute to disease pathogenesis.

Clinical features of PKAN

Disease associated with defects in *PANK2* spans a spectrum of severity. Classical disease has onset in early childhood with dystonia as the predominant feature. This is a rapidly progressive form with loss of ambulation usually in the second decade of life. Retinopathy is common in the classical form of PKAN. Atypical PKAN refers to disease that falls outside of this early-onset and rapidly progressive form. Atypical PKAN can have its onset any time after age 5 years, with the rate of progression being slower than that seen in classical disease. Presenting features may be dystonia but they are more likely to involve behavioural or psychiatric problems, with a movement disorder developing later in the disease. Retinopathy, though present in a significant portion of patients with atypical disease, is less common. The range of features seen in patients with *PANK2* defects is very broad. These features may be non-specific; however, radiographic examination almost always leads to a suspected diagnosis.

Radiographic features of PKAN

Brain magnetic resonance imaging (MRI) changes are virtually pathognomonic for PKAN (Hayflick *et al.*, 2003). The diagnostic changes seen on T2-weighted images include a central hyperintensity of signal in the medial globus pallidus, surrounded by a region of signal hypointensity, called the eye-of-the-tiger sign. The substantia nigra may or may not show an abnormality early in the disease. The correlation is nearly absolute between these MRI changes and the presence of mutations in *PANK2* (Hayflick *et al.*, 2006).

Pathological features of PKAN

The abundant literature on pathological changes is confounded by the heterogeneity of disorders formerly termed Hallervorden-Spatz syndrome. The specific pathology of PKAN is being delineated, though many questions still remain (Kotzbauer *et al.*, 2005).

Iron accumulates abnormally in the brain regions that are normally iron-rich, including the globus pallidus and the substantia nigra pars reticulata. Older neuropathological studies of tissue from patients with neurodegeneration with brain iron accumulation (NBIA) showed that the globus pallidus and substantia nigra contain approximately three times the normal amount of iron, yet the iron content is normal in other regions of the brain and in the retina (Gregory & Hayflick, 2005). Systemic iron metabolism is also normal. Iron uptake studies in NBIA patients suggest that the accumulation of iron in the basal ganglia is secondary to increased iron uptake with normal turnover (Szanto & Gallyas, 1966).

In regions of massive iron accumulation, spheroid bodies – many positive for iron – are also seen (Hallervorden & Spatz, 1922). Axonal spheroids are posited to represent swollen or bloated axons, possibly secondary to defects in axonal transport. They have been observed in normal ageing brains and in various other neurodegenerative disorders, including the neuroaxonal dystrophies. Other neuropathological findings include demyelination, neuronal loss, and gliosis, which occur predominantly within the globus pallidus and substantia nigra, where focal symmetrical destruction may be grossly evident.

Treatment of PKAN

Pharmacological and surgical interventions are aimed at palliation of symptoms. For many of the interventions that offer improvement of clinical symptoms, the period of benefit is limited. Even with these limitations, it is possible for clinicians to work closely with families and make periodic adjustments to maintain as high a quality of life as possible. Baclofen and trihexyphenidyl remain the most effective drugs against disabling dystonia and spasticity. As a rule, patients with PKAN do not benefit from L-dopa, although patients with non-PKAN NBIA and parkinsonism may respond to this agent. Botulinum toxin can be helpful for some patients, especially those whose quality of life is improved by treating a limited body region.

When oral baclofen is no longer able to control the movement disorder adequately, placement of an intrathecal baclofen pump may be considered. Deep brain stimulation (DBS) is also an option for relieving some symptoms. Anecdotal cases suggest that the benefit from these more invasive treatments is relatively short-lived, but they may provide relief to patients experiencing extreme dystonia and spasticity. A recent report on the use of DBS in PKAN suggests that it may hold promise (Castelnau *et al.*, 2005). The patients treated with DBS showed overall improvements in writing, speech, walking, and global measures of motor skills. The length of follow-up time, however, varied from 6 to 42 months at the time of publication. For those who choose to undergo DBS, the chance of a good outcome will be increased by working with an experienced team which specializes in the procedure.

Families of patients with PKAN frequently try pantothenate and other dietary supplements in a quest to improve function or slow disease progression. None of these has been studied formally in a clinical setting, and only anecdotal information is available on their possible effects. Based on the disease mechanism, we speculated that high doses of oral pantothenate may drive any residual enzyme activity in those patients suspected of having low levels of partially functional enzyme, predicted to be patients with later onset, more slowly progressive disease. However, as there is evidence that pantothenate is non-toxic, even in high doses, we have recommended a trial of high dose pantothenate in patients with PKAN. Some patients have reported improvements in speech and balance, though no trials of this compound have yet been developed. The challenge to evaluating this or any treatment for efficacy is the need for outcome measures. We are currently working to define these.

Video – Illustrative case

The appended videoclip (track 1) shows impaired ambulation in a 5-year-old girl with classical PKAN after taking her morning dose of baclofen.

Acknowledgments: I am grateful to the many NBIA families, the NBIA Disorders Association, the National Organization for Rare Disorders and the National Eye Institute for support of this work.

References

Castelnau, P., Cif, L., Valente, E.M., Vayssiere, N., Hemm, S., Gannau, A., Digiorgio, A. & Coubes, P. (2005): Pallidal stimulation improves pantothenate kinase-associated neurodegeneration. *Ann. Neurol.* **57**, 738–741.

Gregory, A. & Hayflick, S.J. (2005): Neurodegeneration with brain iron accumulation. *Folia Neuropathol.* **43**, 286–296.

Hallervorden, J. & Spatz, H. (1922): Eigenartige Erkrankung im extrapyramidalen System mit besonderer Beteiligung des Globus pallidus und der Substantia nigra. *Z. Ges. Neurol. Psychiatr.* **79**, 254–302.

Hayflick, S.J., Westaway, S.K., Levinson, B., Zhou, B., Johnson, M.A., Ching, K.H. & Gitschier, J. (2003): Genetic, clinical, and radiographic delineation of Hallervorden-Spatz syndrome. *N. Engl. J. Med.* **348**, 33–40.

Hayflick, S., Hartman, M., Coryell, J., Gitschier, J. & Rowley, H. (2006): Brain MRI in neurodegeneration with brain iron accumulation with and without PANK2 mutations. *Am. J. Neuroradiol.* **27**, 1230–1233.

Johnson, M.A., Kuo, Y.M., Westaway, S.K., Parker, S.M., Ching, K.H., Gitschier, J. & Hayflick, S.J. (2004): Mitochondrial localization of human PANK2 and hypotheses of secondary iron accumulation in pantothenate kinase-associated neurodegeneration. *Ann. N.Y. Acad. Sci.* **1012**, 282–298.

Kotzbauer, P.T., Truax, A.C., Trojanowski, J.Q. & Lee, V.M. (2005): Altered neuronal mitochondrial coenzyme A synthesis in neurodegeneration with brain iron accumulation caused by abnormal processing, stability, and catalytic activity of mutant pantothenate kinase 2. *J. Neurosci.* **25**, 689–698.

Perry, T.L., Norman, M.G., Yong, V.W., Whiting, S., Crichton, J.U., Hansen, S. & Kish, S.J. (1985): Hallervorden-Spatz disease: cysteine accumulation and cysteine dioxygenase deficiency in the globus pallidus. *Ann. Neurol.* **18**, 482–489.

Szanto, J. & Gallyas, F. (1966): A study of iron metabolism in neuropsychiatric patients. Hallervorden-Spatz disease. *Arch. Neurol.* **14**, 438–442.

Zhou, B., Westaway, S.K., Levinson, B., Johnson, M.A., Gitschier, J. & Hayflick, S.J. (2001): A novel pantothenate kinase gene *(PANK2)* is defective in Hallervorden-Spatz syndrome. *Nat. Genet.* **28**, 345–349.

Chapter 15

Functional (psychogenic) movement disorders in childhood

Robert Surtees

*Neurosciences Unit, Institute of Child Health, University College London,
30 Guilford Street, London WC1N 1EH, UK*
R.Surtees@ich.ucl.ac.uk

Summary

Very little is known about functional (psychogenic) movement disorders in childhood. By contrast, adults with psychogenic movement disorders have been studied, and clinical clues that increase the suspicion that a movement disorder is psychogenic are known. It is likely that very similar clinical clues will pertain to children and adolescents. Here, I briefly describe six cases of children and adolescents with a functional movement disorder and compare these with one child who had an undiagnosed primary dystonia, but who was previously thought to have a functional disorder. From the cases and the limited literature, some conclusions can be drawn: (1) the clinical suspicions do apply to children and adolescents; (2) functional tremor is the most prevalent and is essentially a clinical diagnosis; other functional movement disorders require biochemical, immunological, genetic, and brain structural investigations; (3) most children have pre-existing neurological or psychiatric disorders; (4) treatment with cognitive and behavioural therapy and rehabilitation by a multidisciplinary team causes marked improvement in symptoms and a functional return to school and home life; (5) children are rarely cured.
Terminology and the multidisciplinary approach to treatment are also described.

Introduction

Very little is known about functional (psychogenic) movement disorders in childhood and adolescence that is open to scientific scrutiny. Neurological disorders believed to be of functional origin comprise 4-7 per cent of all referrals to paediatric neurology services (Spierings *et al.*, 1990; Thomas, 2002). Of these, approximately 12 per cent have a motor disorder (Spierings *et al.*, 1990), but the proportion with a movement disorder is not known. However, functional movement disorders in children appear rare (Ozekmekci *et al.*, 2003; Kirsch & Mink, 2004; Fernandez-Alvarez, 2005).

By contrast, psychogenic movement disorders have been extensively studied in adults (Miyasaki *et al.*, 2003). In adults the incidence is around 3 per cent of all movement disorders and their prevalence varies with the type of disorder – for instance, psychogenic dystonia is rare (Pringsheim & Lang, 2003) but psychogenic myoclonus is common (Monday & Jankovic, 1993).

The study of psychogenic movement disorders in adults has led to the identification of clinical clues that increase suspicion that a movement disorder is psychogenic in origin (Tables 1, 2, and 3; modified from Fahn (Fahn, 1994).

In this chapter, I present six brief illustrative cases of children and adolescents presenting with a functional movement disorder and, by way of contrast, one brief case of a child with an undiagnosed primary dystonia, previously thought to be functional in origin. I will then discuss the terminology (psychogenic and functional), therapeutic approach, and outcome.

Table 1. Clinical clues from the history that increase suspicion that a movement disorder is psychogenic in origin

- Abrupt onset
    May follow minor injury
- Rapid progression to maximal severity
- Non-progressive course
    Characteristics may change with time
    Paroxysmal exacerbations
- Spontaneous remissions
- Other medically unexplained symptoms

Table 2. Clinical clues from the examination that increase suspicion that a movement disorder is psychogenic in origin

- Inconsistency
- Incongruity
- Other abnormal movements
    Shaking
    Slowness
    Bizarre gait
    Excessive startle
- Other non-organic sensory or motor signs

Table 3. Clinical clues from the examination of specific movement disorders that increase suspicion that the movement disorder is psychogenic in origin

- Tremor
    Decreases with distraction
    Increases with attention
    Frequency can be entrained
    Absent finger tremor
    Co-activation (tonic muscle contraction with tremor)
- Dystonia
    Begins with fixed posture

Illustrative cases

Case 1

A 12-year-old girl presented with a sudden onset of being unable to walk. At the age of 6 years she had had a sudden onset of an abnormal head position and difficulties using her dominant hand. At the time there was a questionable response to treatment with carbidopa/laevodopa. Investigations then (including mutation analysis of the GTP-cyclohydrolase 1 gene) were all negative and the symptoms resolved spontaneously after approximately 7 months. She remained well for the next 6 years. Examination at the age of 12 showed dystonic posturing of the non-dominant hand as the only abnormality when seated at rest. Attempts to passively flex her hips or passively extend her knees or to get her to stand caused immediate, sustained, and extreme plantar flexion of both feet. Biochemical, immunological, genetic, and brain structural investigations [along the lines of Assmann and colleagues (2003)] revealed no abnormality. Cognitive assessment showed mild-to-moderate global learning difficulties. Treatment included a change in school and cognitive-behavioural therapy and there was a sudden remission 6 months after the second presentation. Despite continuing psychological support and treatment, she has developed a pattern of relapsing-and-remitting symptoms with inconsistent and incongruous signs. A diagnosis of functional dystonia was made.

Case 2

A 14-year-old boy had a sudden onset of tremor affecting his dominant arm and preventing him from writing. This remitted for 2 months during the school summer vacation. The tremor relapsed when he returned to school. On examination within 2 weeks of the tremor relapse, he had a variable tremor of the right arm and hand, but not involving the fingers. The tremor varied in intensity, being more marked when attention was drawn to it, and it also varied in frequency. He was noted to have dystonic head and neck tics (as did his father), and an obsessive personality. He was being bullied at school and he thought that the tremor was 'all in my mind'. After discussion of the nature of functional tremor, his symptoms remitted. The tic disorder was noted but not otherwise commented on.

Case 3

This 14-year-old girl had a sudden onset of abnormal head and dominant arm posture and an inability to stand or walk without the support of another person. She had a previous history of physical and emotional abuse, had longstanding challenging behaviour, and was in the care of the Social Services. On examination she had fixed posturing of her right arm and a fixed torticollis. Lower limb muscular tone and tendon reflexes were normal, but she showed 'give-way' muscular weakness in all groups tested. She was unable to stand or walk without the light support of another person. Magnetic resonance imaging of her brain showed cerebellar hypoplasia. Biochemical, immunological, and genetic investigations were normal. She was admitted for inpatient psychiatric treatment but deteriorated and developed all the features of the pervasive refusal syndrome (Lask *et al.*, 1991).

Case 4

At the age of 12 years, some months after an episode of left otitis media, this boy developed paroxysms of excruciating left facial pain. Infective, brain structural, angiographic, and ear, nose and throat investigations were all negative. His father, to whom he was particularly close, had recently left the family. A diagnosis of atypical facial pain was made and he was treated with amitriptyline and cognitive and behavioural therapy. The paroxysms of pain decreased in frequency and he continued to attend school and do well there. At the age of 14 years, following a paroxysm of facial pain, he became depersonalised, breathless, and fell to the floor. On recovery, after some minutes, he had developed difficulty in walking and had lost sensation in both arms from shoulder to wrist and in both legs from hip to ankle. On examination he had a bizarre, monoplegic gait with his right leg held stiffly extended and externally rotated at the hip. He had circumferential loss of all sensory modalities in both arms from shoulder to wrist and in both legs from hip to ankle. Muscle tone and power were normal, as were deep tendon reflexes. The gait disorder and disordered sensation remitted with rehabilitation and cognitive and behaviour therapy.

Case 5

This 12-year-girl had congenital ataxia and moderate learning difficulties caused by a cerebellar malformation. She had also had a cadaveric renal transplant because of chronic renal failure secondary to nephronophthisis. Two years previously she had had an episode of transient generalized dystonia, thought to be a postinfectious autoimmune phenomenon and associated with circulating anti-basal-ganglia antibodies. She presented with a sudden onset of dominant arm tremor. Anti-basal-ganglia antibodies were again positive. A diagnosis of autoimmune basal ganglia disease was made and she was treated symptomatically with first trihexyphenidyl and later carbamazepine. Despite this, her tremor worsened, spread to involve both arms and her trunk, and she became unable to perform any acts of daily living without assistance. At this stage, examination showed a highly variable tremor affecting her right arm, but not her fingers, at rest. The tremor was not evident when she was distracted but increased in amplitude when attention was drawn to it. The frequency of the tremor could be entrained. A diagnosis of a functional tremor was made and the condition explained to the patient and her family. The tremor remitted following two sessions of cognitive behavioural therapy, but subsequently recurred at times of family stress.

Case 6

A 14-year-old girl had a longstanding needle phobia. Immediately after a routine BCG vaccination she developed a tremor of her head and upper limbs. The tremor was variable in severity when awake and disappeared in sleep. Over the next 2 weeks she also developed some difficulties with gait and balance. On examination the head and upper limb tremor were not noticeable when she was sitting quietly and reading a book, but when not distracted the head and arm tremor were incongruent, of variable frequency, and could be entrained. The tremor involved the fingers. She also had a mild gait disturbance with features reminiscent of astasia-abasia. The rest of the neurological examination was normal. Explanation of the functional nature of the tremor and reassurance that she would get better did not help. She was then treated with carbamazepine as a mood stabiliser and had several sessions of cognitive and behavioural therapy with good results.

Case 7

This 13-year-girl had undiagnosed congenital sensorineural deafness and mild learning difficulties. At the age of 10 years she developed task-specific dystonia of her dominant arm affecting her writing. Extensive brain structural, immunological, biochemical, and genetic investigations were negative. A trial of laevodopa/carbidopa was ineffective. The dystonia remitted spontaneously for a 3-month period but relapsed at the age of 11 years and spread to involve the non-dominant arm. Before this relapse, her father and her brother had left the family home. A diagnosis of a functional movement disorder was made (because of bizarre movements, periods of spontaneous remission, and the relapse occurring at a time of psychological stress) and treatment was started with a selective serotonin reuptake inhibitor and cognitive and behavioural therapy. However, the dystonia progressed and she developed axial involvement by the age of 13 years. Examination at this time showed a generalised dystonia affecting the left arm more than the right, a hyperlordosis, and scoliotic movements concave towards the left. She had a dystonic writer's cramp on the right and an elevating left arm controlled by a sensory trick. There was no clear involvement of the legs, but she had a positive Babinski sign on walking. A diagnosis of an idiopathic (not associated with the common deletion in *DYT1* gene) generalised dystonia was made and she was started on trihexyphenidyl. Over the next two years the dystonia spread to involve both lower limbs and the orobulbar musculature, despite treatment with high doses of trihexyphenidyl, sulpiride, and tetrabenazine. She then developed status dystonicus and underwent urgent bilateral pallidal stimulation. Subsequently, there was a marked improvement in the limb and axial dystonia, she came off all medication and was able to return to school; however, the oro-bulbar dystonia – in particular painful dystonic spasms of the mandibular musculature – remained problematic.

Discussion of cases

These cases were seen in a specialist quaternary movement disorder clinic over the past 3 years, suggesting an incidence of around 3 per cent – very similar to that in adult series. The children were all seen in their teenage or immediate preteen years, although one (case 1) first developed symptoms at 6 years of age. All the children with a functional movement disorder had pre-existing neurological or psychological problems [learning difficulties in two, abuse at home or school in two (and suspected in case 1 also), tic disorder in one, needle phobia in one, and medically unexplained symptoms in one]. Interestingly, case 7, who had an idiopathic dystonia, also had a pre-existing neurological disorder. With the exception of the children with functional tremor, all underwent extensive investigations to exclude structural, biochemical, immunological, and genetic causes of their movement disorder. This suggests that functional tremor is more easily diagnosed on clinical grounds than the other functional movement disorders. All the children with functional movement disorders had clinical features suggestive of the diagnosis (see the tables). A cognitive and behavioural approach to treatment, in the setting of an assessment by a multidisciplinary team – which included a clinical psychologist, physiotherapist, occupational therapist, neurologist, and psychiatrist – proved helpful to all the children except case 3. However, only those children with a relatively brief duration of symptoms (a few months) were cured, though the others, with the exception of case 3, were all rehabilitated back to a normal school and home life.

These findings suggest that early diagnosis should be possible in functional movement disorders in children, where specific psychological interventions offer the prospect of cure. In long-established disease, most children can be rehabilitated, although symptoms persist.

Terminology

The concept of functional movement disorders implies that the disease origins do not lie in an organic neurological disease but rather in a subconscious psychological domain. That is, these disorders are caused by abnormal brain function and not by abnormalities of the biophysical substrate of the brain. Many different terms have been used to describe these disorders, which reflect their perceived origin and the prevalent linguistic culture. Thus, 'hysterical', 'psychosomatic', 'stress-related', 'medically unexplained', 'conversion', 'psychogenic', and 'functional' have all been used. The preferred term should be acceptable to the child and the parents, describe the nature of the disorder, and lead to a discussion of the symptoms and their cause.

An imaginative study from Edinburgh calculated the degree of offensiveness of these labels in adults attending a general neurology clinic (Stone *et al.*, 2002). They found that the label 'functional' was least likely to cause offence (for the time being at least). In addition, the use of this label implies abnormal functioning of the central nervous system but avoids debate about the biological, psychological, and social contributions to the disorder; and leads the way to a transparent explanation of the symptoms to the child and parent. However, in adult practice the term psychogenic is currently preferred. Thus here I have used 'functional' when discussing children and 'psychogenic' when discussing adults.

Management

A clear explanation of the nature of the disorder, understandable by both the child and the parents, is an essential first step in management. First, I stress that there has been no damage to the brain but the symptoms have been produced by abnormal brain function. This implies that there is the potential for recovery. Often an analogy is needed to improve understanding. Examples given by children and parents in roughly ascending sophistication are: a car that is working properly but whose driver doesn't know where to go; an out-of-tune musical instrument; a computer with software problems. Then I introduce the idea that the cause of the brain dysfunction is emotional in origin; but also that we often do not identify a definite triggering stressor. It is also important to state explicitly that we do not think that the child is mad or putting on their symptoms. It is important that the child and the parents understand the multidisciplinary approach to assessment and treatment and that the child will be followed up by the neurologist until there is full recovery.

Almost always the management of functional movement disorders in childhood is multidisciplinary. Assessment will normally involve input from neurology, nursing, psychiatry, clinical psychology, social work, occupational therapy, and physiotherapy. Treatment normally consists of two parallel approaches: rehabilitation (in particular a prompt return to school as soon as the child shows improvement) and cognitive and behavioural therapy. If a coexisting medical or psychiatric condition is also diagnosed and amenable to treatment, this should be treated as well. Underlying psychological and social problems, where identified, should be addressed and ameliorated where possible; this may also involve the child's school.

Outcome

There have been very few scientific studies of the outcome of children with functional neurological disorders. One study found that with treatment over 70 per cent of these children improved, although over half still had the same (or, more rarely, different) symptoms (Spierings et al., 1990). Another study of children with astasia-abasia (a functional inability to stand or walk) found that most recovered over a prolonged period of treatment, but around 30 per cent continued to have symptoms (Stickler & Cheung-Patton, 1989).

There have been no studies on the outcome of functional movement disorders in childhood. Personal experience suggests that almost all children improve with psychological support and the use of cognitive and behavioural techniques to control their symptoms; however, unless symptoms are of short duration, they are rarely cured.

Acknowledgments: I would like to thank the children and their parents who have taught me so much about movement disorders in childhood.

References

Assmann, B., Surtees, R. & Hoffmann, G.F. (2003): Approach to the diagnosis of neurotransmitter diseases exemplified by the differential diagnosis of childhood-onset dystonia. *Ann. Neurol.* **54** (Suppl. 6), S18–S24.

Fahn, S. (1994): Psychogenic movement disorders. In: *Movement disorders 3*, eds. C.D. Marsden & S. Fahn, pp. 359–372. Oxford: Butterworth-Heinemann.

Fernandez-Alvarez, E. (2005): Movement disorders of functional origin (psychogenic) in children. *Rev. Neurol.* **40** (Suppl. 1), S75–S77.

Kirsch, D.B. & Mink, J.W. (2004): Psychogenic movement disorders in children. *Pediatr. Neurol.* **30**, 1–6.

Lask, B., Britten, C., Kroll, L., Magagna, J. & Tranter, M. (1991): Children with pervasive refusal. *Arch. Dis. Child.* **66**, 866–869.

Miyasaki, J.M., Sa, D.S., Galvez-Jimenez, N. & Lang, A.E. (2003): Psychogenic movement disorders. *Can. J. Neurol. Sci.* **30** (Suppl. 1), S94–S100.

Monday, K. & Jankovic, J. (1993): Psychogenic myoclonus. *Neurology* **43**, 349-352.

Ozekmekci, S., Apaydin, H., Ekinci, B. & Yalcinkaya, C. (2003): Psychogenic movement disorders in two children. *Mov. Disord.* **18**, 1395–1397.

Pringsheim, T. & Lang, A.E. (2003): Psychogenic dystonia. *Rev. Neurol. (Paris)* **159**, 885–891.

Spierings, C., Poels, P.J., Sijben, N., Gabreels, F.J. & Renier, W.O. (1990): Conversion disorders in childhood: a retrospective follow-up study of 84 inpatients. *Dev. Med. Child Neurol.* **32**, 865–871.

Stickler, G.B. & Cheung-Patton, A. (1989): Astasia-abasia. A conversion reaction. Prognosis. *Clin. Pediatr. (Phila)* **28**, 12–16.

Stone, J., Wojcik, W., Durrance, D., Carson, A., Lewis, S., MacKenzie, L., Warlow, C.P. & Sharpe, M. (2002): What should we say to patients with symptoms unexplained by disease? The 'number needed to offend'. *BMJ* **325**, 1449–1450.

Thomas, N.H. (2002): Somatic presentation of psychogenic disease in child neurologic practice. *Neurology* **58** (Suppl. 3), A28.

Chapter 16

Movement disorders in Rett syndrome

Teresa Temudo

Neuropaediatric Unit, Service of Paediatrics, Hospital Geral de Santo António, largo Abel Salazar, 4099/001 Porto, Portugal
teresatemudo@netcabo.pt
Video 7

Summary

Rett syndrome is a progressive neurodevelopmental disorder with onset in early childhood, occurring almost exclusively in girls and caused by mutations in methyl-CpG-binding protein 2 (MECp2). It is one of the commonest causes of mental retardation in females. Regression is a defining feature of Rett syndrome, and during the regression period the patients develop autistic behaviour. This is the reason why Rett syndrome has been classified as a pervasive developmental autistic spectrum disorder.

However, movement disorders are so exuberant, characteristic, and unique in Rett syndrome that it is unlikely that an experienced clinician would mistake the two conditions. We can define Rett syndrome as a condition which manifests in the majority of the cases as a hyperkinetic movement disorder and progresses (at varying rates) to a bradykinetic disorder.

My aim in this chapter is to characterize and describe the movement disorders of Rett syndrome, based on a review of published reports and my personal experience.

Introduction

Rett syndrome was discovered by Andreas Rett, a Viennese paediatrician, when he noticed that two girls who were waiting for a consultation with him had the same movement disorder: hand stereotypy. In 1966 he published data on 22 girls with progressive cerebral atrophy, stereotyped hand movements, dementia, alalia, gait apraxia, and a tendency to epileptic fits (Rett, 1966). This disorder was named Rett syndrome in 1983 by Hagberg and his colleagues, who studied 35 female patients from Sweden, France, and Portugal and emphasized autistic behaviour, acquired microcephaly, jerky truncal ataxia, and vasomotor disturbance (Hagberg *et al.*, 1983). Diagnostic criteria for this syndrome were further defined in 1988 (The Rett syndrome Diagnostic Working Group, 1988). It took more than 30 years following Rett's discovery of this syndrome to determine the genetic basis of the condition – mutations in methyl-CpG-binding protein 2 (MeCP2) – largely because the disease is primarily sporadic and familial cases are rare (Amir *et al.*, 1999).

Among the specific diagnostic criteria of Rett syndrome (Tables 1 and 2) are movement disorders such as stereotyped hand movements, gait apraxia, and dystonia (Hagberg *et al.*, 2002). However, other movement disorders can be present and are less well described. These include additional types of stereotyped movements or behaviours apart from hand stereotypies, tremor, chorea, myoclonus, rigidity, and gait abnormalities. It is apparent that Rett syndrome starts as a hyperkinetic disorder and progresses to a hypokinetic one.

Table 1. Revised diagnostic criteria for Rett syndrome

Necessary criteria
1. Apparently normal prenatal and perinatal history
2. Psychomotor development largely normal through the first 6 months or may be delayed from birth
3. Normal head circumference at birth
4. Postnatal deceleration of head growth in the majority
5. Loss of achived purposeful hand skill between ages 1/2 -2 1/2 years
6. Stereotypic hand movements such as hand wringing/squeezing, clapping/tapping, mouthing, and washing/rubbing automatisms
7. Emerging social withdrawal, communication dysfunction, loss of learned words, and cognitive impairment
8. Impaired (dyspraxic) or failing locomotion

Supportive criteria
1. Disturbances of breathing while awake (hyperventilation, breath-holding, forced expulsion of air or saliva, air swallowing)
2. Bruxism
3. Impaired sleep pattern from early infancy
4. Abnormal muscle tone successively associated with muscle wasting and dystonia
5. Peripheral vasomotor disturbances
6. Scoliosis/kyphosis progression through childhood
7. Growth retardation
8. Hypotrophic small and cold feet; small, thin hands

Exclusion criteria
1. Organomegaly or other signs of storage disease
2. Retinopathy, optic atrophy, or cataract
3. Evidence of perinatal or postnatal brain damage
4. Existence of identifiable metabolic or other progressive neurological disorder
5. Acquired neurological disorders resulting from severe infections or head trauma

Clinical presentation

Stereotypies

Definition

Stereotypies may be defined as involuntary rhythmic, patterned, coordinated, repetitive, and seemingly purposeless movements or utterances (Jankovick, 2005). Stereotypies are usually continuous, in contrast to mannerisms or tics. However, the differential diagnosis between stereotypies and tics may be difficult or sometimes impossible, and both movement disorders may coexist in the same patient. The term stereotypy should be used to describe a phenomenological and not an aetiological category of hyperkinetic movement disorder, but in rare situations a particular type of stereotypy may help in making a precise diagnosis (such as hand-washing movements in Rett syndrome). Stereotypies can be transient (physiological) or persistent. Transient stereotypies are common in infants. Thelen has identified 49 patterns of stereotypy in normal infants. The time spent in such activities is variable but increases progressively up to the age of 6 months and then decreases, while at the same time the pattern becomes more varied (Thelen, 1979; 1980).

Table 2. Revised delineation of variant phenotypes

Inclusion criteria
1. Must meet at least three of six main criteria
2. Must meet at least five of 11 supportive criteria

Six main criteria
1. Absence or reduction of hand skills
2. Reduction or loss of babble speech
3. Monotonous pattern to hand stereotypies
4. Reduction or loss of communication skills
5. Deceleration of head growth from the first years of life
6. Rett syndrome disease profile: a regression stage followed by a recovery of interaction contrasting with slow neuromotor regression

Eleven supportive criteria
1. Breathing irregularities
2. Bloating/air swallowing
3. Bruxism (harsh sounding type)
4. Abnormal locomotion
5. Scoliosis/ kyphosis
6. Lower limb atrophy
7. Cold, purplish feet, usually growth impaired
8. Sleep disturbances including night screaming outbursts
9. Laughing/screaming spells
10. Diminished response to pain
11. Intense eye contact/eye pointing

Persistent stereotypies are common in children with sensory deprivation (blindness, deafness) or emotional deprivation (institutionalized infants) (Fernandez-Alvarez & Aicardi, 2001), and they often accompany various psychiatric or neurological disorders such as anxiety, obsessive-compulsive disorders, Tourette syndrome, schizophrenia, autism, Rett syndrome, mental retardation, akathisia, restless legs syndrome, and several neurodegenerative disorders including fronto-temporal dementia (Nyatsanza et al., 2003).

In addition to motor and phonic types, stereotypies can be classified as either simple (for example, tapping, mouthing, clapping) or complex (a sequence of different movements always performed in the same way), or they can be classified by the predominant site of involvement (head, trunk, hand, lower limbs, and so on) (Table 3).

The pathophysiology of stereotypies

The neurophysiological basis of stereotypies is unknown. There is no clear anatomical-clinical correlation for stereotypies, although it is believed that both cortical and subcortical structures are involved (basal ganglia dysfunction, mesolimbic system) (Jankovick, 2005). Stereotypies have also been observed in patients with structural lesions of the central nervous system including bilateral areas of the medial frontoparietal cortices (Sato et al., 2001) and cerebellum (Hottinger-Blanc et al., 2002).

The dopaminergic system in the basal ganglia has been implicated in the production of stereotypies. Intrastriatal injection of dopamine and the systemic administration of both presynaptically active dopamine agonists (such as amphetamine) and postsynaptically active dopamine agonists (such as apomorphine) in rats produce dose-related repetitive sniffing, gnawing, licking, biting, rearing, head bobbing, and other stereotyped learned activities (Costall et al., 1977). These stereotypies can be blocked by neuroleptic drugs (Tschanz & Rebec, 1988). SKF 38393, a D1 agonist, did not induce stereotypies, but it enhanced stereotypies induced by apomorphine (a mixed D1 and D2 agonist) and by PHNO, a selective D2 agonist (Koller

Table 3. Classification of stereotypies, modified from the classification of Jankovick (2005) and Fernandez-Alvarez & Aicardi (2001)

Transient (physiological)
Normal child development
Stress related
Self-gratifying behaviour
Persistent (pathological)
Sensory deprivation (restraining, blindness, deafness)
Mental retardation
Autism
Rett syndrome
Neuroacanthocytosis
Schizophrenia
Catatonia
Obsessive-compulsive disorder
Tourette syndrome
Tardive and other dyskinesias
Akathisia
Restless legs syndrome
Fronto-temporal dementia
Epileptic authomatism
Psychogenic
Motor (body part localization)
Head/neck
Face
Mouth
Eyes
Arm
Hand (visual behaviour present or absent)
Leg
Feet
Body
Phonic
Repetitive sounds
Repetitive words or phrases

& Herbster, 1988). This suggests that D2 receptors mediate stereotypies and D1 receptors potentiate this effect.

Neuropeptides may also modulate stereotyped behaviour. Microinjection of cholecystokinin and neurotensin into the medial nucleus accumbens potentiates apomorphine-induced stereotypy (Blumstein et al., 1987). Injection of these peptides into the striatum had no effect on the apomorphine-induced stereotypy, providing additional evidence for the involvement of the limbic system in the pathogenesis of this movement disorder.

Endogenous opiates (for example β-endorphins) may also be involved in the pathogenesis of stereotypies because some autistic children with self-injurious movements improve their behaviour after administration of opiate blockers (naloxone and naltrexone), and raised plasma and cerebrospinal fluid levels of β-endorphins were found in these patients (Sandman, 1988).

More recently the serotonin system has also been implicated, supported by the observation that certain animal behaviours improve with serotonin uptake inhibitors (Hugo et al., 2003).

Clinical presentation of stereotypies in Rett syndrome

The most striking core symptom of Rett syndrome is the stereotyped movement of the hands. These movements are associated with or follow the disappearance of purposeful prehension.

However, a video analysis of 22 cases of Rett syndrome in the first 6 months of life, before the beginning of regression, showed stereotyped hand movements in 42 per cent (Einspieler *et al.*, 2005). The voluntary hand movements seen in Rett syndrome are limited to gross hand manipulation, and fine movements are not possible. A previous report showed that voluntary movements in Rett syndrome reach the level of the 4th month at most (Nomura & Segawa, 1990).

The almost continuous, repetitive, and compulsive automatisms disappear during sleep, and environmental manipulation has been shown to have a relatively limited effect on the frequency of the repetitive hand movements, suggesting that the movements are a manifestation of automatic reinforcement or neurochemical processes (Wales *et al.*, 2004).

The most characteristic hand movement is the wringing, washing-like movement of both hands, usually in the midline, often in front of the body, and often without crossing the midline. There can also be symmetrical movements of both hands of other types, for example clapping, tapping, or putting their hands in their mouths (see the videoclip on the accompanying DVD, video 7, track 1).

Hand stereotypies may manifest with the hands apart and most often with each hand carrying out a different movement: hair pulling with one hand, trunk tapping with the other; hair pulling with one hand and putting the other in the mouth; flapping one hand, pill-rolling with the other; raising one hand above the head and making gestures like a Seville dance, making castanet movements with the fingers of one hand to produce a sound; twisting two or three fingers in a complex way, and so on (personal observations) (video 7, track 1). When they put their hands into their mouths, they often bite them and cause hand mutilations; stereotypies therefore have to be inhibited by mechanical methods or by using low doses of risperidone (Nyatsanza *et al.*, 2003).

One of the peculiarities of hand stereotypies in Rett syndrome is that the patients do not look at their hands when they are carrying out the movements, perhaps because they have very poor eye-hand coordination. I believe this feature may help clinicians to differentiate the hand stereotypies of Rett syndrome from those of other conditions such as mental retardation or autism (personal observation).

The second most common stereotypy in Rett syndrome is bruxism. In a series of 65 Rett syndrome patients I found bruxism in 82 per cent (Temudo, 2005). It occurs in the waking state and ceases in sleep (Hagberg *et al.*, 1983; Naidu *et al.*, 1986), is very common in mentally retarded individuals (Blount *et al.*, 1982), and may be associated with dental and psychological disturbances (Glaros & Rao, 1977; Rugh & Harlan, 1988).

FitzGerald *et al.* (1990) considered that bruxism might be a form of focal dystonia, but other investigators – including myself – consider that it is a type of self-injurious stereotypy. Some older Rett syndrome girls with bruxism have a particular maxillary morphology with prognathism, maybe as a result of this particular type of continuous movement (personal observation).

Apart from hand stereotypies and bruxism, there are additional types of stereotypy involving other parts of the body (personal observations): rhythmical head rolling, cervical retropulsion, eye rolling, eye closure, facial grimacing, lip sucking, repetitive sounds or words, trunk rocking, intermittent leg elevation and tapping of the floor, toe walking, feet stereotypies, and swaying movements of the body with the weight shifting from one leg to the other. Stereotypies can also be very complex at the onset of the disease, some girls exhibiting a form of 'stereotyped dance' involving many areas of the body (personal observation; video 7, track 2).

With the progress of the disease, stereotypies diminish and became simpler and slower with age, with the patients becoming hypokinetic and rigid. Generally, however, patients maintain the same types of hand movement throughout their lives. Stereotypies involving other parts of the body tend to disappear and behave like tics, while new movements substitute preceding movements over time (personal observation).

Dystonia

Postural asymmetry is a common finding in Rett syndrome and at late stages of the disease is always present in the lower limbs. A discrete dystonia of the halux is a very common and early sign of Rett syndrome (Temudo et al., 2005) (Figs. 1-2).

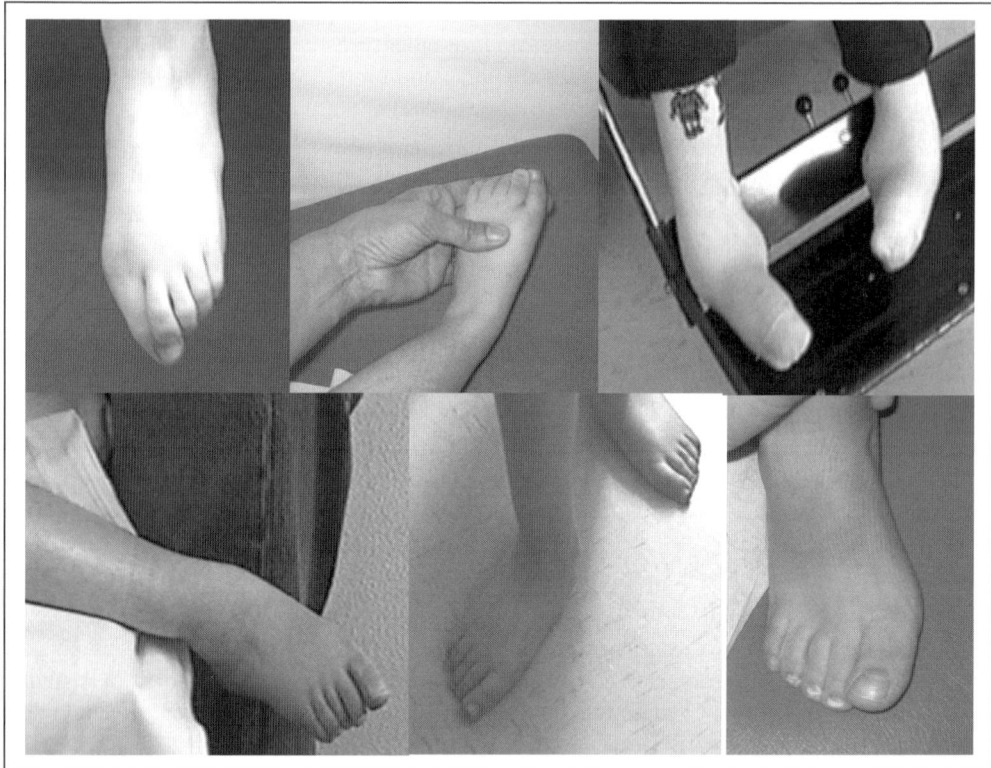

Fig. 1. Foot dystonia in Rett syndrome.

FitzGerald et al. (1990) reported dystonia in 19 of 32 patients (59 per cent), usually crural or generalized but sometimes focal, involving the upper or lower extremities. In a series of 71 Rett syndrome patients, Temudo et al. found dystonia in 69 per cent (unpublished data). Usually the impairments are asymmetrical, the right side of the body being most affected (Nomura et al., 1984; Hagberg & Romell, 2002).

Scoliosis, which is a common feature of Rett syndrome, may be a sign of truncal dystonia and in those severe cases who never achieve ambulation it is present from the earliest stages of the disease. Temudo et al. found scoliosis in 70 per cent of 71 Rett syndrome, patients and in 42 per cent of those with scoliosis it was present before the age of 10 (unpublished data).

Rigid-akinetic syndrome

The facial features in Rett syndrome patients are usually animated in the early stages of the disease but the face later becomes expressionless. However, an inexpressive 'mask-like' face may be an early clinical sign, accompanied by a disproportionate ability to communicate with the eyes and by normal eye blinking. In a series of 32 Rett syndrome patients analysed by FitzGerald *et al.* (1990), hypomimia was more severe and more common in the older girls.

Bradykinesia and rigidity are also common in older girls (FitzGerald *et al.*, 1990) and some severe cases who never acquire independent ambulation show rigidity very early in life. In a series of 71 patients with Rett syndrome, Temudo *et al.* found rigidity in 25 per cent at a mean age of 12.5 years (unpublished). Rigidity was not related entirely to the age of the patients.

Rett syndrome gait

The majority of the patients acquire independent ambulation and this feature is correlated with the type of the mutation in the MECP2 gene (Huppke *et al.*, 2002; Schanen *et al.*, 2004). The gait can be normal but purposeless, or have peculiar characteristics which were described as apraxic by Rett (1966). This apraxic gait consists of a wide base with extended knees and rigid legs and contraction of the gluteal and abdominal muscles (video 7, track 3). When these girls walk, the stereotyped hand movements continue and the normal arm balance, essential to equilibrium, is absent, provoking retropulsion of the body (video 7, track 4). Some girls have particular stereotypies, with tiptoe gate, shifting of body weight from one leg to the other, or tapping the floor with one leg.

With the progression of the disease (the rate being variable), neuromotor functions decline in most patients and the majority lose their gait and became wheelchair-dependent. However, 15 to 20 per cent of these patients remain ambulatory well into middle age (Witt-Engerström & Hagberg, 1990). In such patients, the gait becomes more rigid and some may have freezing when they try to initiate a movement.

Tremor

FitzGerald *et al.* (1990) did not find rest or postural tremor in 32 Rett syndrome girls, but they found kinetic tremor in those who were predominantly ataxic. Postural tremor may also be present in some rigid and akinetic cases. In a series of 71 patients, 41 per cent had tremor and in 66 per cent of these the tremor was postural (Temudo *et al.*, unpublished data) (video 7, track 5).

Chorea

Choreoathetoid movements usually involve the hands (FitzGerald *et al.*, 1990) but in my experience this is not a common finding in Rett syndrome patients. In a series of 71 cases I observed only one girl with generalized choreoathetosis and one other with hand athetosis (Temudo *et al.*, unpublished data).

Myoclonus

Myoclonus was reported in 34 per cent of 32 Rett syndrome patients examined by FitzGerald *et al.* (1990), and predominantly involved the head or the trunk. Guerrini *et al.* (1998) studied 10 patients with Rett syndrome and observed myoclonus involving the distal limbs in nine. The

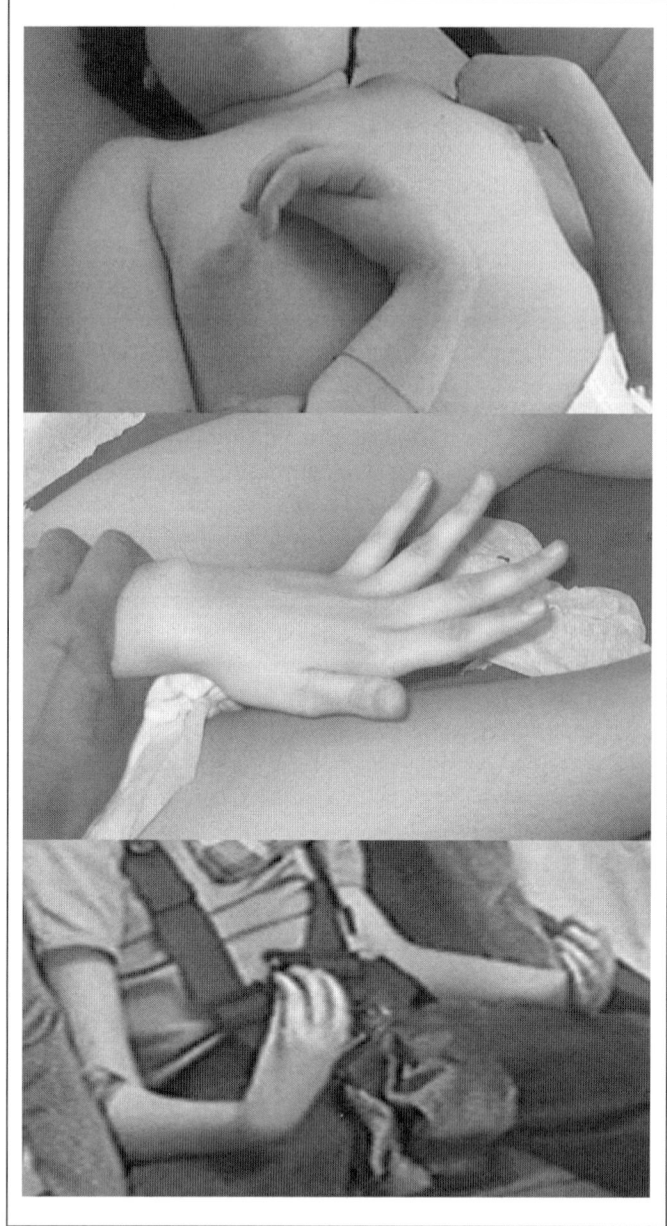

Fig. 2. Hand dystonia or athetosis in Rett syndrome.

severity of the myoclonus was not correlated with other symptoms or with age. These investigators undertook neurophysiological studies and concluded that their Rett syndrome patients had a distinctive pattern of cortical reflex myoclonus.

I observed one girl with Rett syndrome with generalized continuous myoclonus. During this state she maintained normal interpersonal contact but there was cessation of her usual continuous hand stereotypies. The myoclonic movements did not respond to benzodiazepines, valproate, lamotrigine, or topiramate, and they disappeared with sleep or spontaneously (video 7, track 6).

Biochemical studies

Assays of biogenic amines and their metabolites have given conflicting results, showing either decreased levels of homovanillic acid (HVA), 3-methoxy-4-hydroxyphenylglycol (MHPG), and 5-hydroxyindoleacetic acid (5-HIAA) (Zoghbi et al., 1989; Ramaekers & Blau, 2001), or no significant changes in these metabolites (Lekman et al., 1990). Decreased CSF levels of 5-HIAA are accompanied by low levels of 5-methyltetrahydrofolate (5-MTHF), in contrast to normal serum folate levels, while oral supplementation with folinic acid restores 5-MTHF values and serotonin turnover (Ramaekers & Blau, 2001). The CSF concentrations of γ-butyric acid (GABA) and other amino-acids are normal (Perry et al., 1988), while glutamate is markedly raised (Lappalainen et al., 1996). Decreased CSF levels of β-phenylalanine – an endogenous amine synthesized by decarboxylation of phenylalanine – may reflect impairment of the nigro-striatal dopaminergic system (Satoi et al., 2000). Plasma levels of β-endorphin and prolactin are mildly decreased (Fanchetti et al., 1986), with increased CSF β-endorphin in some but not in all cases (Budden et al., 1990). CSF levels of substance P are decreased (Matsuishi et al., 1977). Biopterin, a cofactor in the synthesis of biogenic amines found in blood and urine, is normal, with a mild decrease in the CSF but no deficiency of the critical enzyme dihydropteridine reductase (Zoghbi et al., 1989). Membrane cerebral lipids are decreased in the CSF (Lekman et al., 1991). Necropsy studies showed reduced levels of dopamine, serotonin, and their respective metabolites HVA and 5-HIAA in the substantia nigra of older girls with Rett syndrome, but no generalized deficiency of dopamine (Lekman et al., 1990), while others reported decreased levels of dopamine, norepinephrine, serotonin, and their metabolites in most brain regions (Riederer et al., 1986). An increased striatal dopamine-to-HVA ratio and raised 3,4-dihydroxyphenylacetic acid indicate increased dopamine turnover in the brain, with reduced serotonin and a regional increase in its precursor tryptophan in the striopallidum and substantia nigra (Lekman et al., 1990). A reduction in cortical choline acetyltransferase (ChAT) suggests a dysfunction of the cholinergic forebrain system (Lekman et al., 1990).

Neuropathology

There is a generalized reduction in neuronal size with increased cell-packing density in the cerebral cortex, thalamus, basal ganglia, amygdala, and hippocampus (Bauman et al., 1995). Other studies have revealed a decline in neuronal numbers in the frontal and temporal cortex but no decrease in cortical thickness. The decrease in cell numbers primarily involves the large pyramidal cells, more prominent in layers II and III than in the deep layers, with preservation of the visual cortex (Belichenko et al., 1994). These changes are associated with abnormalities in the orientation pattern of dendrites and axons, decreased dendritic branching (Armstrong, 1997), small neurons with increased neuronal packing (Armstrong, 2002), loss of dendrites of pyramidal cells in the frontal, motor, and subicular areas (Cornford et al., 1994), shortening of the apical and basilar dendritic branches in layers 3 and 5 of the frontal, motor, and inferior temporal cortex (Armstrong et al., 1998), and 'naked dendrites' without spines in pyramidal neurons, indicating a reduction in synaptic contacts from afferent neurons (Belichenko et al., 1994). Golgi studies showed a selective alteration in the size of dendrites of pyramidal neurons in the frontal, motor, and temporal cortices, while the dendrites in the pyramidal neurons in the hippocampus and visual cortex showed no changes. Similar abnormalities characterize the medial temporal structures in infantile autism (Bauman & Kemper, 1994).

Mild hypochromasia has been observed in the striatum, and hyperchromia of large neurons in the striatum and internal pallidum – here with abnormal dendrites and degeneration of thick myelinated fibres (Belichenko et al., 1994; Leontovich et al., 1999), and mild diffuse gliosis.

Another finding is hypomelanation of the substantia nigra pars compacta without definite neuronal loss – the majority of large nigral neurons containing little or no neuromelanin (Kitt & Wilcox, 1995; Jellinger et al., 1988). In one Rett syndrome patient only, aged 21 years, nigral cells were reduced by about 30 per cent of age-matched controls, and there were free pigment granules in the neuropils, as in Parkinson's disease. These and preliminary data showing labelling of fragmented intranucleosomal DNA using the TUNEL (TdT-mediated dUTP-biotin 3'-OH nick-end labelling) method in substantia nigra neurons suggest that they undergo active degeneration (Kitt & Wilcox, 1995). No apparent abnormalities in other pigmented brain stem nuclei are seen; morphometric studies of the serotonergic dorsal raphé nuclei showed no neuronal decrease, though reduced cell numbers have been reported in the cholinergic nucleus basalis of Meynert (Kitt et al., 1990).

The cerebellum may show gross atrophy of all lobules of the vermis and progressive loss of Purkinje cells with preservation of the basket and stellate cells independent of age (Oldfors et al., 1990), and simplification of the inferior olivary nucleus without cell loss or with gliosis. These findings, which are also seen in infantile autism (Bauman & Kemper, 1994), suggest arrested development beginning before birth (Bauman et al., 1995).

Drug trials

The benefit of dopaminomimetic drugs – for example, L-dopa and dopamine agonists – is controversial but may improve motor abilities (Zappella, 1990), while naltrexone, an opiate antagonist, may help to stabilize breathing irregularities (Percy et al., 1994). Drugs that block postsynaptic dopamine and serotonin receptors – such as risperidone – have been found to be effective in the treatment of tantrums, aggression, and self-injurious behaviours in patients with autistic disorders (Percy, 2002; Research Units on Pediatric Psychopharmacology Autism Network, 2002; Gagliano et al., 2004).

Conclusions

The motor symptoms seen in Rett syndrome are unique. The core motor symptoms of the condition are considered to be an abnormality of muscle tone, posture, locomotion, and voluntary movement. Each symptom may be observed in other diseases, but the prototypical symptoms of Rett syndrome and their combination are seen only in this disorder.

Though Rett syndrome has been studied for almost 40 years, little is known about the pathophysiology of this neurodevelopmental disease. Recent studies point to a deficiency of the dendritic and synaptic apparatus in selected neurons, their neurotransmitters, and possibly some cellular proteins. The cause of these deficiencies is not yet understood.

References

Amir, R.E., Veyver, I.B., Wan, M., Tran, C.Q., Francke, U. & Zoghbi, H.Y. (1999): Rett syndrome is caused by mutations in X-linked MECP2, encoding methyl.CpG-binding protein 2. *Nat. Genet.* **23**, 1885–1887.

Armstrong, D.D. (1997): Review of Rett syndrome. *J. Neuropathol. Exp. Neurol.* **56**, 843–849.

Armstrong, D.D. (2002): Neuropathology of Rett syndrome. *Ment. Retard. Dev. Disabil. Res. Rev.* **8**, 72–76.

Armstrong, D.D., Dunn, K. & Antalffy, B. (1998): Decreased dendritic branching in frontal, motor and limbic cortex in Rett syndrome compared with trisomy 21. *J. Neuropathol. Exp. Neurol.* **57**, 1013–1017.

Bauman, M.L. & Kemper, T.L. (1994): Neuroanatomic observations of the brain in autism. In: *The neurobiology of autism*, eds. M.L. Bauman & T.L Kemper, pp. 116–147. Baltimore: Johns Hopkins University Press.

Bauman, M.L., Kemper, T.L. & Arin, D.M. (1995): Pervasive neuroanatomic abnormalities of the brain in three cases of Rett syndrome. *Neurology* **45**, 1581–1586.

Belichenko, P.V., Oldfors, A., Hagberg, B. & Dahlstrom, A. (1994): Rett syndrome: 3-D confocal microscopy of cortical pyramidal dendrites and afferents. *NeuroReport* **5**, 1509–1513.

Blount, R.L., Drabman, R.S., Wilson, N. & Stewart, D. (1982): Reducing severe diurnal bruxism in two profoundly retarded females. *J. Appl. Behav. Anal.* **15**, 565–571.

Blumstein, L.K., Crawley, J.N., Davis, L.G. & Baldino, F. (1987): Neuropeptide modulation of apomorphine-induced stereotyped behaviour. *Brain Res.* **404**, 293–300.

Budden, S.S., Myer, E.C. & Butler, I.J. (1990): Cerebrospinal fluid studies in Rett syndrome: biogenic amines and P-endorphines. *Brain Dev.* **12**, 81–84.

Cornford, M.E., Philippart, M., Jacobs, B., Scheibel, A.B. & Vinters, H.V. (1994): Neuropathology of Rett syndrome: case report with neuronal and mitochondrial abnormalities in the brain. *J. Child Neurol.* **9**, 424–431.

Costall, B., Marsden, C.D., Naylor, R.J. & Pycock, C.J. (1977): Stereotyped behaviour patterns and hyperactivity induced by amphetamine and apomorphine after discrete 6-hydroxydopamine lesions of extrapyramidal and mesolimbic nuclei. *Brain Res.* **123**, 89–111.

Einspieler, C., Kerr, A.M. & Prechtl, H.F. (2005): Is the early development of girls with Rett disorder really normal? *Pediatr. Res.* **57**, 1–5.

Fanchetti, E., Zappela, M., Nalin, A. & Petroglia, F. (1986): Plasmaendorphines in Rett syndrome. Preliminary data. *Am. J. Med. Genet.* **24**, 331–338.

Fernandez-Alvarez, E. & Aicardi, J. (2001): Miscellaneous movement disorders in childhood. In: *Movement disorders in children*, eds. E. Fernandez-Alvarez & J. Aicardi, pp. 216–227. London: MacKeith Press for the International Child Neurology Association.

FitzGerald, P.M., Jankovic, J., Glaze, D.G., Schultz, R. & Percy, A.K. (1990): Extrapyramidal involvement in Rett syndrome. *Neurology* **40**, 293–295.

Gagliano, A., Germano, E., Pustorino, G., Impallomeni, C., D'Arrigo, C., Calamoneri, F. & Spina, E. (2004): Risperidone treatment in children with autistic disorder: effectiveness, tolerability, and pharmacokinetic implications. *J. Child Adolesc. Psychopharmacol.* **14**, 39–47.

Glaros, A.G. & Rao, S.M. (1977): Bruxism: a critical review. *Psychol. Bull.* **84**, 767–781.

Guerrini, R., Bonanni, P., Parmeggiani, L., Santucci, M., Parmeggiani, A. & Santucci, F. (1998): Cortical reflex myoclonus in Rett syndrome. *Ann. Neurol.* **43**, 472–479.

Hagberg, B. & Romell, M. (2002): Rett females: patterns of characteristic side-asymmetric neuroimpairments at long-term follow-up. *Neuropediatrics* **33**, 324–326.

Hagberg, B., Aicardi, J., Dias, K. & Ramos, O. (1983): Progressive syndrome of autism, dementia, ataxia and loss of purposeful hand use in girls: Rett syndrome: report of 35 cases. *Ann. Neurol.* **14**, 471–479.

Hagberg, B., Hanefeld, F., Percy, A. & Skjeldal, O. (2002): An update on clinically applicable diagnostic criteria in Rett syndrome. *Eur. J. Pediatr. Neurol.* **6**, 293–297.

Hottinger-Blanc, P.M., Ziegler, A.L. & Deonna, T. (2002): A special type of head stereotypies in children with developmental (?cerebellar) disorder: description of 8 cases and literature review. *Eur. J. Paediatr. Neurol.* **6**, 143–152.

Hugo, C., Seier, J., Mdhluli, C., Daniels, W., Harvey, B.H., Du Toit, D., Wolfe-Coote, S., Nel, D. & Stein, D.J. (2003): Fluoxetine decreases stereotypic behaviour in primates. *Prog. Neuropsychopharmacol. Biol. Psychiatry* **27**, 639–643.

Huppke, P., Held, M., Hanefeld, F., Engel, W. & Laccone, F. (2002): Influence of mutation type and location on phenotype in 123 patients with Rett syndrome. *Neuropediatrics* **33**, 63–68.

Jankovick, J. (2005): Stereotypies in autistic and other childhood disorders. In: *Paediatric movement disorders: progress in understanding*, eds. E. Fernandez-Alvarez, A. Arzimanoglou & E. Tolosa, pp. 247–260. Paris: John Libbey Eurotext.

Jellinger, K., Armstrong, D., Zoghbi, H. & Percy, K.A. (1988): Neuropathology of Rett syndrome. *Acta Neuropathol.* **76**, 142–158.

Kitt, C.A. & Wilcox, B.J. (1995): Preliminary evidence for neurodegenerative changes in the substantia nigra of Rett syndrome. *Neuropediatrics* **26**, 114–118.

Kitt, C.A., Troncoso, J.C., Priece, D.L., Naidu, S. & Moser, W.J. (1990): Pathological changes in substantia nigra and basal forebrain neurons in Rett syndrome. *Ann. Neurol.* **28**, 416–417.

Koller, W.C. & Herbster, G. (1988): D_1 and D_2 dopamine receptor mechanisms in dopaminergic behaviours. *Clin. Neuropharmacol.* **11**, 221–231.

Lappalainen, R., Lindholm, D. & Riikonen, R. (1996): Low levels of nerve growth factor in cerebrospinal fluid of children with Rett syndrome. *J. Child Neurol.* **11**, 296–300.

Lekman, A., Witt-Engerstrom, I., Holmberg, B., Percy, A., Svennerholm, L. & Hagberg, B. (1990): CSF and urine biogenic amine metabolites in Rett syndrome. *Clin. Genet.* **37**, 173–178.

Lekman, A., Hagberg, B. & Svennerholm, L. (1991): Membrane cerebral lipids in Rett syndrome. *Pediatr. Neurol.* **7**, 186–190.

Leontovich, T.A., Mukhina, J.K., Fedorov, A.A. & Belichenko, P.V. (1999): Morphological study of the entorhinal cortex, hippocampal formation, and basal ganglia in Rett syndrome patients. *Neurobiol. Dis.* **6**, 77–91.

Matsuishi, T., Nagamitsu, S., Yamashita, Y., Murakami, Y., Kimura, A., Sakai, T., Shoji, H., Kato, H. & Percy, A.K. (1977): Decreased cerebrospinal fluid levels of substance P in patients with Rett syndrome. *Ann. Neurol.* **42**, 978–981.

Naidu, S., Murphy, M., Moser, H.W. & Rett, A. (1986): Rett syndrome: natural history in 70 cases. *Am. J. Med. Genet.* **24**, 61–72.

Nomura, Y. & Segawa, M. (1990): Characteristics of motor disturbances in the Rett syndrome. *Brain Dev.* **12**, 27–30.

Nomura, Y., Segawa, M. & Hasegawa, M. (1984): Rett syndrome – clinical studies and pathophysiological considerations. *Brain Dev.* **6**, 475–486.

Nyatsanza, S., Shetty, T., Gregory, C., Lough, S., Dawson, K. & Hodges, J.R. (2003): A study of stereotypic behaviours in Alzheimer's disease and frontal and temporal variant frontotemporal dementia. *J. Neurol. Neurosurg. Psychiatry* **74**, 1398–1402.

Oldfors, A., Sourander, P., Armstrong, D.L., Percy, A.K., Witt-Engerstrom, I. & Hagberg, B. (1990): Rett syndrome: cerebellar pathology. *Pediatr. Neurol.* **6**, 310–331.

Percy, A.K. (2002): Clinical trials and treatment prospects. *Ment. Retard. Dev. Disabil. Res. Rev.* **8**, 106–111.

Percy, A.K., Glaze, D.G., Schultz, R.J., Zoghbi, H.Y., Williamson, D., Frost, J.D., Jankovic, J.J., del Junco, D., Skender, M., Waring, S. et al. (1994): Rett syndrome: controlled study of an oral opiate antagonist, naltrexone. *Ann. Neurol.* **35**, 464–470.

Perry, T.L., Dunn, H.G., Ho, H.H. & Crichton, J.U. (1988): Cerebrospinal fluid values for monoamine metabolites, gamma-aminobutyric acid and other amino compounds in Rett syndrome. *J. Pediatr.* **112**, 234–238.

Ramaekers, V.T. & Blau, N. (2001): Reduced folate transport to the brain in Rett syndrome. *Ann. Neurol.* **50** (3S), S117.

Research Units on Paediatric Psychopharmacology Autism Network (2002): Risperidone in children with autism and serious behavioural problems. *N. Engl. J. Med.* **347**, 314–321.

Rett, A. (1966): Über ein eigarties hinartrophisches Syndrom bei Hyperammoniämie in Kindesalter. *Wien Med. Wochenschr.* **116**, 723.

Riederer, P., Weiser, M., Wichart, I., Schmidt, B., Killian, W. & Rett, A. (1986): Preliminary brain autopsy findings in progredient Rett syndrome. *Am. J. Med. Genet.* **24**, 305–315.

Rugh, J.D. & Harlan, J. (1988): Nocturnal bruxism and temporomandibular disorders. In: *Advances in neurology 49: facial dyskinesias*, eds. J. Jankovic & E. Tolosa, pp. 329–334. New York: Raven Press.

Sandman, C.A. (1988): β-Endorphin disregulation in autistic and self-injurious behaviour: a neurodevelopmental hypothesis. *Synapse* **2**, 193–199.

Sato, S., Hashimoto, T., Nakamura, A. & Ikeda, S. (2001): Stereotyped stepping associated with lesions in the bilateral medial frontoparietal cortices. *Neurology* **51**, 711–713.

Satoi, M., Matsuishi, T., Yamada, S., Yamashita, Y., Ohtaki, E., Mori, K., Riikonen, R., Kato, H. & Percy, A.K. (2000): Decreased cerebrospinal fluid levels of β-phenylethylamine in patients with Rett syndrome. *Ann. Neurol.* **47**, 801–803.

Schanen, C., Houwink, E.J.F., Dorrani, N., Lane, J., Everett, R., Feng, A., Cantor, R.M. & Percy, A. (2004): Phenotypic manifestations of MECP2 mutations in classical and atypical Rett syndrome. *Am. J. Med. Genet.* **126A**, 129–140.

Temudo, T. (2005): Focal and segmental dystonia in children. In: *Paediatric movement disorders: progress in understanding*, eds. E. Fernandez-Alvarez, A. Arzimanoglou & E. Tolosa, pp. 57-70. Paris: John Libbey Eurotext.

Temudo, T., Santos, M.J., Dias, K., Moreira, A.,Vieira, J.P., Barbot, C., Oliveira, G., Calado, E., Levy, A., Carrilho, I., Fonseca, M.J., Dias, A., Lobo Antunes, N., Cabral, P., Monteiro, J., Gomes, R., Barbosa, C., Andrada, G., Santos, M., Sequeiros, J. & Maciel, P. (2005): Stereotypies in Rett syndrome – analysis of 65 Portuguese patients [abstract]. *Eur. J. Pediatr Neurol.* **9,** 177.

The Rett syndrome Diagnostic Working Group (1988): Diagnostic criteria for Rett syndrome. *Ann. Neurol.* **23**, 425–428.

Thelen, E. (1979): Rhythmical stereotypies in normal human infants. *Anim. Behav.* **27**, 699-715.

Thelen, E. (1980): Determinants of stereotyped behaviour in normal human infants. *Ethol. Sociobiol.* **1**, 141–150.

Tschanz, J.T. & Rebec, G.V. (1988): Atypical antipsychotic drugs block selective components of amphetamine-induced stereotypy. *Pharmacol. Biochem. Behav.* **31**, 519–522.

Wales, L., Charman, T. & Mount, R.H. (2004): An analogue assessment of repetitive hand behaviours in girls and young woman with Rett syndrome. *J. Intellect. Disabil. Res.* **48**, 672–678.

Witt-Engerström, I. & Hagberg, B. (1990): The Rett syndrome: gross motor disability and neural impairments in adults. *Brain Dev.* **12**, 33–36.

Zappella, M. (1990): A double blind trial of bromocriptine in the Rett syndrome. *Brain Dev.* **12**, 148–150.

Zoghbi, H.Y., Milstien, S., Butler, I.J., Smith, O.B., Kaufman, S., Glaze, D.G. & Percy, A.K. (1989): Cerebrospinal fluid biogenic amines and biopterin in Rett syndrome. *Ann. Neurol.* **25**, 56–60.

Chapter 17

Rapid-onset dystonia-parkinsonism

Andrew McKeon and Mary D. King

*Department of Neurology, Temple Street Children's Hospital, Temple Street,
Dublin 1, Republic of Ireland*
Mary.King@tsch.ie

Summary

Rapid-onset dystonia-parkinsonism (RDP, DYT12) is characterized classically by the abrupt onset of bulbar and limb dystonia, a stable course, and a lack of response to levodopa. Six different mutations in the Na^+/K^+-ATPase alpha 3 subunit *(ATP1A3)* gene have recently been demonstrated in RDP families. We describe in detail the clinical presentation and outcome of the youngest member of the Irish RDP kindred, who presented at age 7 years. The key features in her case were the acute onset of predominantly bulbar and upper limb dystonia, occurring in the context of an emotionally traumatic family event, and the lack of progression. We also discuss the clinical features in previously described kindreds, and what is known about the pathophysiology of the disorder. While treatment of RDP has been disappointing to date, the hope for reversibility lies in treatment directed at Na^+/K^+-ATPase.

Introduction

Rapid-onset dystonia-parkinsonism (RDP, DYT12) is a rare autosomal dominant inherited movement disorder characterized by the acute onset of dystonia and parkinsonism over hours to weeks. In many cases this manifests as the abrupt development of orofacial, bulbar, and limb dystonia, rigidity, bradykinesia, and loss of postural reflexes, usually reaching a plateau quickly, leaving the patient with chronic severe disability. This disorder has received much attention in recent times since the description of mutations in the gene for Na^+/K^+-ATPase alpha 3 subunit in families with RDP.

Case report

A 7-year-old girl, the first of two children of unrelated parents with no significant past medical history, presented to the emergency department with abnormal posturing and whispering. She had had a mild upper respiratory tract infection for a few days. While on a school trip to a leisure centre she got stuck on a climbing net and had a minor fall. She began whispering within minutes and appeared distressed. She was sent home from school and missed her usual collection by her mother who, on return home, found the child twisting her arms and whispering.

The social history was complex with her parents separated because of alleged sexual abuse by her father several years earlier. Her father was denied access but this was being disputed at the time of presentation. There was a family holiday with the mother's new partner one week earlier, following which the child was noted to be anxious and slept poorly. Finally, there was an unwelcome visit by a paternal aunt and grandfather two days before presentation.

A diagnosis of possible conversion disorder was considered in the emergency department and a referral was made to the child psychiatrist.

Over the following two weeks, she became withdrawn and anarthric with dystonic spasms of the upper limbs, slow movements, dysphagia, drooling, and an expressionless face. On examination, there were whispering monosyllabic responses, dystonic posturing of the limbs with flexion at the elbows and wrists, extension at the metacarpal phalangeal joints, inability to protrude the tongue, and drooling of saliva.

Investigations were all negative. These included brain magnetic resonance imaging, electroencephalography, metabolic tests of blood, urine, and CSF (including neurotransmitter metabolites), toxicology, and molecular genetics (Huntington's disease and DYT1).

There was no response to a trial of levodopa, benzhexol, clonazepam, or baclofen.

During admission for evaluation, details of the family history were revealed (Fig. 1). A paternal uncle (case II:2) died at 32 years from an unexplained movement disorder attributed to an injury at 20 years but characterized by abrupt deterioration at age 30. Several family members were described as having shakes, unsteadiness, strokes, or stiffness, sometimes attributed to injury, drug, or alcohol abuse. Following presentation of a paternal cousin (case III:2), a diagnosis of RDP was made.

Eight years later, there has not been any further deterioration. The patient remains ambulant with bradykinesia, dystonia of upper limbs, and anarthria. She feeds orally, communicates using a computerized system, and is in mainstream second level education.

Genetic studies are ongoing in the family.

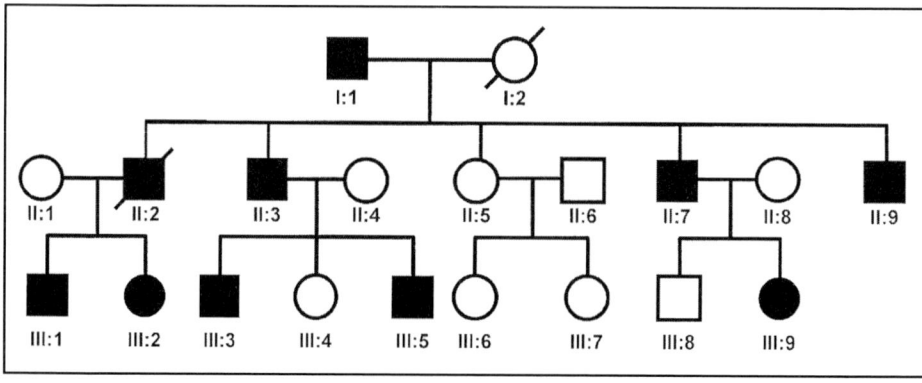

Fig. 1. The Irish RDP pedigree.

Discussion

Dobyns *et al.* (1993) first described RDP in 12 members of a large Midwestern American family. These patients had, for the most part, acute onset of dystonia affecting any muscle group, but with a tendency to progress over hours to days to involve muscles of speech, swallowing, and all limbs. All patients had moderate to severe dystonia combined with manifestations of parkinsonism, such as postural instability, bradykinesia, masked facies, and hypomimia. While any muscle group could be involved, bulbar and upper limbs were always more severely affected than lower limbs. This has been described as classic RDP. However, there tended to be heterogeneity of progression in this family, with some patients stabilizing within weeks and others reporting progression over years. The role of traumatic physical or psychological events in precipitating the disorder was postulated from early on. One patient developed the syndrome within an hour of delivering her fourth child. Dobyns *et al.* also reported two patients who were less severely affected, with segmental symptoms (writer's cramp and mild leg dystonia) which remained stable over time. One member of this family had acute deterioration in his condition 2 years after initial stabilization (Brashear *et al.*, 1996). CSF analysis showed low levels of the dopamine metabolite homovallinic acid (HVA). However, there was at best a minimal and unsustained improvement in symptoms with levodopa and dopamine agonists. Data from positron emission tomographic imaging of dopamine reuptake sites in RDP (Brashear *et al.*, 1999) suggest that the low CSF HVA is not a result of degeneration of striatal dopamine terminals or loss of dopamine reuptake sites.

A second Midwestern American family was described by the same group (Brashear *et al.*, 1997). Again, the four affected individuals had an abrupt onset of dystonia and parkinsonism, predominantly affecting bulbar and upper limb muscles. In three of the four affected individuals, abrupt onset of severe symptoms was preceded by mild limb dystonia. Hyperreflexia was noted in one patient. Direct parent-to-child transmission and poor response to levodopa were also seen.

A detailed description of the proband in the Irish kindred was published by Webb and colleagues (Webb *et al.*, 1999). A first cousin of the patient described above presented with an initial focal dystonia affecting the left upper limb, her condition evolving over 2 weeks to cause severe disability, leaving the patient non-ambulant, dysarthric, requiring nasogastric feeding, and suffering from painful dystonic spasms. The three generations of the Irish kindred (Fig. 1) were subsequently described by Pittock *et al.* (2000). Again heterogeneity of presentation and outcome is characteristic. Three of four affected members from the first two generations were relatively mildly affected with focal limb dystonia, with the fourth developing an acute severe disorder 10 years after the onset and stabilization of a limb dystonia. The third generation of the family was more severely affected, with three of the four suffering from an acute onset of a severe disorder as described above, causing loss of ambulation, flexion contractures, spasms, and severe bulbar symptoms often mandating the introduction of enteral nutritional support. Psychiatric morbidity is common in this kindred and may be part of the phenotype. Half the patients in the kindred suffered an episode of anxiety or panic at the onset of the disorder. Three individuals had features of depression, one with a severe depressive episode responsive to a selective serotonin reuptake inhibitor. Others suffered from social phobia. Low CSF HVA was found in only one patient, who had classic RDP, social phobia, and a major depressive episode. Low levels of CSF HVA had previously been associated with severity in RDP (Brashear *et al.*, 1998). One patient had a baseline mild focal dystonia affecting the left hand and foot, which became severely exacerbated under conditions of heightened emotion or stress.

Seven years on from the original description, further details have emerged from the Irish kindred (McKeon *et al.*, in press). The father of the patient described above, an obligate carrier suffering from social phobia, has developed a mild right-sided focal arm and leg dystonia. Also, one patient with classic RDP has had a progressive course resulting in gait deterioration and the requirement for nasogastric feeding, despite good resolution of his major depressive episode. His younger brother has also developed a relatively mild disorder with a predominant focal right hand dystonia. The Irish kindred is illustrated in Fig. 1.

The father of the proband, who died, provides the only pathological study to date. No pathological changes were found at necropsy.

The American and Irish kindred – and more recently the Polish RDP kindred described by Zaremba *et al.* (2004) – have been linked to chromosome 19q13. Subsequently, de Carvalho Aguiar *et al.* (2004) reported six missense mutations in the gene for the Na^+/K^+-ATPase alpha 3 subunit *(ATP1A3)* in seven unrelated families with RDP. This same mutation has also been described in a sporadic case of RDP initially thought to have had idiopathic Parkinson's disease (Kamphuis *et al.*, 2005). However, the *ATP1A3* mutation has not been described in unaffected or non-penetrant members of RDP families. The α3 subunit of Na^+/K^+-ATPase is present throughout the central nervous system and is responsible for the restoration of resting membrane potential after the firing of voltage-gated sodium channels. This is obviously an exciting development in a disorder characterized by fluctuations, sudden deteriorations, and onset during states of anxiety. Furthermore, this supports the concept of reversibility in RDP. A trial of phenytoin therapy was unsuccessful in the Irish proband; however, treatment with other drugs that have activity at sodium channels such as valproic acid, carbamazepine, and lithium has not been reported. Genetic heterogeneity may also be a feature of this disorder, with the recent description of a German family with predominant cranial-cervical involvement of dystonia, but not linked to 19q13 and with no mutations in *ATP1A3* (Kabakci *et al.*, 2005).

Other treatments are symptomatic and include baclofen, diazepam, and botulinum toxin for painful spasms and flexion contractures; nasogastric feeding for severe dysphagia; and speech therapy, physical therapy, and occupational therapy. One patient from the Irish kindred had an unsuccessful pallidotomy before recognition of the disorder in the kindred. More recently (Deutschlander *et al.*, 2005), a patient with apparent sporadic RDP was treated with bilateral deep brain stimulation of the globus pallidus, but had no improvement in her symptoms.

Conclusions

While RDP is a rare disorder, it is increasingly recognised as more reports of sporadic cases come through (Linazasoro *et al.*, 2002). While the classic presentation of acute onset dystonia and parkinsonism – with predominant upper limb and bulbar involvement – is the most dramatic, the presentation and outcome of this disorder is heterogeneous. In suspected cases, testing for missense mutations in *ATP1A3* will be helpful. As our understanding of the underlying pathophysiology of the condition grows, this may give future insight into other forms of idiopathic dystonia and lead to the development of treatments for this often severely debilitating disorder.

References

Brashear, A., Farlow, M.R., Butler, I.J., Kasarskis, E.J. & Dobyns, W.B. (1996): Variable phenotype of rapid-onset dystonia-parkinsonism. *Mov. Disord.* **11**, 151–156.

Brashear, A., Deleon, D., Bressman, S.B., Thyagarajan, D., Farlow, M.R. & Dobyns, W.B. (1997): Rapid-onset dystonia-parkinsonism in a second family. *Neurology* **48**, 1066–1069.

Brashear, A., Butler, I.J., Hyland, K., Farlow, M.R. & Dobyns, W.B. (1998): Cerebrospinal fluid homovanillic acid levels in rapid-onset dystonia-parkinsonism. *Ann. Neurol.* **43**, 521–526.

Brashear, A., Mulholland, G.K., Zheng, Q.H., Farlow, M.R., Siemers, E.R. & Hutchins, G.D. (1999): PET imaging of the pre-synaptic dopamine uptake sites in rapid-onset dystonia-parkinsonism (RDP). *Mov. Disord.* **14**, 132–137.

De Carvalho Aguiar, P., Sweadner, K.J., Penniston, J.T., Zaremba, J., Liu, L., Caton, M., Linazasoro, G., Borg, M., Tijssen, M.A., Bressman, S.B., Dobyns, W.B., Brashear, A. & Ozelius, L.J. (2004): Mutations in the Na+/K+-ATPase alpha3 gene ATP1A3 are associated with rapid-onset dystonia parkinsonism. *Neuron* **43**, 169–175.

Deutschlander, A., Asmus, F., Gasser, T., Steude, U. & Botzel, K. (2005): Sporadic rapid-onset dystonia-parkinsonism syndrome: failure of bilateral pallidal stimulation. *Mov. Disord.* **20**, 254–257.

Dobyns, W.B., Ozelius, L.J., Kramer, P.L., Brashear, A., Farlow, M.R., Perry, T.R., Walsh, L.E., Kasarskis, E.J., Butler, I.J. & Breakefield, X.O. (1993): Rapid-onset dystonia-parkinsonism. *Neurology* **43**, 2596–2602.

Kabakci, K., Isbruch, K., Schilling, K., Hedrich, K., De Carvalho Aguiar, P., Ozelius, L.J., Kramer, P.L., Schwarz, M.H. & Klein, C. (2005): Genetic heterogeneity in rapid onset dystonia-parkinsonism: description of a new family. *J. Neurol. Neurosurg. Psychiatry* **76**, 860–862.

Kamphuis, D.J., Koelman, H., Lees, A.J. & Tijssen, M.A. (2006): Sporadic rapid-onset dystonia-parkinsonism presenting as Parkinson's disease. *Mov. Disord.* **21**, 118–119.

Linazasoro, G., Indakoetxea, B., Ruiz, J., Van Blercom, N. & Lasa, A. (2002): Possible sporadic rapid-onset dystonia-parkinsonism. *Mov. Disord.* **17**, 608–609.

Pittock, S.J., Joyce, C., O'Keane, V., Hugle, B., Hardiman, M.O., Brett, F., Green, A.J., Barton, D.E., King, M.D. & Webb, D.W. (2000): Rapid-onset dystonia-parkinsonism: a clinical and genetic analysis of a new kindred. *Neurology* **55**, 991–995.

Webb, D.W., Broderick, A., Brashear, A. & Dobyns, W.B. (1999): Rapid onset dystonia-parkinsonism in a 14-year-old girl. *Eur. J. Paediatr. Neurol.* **3**, 171–173.

Zaremba, J., Mierzewska, H., Lysiak, Z., Kramer, P., Ozelius, L.J. & Brashear, A. (2004): Rapid-onset dystonia-parkinsonism: a fourth family consistent with linkage to chromosome 19q13. *Mov. Disord.* **19**, 1506–1510.

Chapter 18

Alternating hemiplegia of childhood (AHC)

Giuseppe Gobbi[*], Melania Giannotta[*], Tiziana Granata[#], Fiorella Gurrieri[°], Edvige Veneselli[§], Federico Vigevano[¶], Claudio Zucca[**], Nardo Nardocci[#] and Emilio Fernandez-Alvarez[^]

[*] Child Neurology Unit, Hospital Maggiore, largo Nigrisoli 2, 40133 Bologna, Italy;
[#] Division of Child Neurology, Fondazione IRCCS Istituto Neurologico 'C.Besta', via Celoria 11, 20133 Milan, Italy;
[°] Institute of Medical Genetics, Catholic University of Rome, largo F. Vito 1, 00168 Rome, Italy;
[§] Child Neuropsychiatry Unit, Department of Neuroscience, IRCCS G. Gaslini Institute, University of Genova, largo G. Gaslini 5, 16147 Genova, Italy;
[¶] Division of Neurology, IRCCS Bambino Gesù Children's Hospital, piazza Sant'Onofrio 4, 00165 Rome, Italy;
[**] Neurophysiopathology Unit, IRCCS E. Medea, via D.L. Monza 20, 23842 Bosisio Parini (LC), Italy;
[^] Neuropaediatric Department, Hospital Sant Joan de Déu, University of Barcelona, 08950 Esplugues de Llobregat, Barcelona, Spain
giuseppe.gobbi@ausl.bologna.it
Video 8

Summary

Alternating hemiplegia of childhood (AHC) is a rare disease with onset before 18 months, characterized by the association of paroxysmal events with chronic motor and cognitive abnormalities. The most striking and specific symptom is the recurrence of hemiplegic or tetraplegic attacks.
Cognitive impairment and stable neurological deficits of varying severity appear during the disease course. The aetiology is unknown. A cerebrovascular disorder, a mitochondrial disorder, and ion channel dysfunction have been hypothesized. Laboratory investigations are unrevealing, and the diagnosis rests on the clinical features. In this chapter we summarize the clinical features of the disease and the current hypothesis on its aetiology and pathogenesis.
Video recordings of five patients selected from among the series of 31 patients collected by the Italian Association of AHC (AISEA) in a clinical database are presented in the accompanying DVD to illustrate the main clinical features of the disease

Introduction

Alternating hemiplegia of childhood (AHC) is a rare disease of infancy of unknown aetiology, characterized by the association of paroxysmal phenomena and persistent neurological deficits. First described by Verret and Steele (1971), the disease was later better characterized by Krogaloh and Aicardi (1980) and then by Bougeois (Bougeois et al., 1993). The syndrome typically has its onset before the age of 18 months and runs a slowly progressive course. The most striking and specific symptom is the recurrence of hemiplegic or tetraplegic attacks, although other types of paroxysmal phenomena are also usually present. These include paroxysmal dystonia, paroxysmal strabismus or nystagmus, dyspnoea, and autonomic symptoms, occurring either in the course of the episodes of hypomobility or independently. Cognitive impairment and stable neurological deficits of varying severity almost always appear during the disease course.

Clinical features

Paroxysmal symptoms

Each of the paroxysmal phenomena described below may appear as an isolated manifestation, but more often they combine in a complex fashion and result in multifarious events that are difficult to describe. The attacks may be triggered by sudden temperature variations (such as hot or cold water), physical exercise, excitement, emotional stress, trauma, intercurrent illness, loud noise, bright light, and menstruation.

Abnormal ocular movements in the form of paroxysmal strabismus or nystagmus are an early symptom but seldom the presenting one. Paroxysmal strabismus usually consists of transient supranuclear ophthalmoplegia. Nystagmus is of large amplitude. It may be horizontal or pendular, and its direction can change even during a single attack. When associated with a hemiplegic attack, nystagmus may be unilateral.

Tonic attacks often mark the onset of the disease. Although the attack may affect only one limb, more often both the arm and the ipsilateral leg are involved. Stiffness and extension of limbs are sometimes associated with head-and-eye deviation towards the affected side. Extreme tonic contraction may result in a rapid vibratory tremor. During the less common bilateral tonic attacks, intense crying is associated with abnormal postures such as painful arching of the back, lateral flexion of the trunk or opisthotonus, trisma, drooling, and upward deviation of gaze. Nystagmus, autonomic changes, and dyspnoea may also be associated.

The hemiplegic attacks can be absent at the onset of disease, but rapidly become the predominant and most specific paroxysmal phenomenon. During the hemiplegic fit, hypomobility is associated with hypotonia and may involve the limbs, neck, trunk, and facial muscles of one side of the body. A shift of the motor deficit to the contralateral side may be observed during a single episode. The severity of the paralysis can fluctuate during the fits. Flaccid weakness is often intermingled with brief episodes of dystonic posturing. Consciousness is usually preserved or only slightly reduced (Bourgeois et al., 1993). Episodes last from minutes to days, and are typically interrupted by sleep. Tetraplegic attacks may appear as an isolated manifestation or as the result of the shifting of hypomobility from one side of the body to the other. Autonomic phenomena consist of irregular breathing, vasomotor changes, drooling, and hiccups.

Epileptic seizures are common, mainly in older patients. Both generalized (tonic, atonic, and atypical absence) and focal seizures may be observed, and status epilepticus has also been reported. Epileptic tonic seizures, particularly in infants, are often difficult to differentiate from non-epileptic tonic attacks.

Non-paroxysmal symptoms

Hypotonia and delay in motor and cognitive milestones are often present before the onset of paroxysmal symptoms. Movement disorders – including choreoathetosis, dystonia, and tremor – appear at the age of 2 to 5 years. Choreoathetosis is the most consistently reported disorder, present in virtually all cases. Ataxia may appear at different ages, it is usually mild and non-progressive. Paresis may affect the side of the body most often involved in the hemiplegic or tetraplegic attacks. Cognitive deficits of varying severity are present in all patients. In some children mental deterioration has been reported (Bourgeois et al., 1995). Finally, behavioural and psychiatric disorders characterized by aggressiveness, depression, and low self-esteem have been described (Bourgeois et al., 1993).

The disease takes a slowly progressive course in which three phases have been described (Mikati et al., 2000). The first phase, lasting about one year from the onset, is mainly characterized by the presence of abnormal ocular movements, tonic head deviation, and tonic attacks. Mild developmental delay may precede or be concomitant with the onset of the paroxysmal symptoms. In phase 2, which evolves over 1 to 5 years, hemiplegic or tetraplegic attacks dominate the clinical picture, psychomotor delay becomes more evident, and non-paroxysmal neurological disturbances appear. In phase 3, the severity and frequency of the paroxysmal disorders decrease and the neurological deficits slowly stabilize. The outcome is characterized mainly by mental retardation of varying degree and by the motor disability. The severity of functional disability is variable, but as a rule the presence of movement disorders and ataxia impair fine motor skills and gait. By contrast, paroxysmal phenomena and epileptic seizures become less frequent.

Laboratory investigations

The diagnosis of AHC rest on the clinical features, as laboratory investigation are unrevealing. Interictal EEG is usually normal at onset, while slow activity with variable localization may appear during evolution. Rare epileptic abnormalities such as focal spike-and-wave discharges have been reported. During the hemiplegic attack, the EEG may show non-specific theta-delta activity on the hemisphere contralateral to the attack, sometimes predominant in the temporo-occipital regions, which disappears during sleep (Dalla Bernardina et al., 1995). Evoked potentials have been reported as normal. Recently, blink reflex abnormalities pointing to brain stem dysfunction have been demonstrated in six patients (Rinalduzzi et al., 2006). Magnetic resonance imaging (MRI) is unrevealing, while 'ictal' positron emission tomography (PET) and single photon emission computed tomography (SPECT) studies have shown asymmetrical perfusion or captation between the hemispheres, but these results are controversial and non-conclusive.

Searches for metabolic disorders (for example, serum and CSF lactate, amino-acids, urinary organic acids, biogenic amines) are unrevealing.

Few pathological studies have been reported. Extensive bilateral involvement of the hippocampus has been described in one patient (Becker, 1995). According to this investigator, the location of the lesion would explain a progressive cognitive decline in that patient.

Aetiopathogenesis

The aetiology remains unknown. Different hypotheses on the pathogenesis of the disease have been proposed, including migraine, cerebrovascular dysfunction, mitochondriopathy, and channelopathies (Rho and Chugani, 1998).

The hypothesis of a *cerebrovascular dysfunction* has been tested by cerebral blood flow studies (Zupanc et al 1991; Mikati et al 1992; Nevsimalova et al 1994; Dangond et al 1997). Results from SPECT are, however, inconsistent. Regional or hemispheric changes – either hyper- or hypoperfusion, and related or unrelated to the side of the hemiplegia – have been reported (Wong *et al.*, 1993). The inconsistency of the results may reflect differences in the timing of the perfusion studies in relation to the course of the attack.

Dysfunction of brain metabolism has been demonstrated in PET studies (Pfund et al, 2002, Nemsimalova et al, 2005). In 2002, Pfund and colleagues reported unilaterally increased serotonin synthesis in the basal ganglia and the fronto-parietal regions in the ictal and post-ictal phase (Pfund *et al.*, 2002).

Excessive activation or expression of NMDA receptors with a subsequent increase in nitric oxide as a result of a hypoxic-ischaemic event with direct neuronal damage has also been proposed (Korinthenberg, 1996).

The hypothesis of a mitochondriopathy was suggested by cerebral MRI spectroscopy studies which showed a decrease in N-acetyl aspartate (NAA), phosphocreatine (CR), and cytosolic phosphorylation potential, coupled with increased intensities of inorganic phosphate (Arnold *et al.*, 1993). It has been suggested that a low NAA/CR ratio might reflect neuronal loss as a result of mitochondrial dysfunction (Arnold *et al.*, 1993). Increased plasma lactate concentration, an increased pyruvate to lactate ratio, accompanied by elevated inorganic phosphate values in muscle MRI spectroscopy have also been reported (Nevsimalova *et al.*, 1994). In no case, however, have morphological or biochemical changes consistent with mitochondrial dysfunction ever been observed. Recently, dysfunction of ion channels has been proposed. This hypothesis is suggested by the abrupt onset and episodic recurrence of symptoms, by some clinical features that resemble those of hemiplegic migraine, and by the efficacy of drugs targeted at ion channels (for example, flunarizine, which is a calcium channel antagonist). Studies have mostly focused on those genes implicated in familial hemiplegic migraine: *CACNA1A* and *ATP1A2*. *CACNA1A* is located on chromosome 19p13 and has been considered a good candidate as its mutations are associated with both paroxysmal and progressive symptoms. *CACNA1A* mutations are associated with familial hemiplegic migraine and episodic ataxia type 2, whereas a pathological triple repeat causes spinocerebellar ataxia type 6. To date, however, while several polymorphisms have been identified, no mutations or triple repeats have been found in patients with AHC (Haan *et al.*, 2000). The *ATP1A2* gene for familial hemiplegic migraine type 2 is located on chromosome 1q23 and codes for the alpha-2 subunit of Na^+/K^+-ATPase. A mutation of this gene has been identified in a Greek family with four members, in two generations, affected by a 'mild' phenotype of AHC (Bassi *et al.*, 2004; Swoboda *et al.*, 2004). Mutation analysis of the same gene in six sporadic patients with the classic phenotype again detected several polymorphisms but no mutation in the coding region (Kors *et al.*, 2004).

Although mostly sporadic, a few familial cases of AHC have been reported (Mikati *et al.*, 1992; Kramer *et al.*, 2000). In one of these families, the pedigree was consistent with autosomal dominant inheritance (Mikati *et al.*, 1992) and a balanced reciprocal translocation (46,XY,t(3;9)(p26;q34)) was found.

Video – Illustrative cases

The videoclips on the accompanying DVD (video 8, tracks 1-5) show examples of paroxysmal phenomena: a tetraplegic attack (Patient 1), abnormal eye movements (Patient 2), and a complex paroxysmal attack (Patient 3), as well as the presence of movement disorders such as tremor and choreoathetosis (Patients 4 and 5).

The cases presented have been selected from among the series of 31 patients collected in an Italian collaborative study, which started in 2002 and was supported by the Italian Association of AHC (AISEA).

Video 8, track 1 – 5-year-old boy. Born by caesarean section after a normal pregnancy. At birth mild respiratory distress was reported. Tetraplegic attacks associated with drooling, breathing difficulties, and swallowing dysfunction began at 9 days of age. Hemiplegic attacks, associated with horizontal nystagmus and torticollis, appeared during the disease course. No impairment of consciousness has ever been observed during the fits, which usually last several hours and recur about twice a week. A typical tetraplegic attack is shown in track 1.

Video 8, track 2 – 3-year-old boy. Pregnancy and delivery were normal. Two days after birth, the infant presented episodes of diffuse hypotonia, with breathing difficulties, autonomic dysfunction, and monocular nystagmus, lasting a few hours. From 2 years of age hemiplegic or tetraplegic events appeared, combined with hypertonia and dystonia. Severe mental impairment, hypotonia, pyramidal signs, and dystonia characterized the disease course. Monocular nystagmus is shown in track 2. In the first attack, predominant on the left side, the nystagmus involves the left eye. In the second, the nystagmus is associated with upward deviation of the gaze and involves the right eye.

Video 8, track 3 – 4-year-old boy. Delivery was normal. Hemiplegic attacks began at 4 months of age. They were hemi- or tetraplegic, associated with nystagmus. Mild developmental delay appeared during the evolution of the disease. Neurological examination at the age of 4 revealed hypotonia and choreoathetosis. Track 3 shows a hemiplegic attack.

Video 8, track 4 – 10-year-old boy. Delivery was at term after normal pregnancy. At birth, paroxysmal abnormal ocular movements and strabismus were noted. At 5 months of age, hemiplegic attacks appeared, frequently spreading to the whole body. The clinical course was characterized by mental retardation and the appearance of a complex movement disorder. At the age of 10, neurological examination revealed dysarthria, pyramidal tract signs, ataxia, and tremor.

Video 8, track 5 – 8-year-old girl. Normal pregnancy and delivery. Paroxysmal events appeared at the age of 3 months, characterized by hypotonia and weakness involving the whole body, or by mono- or hemiplegic attacks associated with head deviation toward the affected side, sweating, and nystagmus. She also developed tonic attacks with opisthotonus and dystonic posturing of the upper limbs. Developmental delay and cognitive impairment appeared during the course of the disease. Dystonia and myoclonus are shown in track 5.

Acknowledgments: We thank the AISEA for financial support in setting up the database, for the organization of the clinical sessions in Bologna and Rome in 2002 and 2003, and of a workshop in Foligno in 2004.

References

Arnold, D.L., Silver, K. & Andermann, F. (1993): Evidence for mitochondrial dysfunction in patients with alternating hemiplegia of childhood. *Ann. Neurol.* **33**, 604–607.

Bassi, M.T., Bresolin, N., Tonelli, A., Nazos, K., Crippa, F., Baschirotto, C., Zucca, C., Bersano, A., Dolcetta, D., Boneschi, F.M., Barone, V. & Casari, G. (2004): A novel mutation in the ATP1A2 gene causes alternating hemiplegia of childhood. *J. Med. Genet.* **41**, 621–628.

Becker, L.E. (1995): Neuropathology of alternating hemiplegia of childhood. In: *Alternating hemiplegia of childhood*, eds. F. Andermann, J. Aicardi & F. Vigevano, pp. 57-65. New York: Raven Press.

Bourgeois, M., Aicardi, J. & Goutières, F. (1993): Alternating hemiplegia of childhood. *J. Pediatr.* **122**, 673–679.

Bourgeois, M., Nevsimalova, X., Aicardi, J. & Andermann, F. (1995): Alternating hemiplegia of childhood: long-term outcome. In: *Alternating hemiplegia of childhood*, eds. F. Andermann, J. Aicardi & F. Vigevano, pp. 49–54. New York: Raven Press.

Dalla Bernardina, B., Fontana, E., Colamaria, V., Zullini, E., Darra, F., Giardina, L., Franco, A. & Montagnini, A. (1995): Alternating hemiplegia of childhood: epilepsy and electroencephalographic investigations. In: *Alternating hemiplegia of childhood*, eds. F. Andermann, J. Aicardi & F. Vigevano, pp. 75-87. New York: Raven Press.

Dangond, F., Garada, B., Murawski, B.J., Rey-Casserly, C., Holman, B.L. & Mikati, M.A. (1997): Focal brain dysfunction in a 41-year-old man with familial alternating hemiplegia. *Eur. Arch. Psychiatry Clin. Neurosci.* **247**, 35–41.

Haan, J., Kors, E.E., Terwindt, G.M., Vermeulen, F.L.M.G., Vergouwe, M.N., van den Maagdenberg, A.M.J.M., Gill, D.S., Pascual, J., Ophoff, R.A., Frants, R.R. & Ferrari, M.D. (2000): Alternating hemiplegia of childhood: no mutations in the familial hemiplegic migraine CACNA1A gene. *Cephalalgia* **20**, 696–700.

Korinthenberg, R. (1996): Is infantile alternating hemiplegia mediated by glutamate toxicity and can it be treated with nemantine? *Neuropediatrics* **27**, 277–278.

Kors, E.E., Vanmolkot, K.R.J., Haan, J., Kheradmand Kia, S., Stroink, H., Laan, L.A.E.M., Gill, D.S., Pascual, J., van den Maagdenberg, A.M.J.M., Frants, R.R. & Ferrari, M.D. (2004): Alternating hemiplegia of childhood: no mutations in the second familial hemiplegic migraine gene ATP1A2. *Neuropediatrics* **35**, 293–296.

Krageloh, I. & Aicardi, J. (1980): Alternating hemiplegia of infants: report of five cases. *Dev. Med. Child Neurol.* **22**, 784–791.

Kramer, U., Nevo, Y., Margalit, D., Shorer, Z. & Harel, S. (2000): Alternating hemiplegia of childhood in half sisters. *J. Child Neurol.* **15**, 128–130.

Mikati, M.A., Maguire, H., Barlow, C.F., Ozelius, L., Breakfield, X.O., Klauck, S.M., Korf, B., O'Tuama, S.L. & Dangond, F. (1992): A syndrome of autosomal dominant alternating hemiplegia: clinical presentation mimicking intractable epilepsy; chromosomal studies; and physiologic investigation. *Neurology* **42**, 2251–2257.

Mikati, M.A., Kramer, U., Zupanc, M.L. & Shanahan, R.J. (2000): Alternating hemiplegia of childhood: clinical manifestations and long-term outcome. *Pediatr. Neurol.* **23**, 134–141.

Nevsimalova, S., Dittrich, J., Havlova, M. & Tauberova, A. (1994): Alternating hemiplegia in childhood: a cross-sectional study. *Brain Dev.* **16**, 189–194.

Nevsimalova, S., Havlova, M., Tauberova, A. & Prihodova, I. (2005): Alternating hemiplegia of childhood (AHC). *Cas. Lek. Cesk.* **144**, 692–696.

Pfund, Z., Chugani, D.C., Muzik, O., Juhasz, C., Behen, M.E., Lee, J., Chakraborty, P., Mangner, T. & Chugani, H.T. (2002): Alpha[11C] methyl-L-tryptophan positron emission tomography in patients with alternating hemiplegia of childhood. *J. Child Neurol.* **174**, 253–260.

Rinalduzzi, S., Valeriani, M. & Vigevano, F. (2006): Brainstem dysfunction in alternating hemiplegia of childhood: a neurophysiological study. *Cephalalgia* **26**, 511–516.

Rho, J.M. & Chugani, H.T. (1998): Alternating hemiplegia of childhood: insight into its pathophysiology. *J. Child Neurol.* **13**, 39–45.

Swoboda, K.J., Kanavkis, E., Xaidara, A., Johnson, J.E., Leppert, M.F., Schlesinger-Massart, M.B., Ptacek, L.J., Silver, K. & Yoroukos, S. (2004): Alternating hemiplegia of childhood or familial hemiplegic migraine. *Ann. Neurol.* **55**, 884–887.

Verret, S. & Steele, J.C. (1971): Alternating hemiplegia in childhood: a report of eight patients with complicated migraine beginning in infancy. *Pediatrics* **47**, 675–680.

Wong, V., Ho, G.C., Yeung, H.W. & Ma, K.M. (1993): Alternating hemiplegia syndrome: electroencephalogram, brain mapping, brain perfusion SPECT scan study in a Chinese girl. *J. Child Neurol.* **8**, 221–226.

Zupanc, M.L., Dobkin, J.A. & Perlman, S.B.(1991): 123I-Iodoamphetamine SPECT brain imaging in alternating hemiplegia. *Pediatr. Neurol.* **7**, 35838.

Achevé d'imprimer par Corlet, Imprimeur, S.A.
14110 Condé-sur-Noireau
N° d'Imprimeur : 96884 - Dépôt légal : avril 2007
Imprimé en France